T0140157

Studies in Computational Intelligence

Volume 491

Series Editor

Janusz Kacprzyk, Polish Academy of Sciences, Warsaw, Poland
e-mail: kacprzyk@ibspan.waw.pl

For further volumes:
http://www.springer.com/series/7092

About this Series

The series "Studies in Computational Intelligence" (SCI) publishes new developments and advances in the various areas of computational intelligence—quickly and with a high quality. The intent is to cover the theory, applications, and design methods of computational intelligence, as embedded in the fields of engineering, computer science, physics and life sciences, as well as the methodologies behind them. The series contains monographs, lecture notes and edited volumes in computational intelligence spanning the areas of neural networks, connectionist systems, genetic algorithms, evolutionary computation, artificial intelligence, cellular automata, self-organizing systems, soft computing, fuzzy systems, and hybrid intelligent systems. Of particular value to both the contributors and the readership are the short publication timeframe and the world-wide distribution, which enable both wide and rapid dissemination of research output.

Margaret Lech · Insu Song
Peter Yellowlees · Joachim Diederich
Editors

Mental Health Informatics

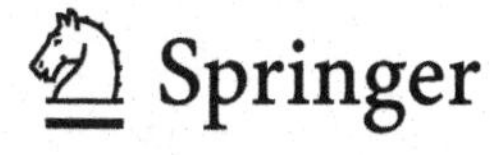

Editors
Margaret Lech
School of Electrical and Computer Engineering
RMIT University
Melbourne
Australia

Insu Song
School of Business and IT
James Cook University Australia
Singapore

Peter Yellowlees
Department of Psychiatry and Behavioral Sciences
University of California, Davis
Sacramento
USA

Joachim Diederich
Psychology Network Pty Ltd
Brisbane
Australia

ISSN 1860-949X ISSN 1860-9503 (electronic)
ISBN 978-3-662-50838-1 ISBN 978-3-642-38550-6 (eBook)
DOI 10.1007/978-3-642-38550-6
Springer Heidelberg New York Dordrecht London

Softcover reprint of the hardcover 1st edition 2014

Printed on acid-free paper

Springer is part of Springer Science+Business Media (www.springer.com)

Preface

Over the last years, the practice of delivering mental health services has changed dramatically. Information on mental health problems is widely available online and indexed for search, mobile devices are being used in large numbers worldwide, the consumers of health services self-organise by use of social networks, medical and psychological assessment is being automated step-by-step and consultation is increasingly conducted via the Internet. Given the prevalence of mental health disorders and the burden on economies worldwide, mental health informatics should be a dedicated branch of Information and Communication Technology (ICT) or applied computer science.

This book introduces a number of approaches that have the potential to transform the daily practice of psychiatrists and psychologists. This includes the asynchronous communication between mental health care providers and clients as well as the automation of assessment and therapy. Fully automated versions of cognitive behaviour therapy are currently available over the Internet and are being used by millions of users worldwide. While the origins of psychometric testing go back to the nineteenth century and the methodology of psychological measurement is highly developed, the Internet revolution has advanced the science of psychological assessment not significantly beyond paper and pencil tests. A significant number of psychological tests are based on self-report or the observation of parents and relatives as well as clinicians. While paper and pencil have been replaced by input devices and tests are scored automatically, the very nature of psychological and cognitive testing has not changed significantly.

This book offers a glimpse at the radical transformations that are awaiting the field of psychological assessment. Even in developing countries, many individuals use mobile phones (most people still have one mobile phone only, some have several devices for professional and private purposes). Mobile phones record and transmit speech, text and movement data. They store and communicate personal information, including search data, shopping behaviour and items identifying cultural, social and other beliefs. Mobile devices are essential for social networking—the organisation of social tribes—and, consequently, the participation of individuals in physical or online groups. For the first time in history, the behaviour of hundreds of millions of individuals is being recorded, stored and analysed. For the first time ever, objective data about the behaviour of a significant portion of the worldwide population is available.

Most psychologists and psychiatrists would agree that these data are valuable for assessment purposes. Clearly, however, there are significant ethical and privacy concerns that must be addressed while methods for the computational assessment and treatment of mental health problems are being developed. Nevertheless, the information on movement and communication patterns, constantly recorded by mobile phones, has significant value beyond that of the traditional psychometric testing techniques. As in other areas of information technology, these data (with permission of the participants) can be used for the benefits of individuals and their families (i.e., assessment and treatment) and for a multitude of purposes in support of the health and personal interests of consumers.

Speech and language are particularly interesting from the viewpoint of psychological assessment. For instance, depression may change the characteristics of voice in individuals and these changes can be detected by a special form of speech analysis. Some psychological problems result in changes in the use of language, such as the use of certain words and the avoidance of others, the inappropriate introduction of new words to a language and a reduction of the overall vocabulary (e.g., schizophrenia). Computational screening methods that utilise speech and language can detect subtle changes and alert clinicians as well as individuals and caregivers.

The importance of speech and language is further emphasised by the redefinition of some mental health categories that is currently underway. This preface is written a few weeks before the introduction of DSM-5, the fifth edition of the American Psychiatric Association's (APA) Diagnostic and Statistical Manual of Mental Disorders (DSM). It is currently assumed that Aspergers will not be part of this edition, which will be published in May 2013. DSM-5 will introduce a new category, Social Communication Disorder (SCD), which is a language disorder and as such different from Autism Spectrum Disorder (ASD) as defined in DSM-5. While the exact criteria for SCD are still unavailable at this point in time, it is assumed that this disorder will focus on a "qualitative impairment in social interaction". This moves the pragmatic aspect of language—the use in social interactions—to centre stage. Hence, the analysis of social interactions by computational methods will be essential for research on SCD and the development of psychological tests.

As stated above, there is an abundance of data that can be used for the assessment and treatment of mental health problems. The use of these data, however, poses ethical problems that will occupy concerned individuals, governments and the wider public for a long time. Assuming that these ethical problems can be solved, it should be possible in principle to diagnose and treat mental health disorders completely online (naturally, this excludes the use of medication). The long-term objective of this line of research is the assessment and treatment of individuals with mental health disorders within a virtual environment.

Brisbane, March 2013 Joachim Diederich

Contents

Chapter 1
Mental Health Informatics: Current Approaches

Joachim Diederich and Insu Song

1.1 Introduction

According to an AHRQ report [60], mental health disorder is one of the five most costly medical conditions in the U.S., with expenditures almost doubling from 1996 to 2006. The number of people with mental health disorders to a similar degree. This has led to mental illness becoming one of most societies' largest public health burdens. The major challenges in mental health care can be grouped as follows: (1) availability of health care for remote and underserved population; and (2) making health care more cost-effective and adequate. Developed mental health informatics technologies include traditional information management systems, such as electronic repository of patient information, electronic clinical summaries, and patients' care plans. These technologies have become critical as network of varying organizations (day hospitals, mental health centres, and small residential units) are involved in the management of mental health patients including chronically disabled patients [30]. One of the main challenges for mental health information management systems is the secure transfer of patient information.

Most notable support in the advancement of mental health informatics has come from the Internet, in particular Web 2.0. The massive production of social media enabled by Web 2.0 drives a wealth of clinical knowledge, thereby providing an efficient platform for patients to support each other. According to a 2008 survey, most Americans (up to 80 %) rely on the Internet to find health information in order to make their health care decisions [22]. This trend rivalled physicians as of

J. Diederich (✉)
School of Information Technology and Electrical Engineering, The University of Queensland, Brisbane Q4072, Australia
e-mail: j.diederich@uq.edu.au

I. Song
School of Business and IT, James Cook University Australia, Singapore Campus 574421, Singapore
e-mail: insu.song@jcu.edu.au

M. Lech et al. (eds.), *Mental Health Informatics*, Studies in Computational Intelligence 491, DOI: 10.1007/978-3-642-38550-6_1,

2008 [56]. An increasing number of patients (and families of patients) are also relying on the Internet for emotional support and to find clinical knowledge for self-care.

Slow but steady progress has been made on automated/assisted assessment technologies of mental health ranging from image based automated assessment of stress and anxiety [13], acoustic speech analysis of depressed patients [40, 44], and text analysis for the assessment of autism [59]. We do not expect to see fully automated mental health assessment and treatment systems in the near future, but many clinical trials indicate their potential to be integrated into relatively well established telepsychiatry (e.g., [68]).

Except for health social networks (e.g., Health 2.0), which are mainly driven by communities, more extensive and structured clinical trials for quantitative analysis are required to bring about wider acceptance, as most studies still report anecdotal qualitative analysis [68] or studies based on small numbers of subjects.

In this paper, we review current approaches to mental health informatics focusing on automated assessment methods, as we believe this is the current bottleneck for providing more objective and efficient mental health care.

1.2 Telemental Health

Telemedicine is the use of communication technologies, such as telephone, video conferencing, or the Internet, to provide and support health care to remote regions. Telemedicine was initially developed to provide health care to rural and underserved populations [4], but distance is no longer the major factor that defines the term. In fact, its applications have been extended to all types of health care including psychiatry consultations in inner cities [34, 35, 68]. While the greatest benefits come from its use in rural and underserved populations, as it makes otherwise unavailable health care available to many patients, its driving force is now more on making health care more cost-effective, affordable, accessible, efficient, and convenient for both health care providers and consumers. For instance, Harrison et al. [33] evaluated teleconferences between doctors for improving communication between primary and secondary health care, [68] reported case studies of telepsychiatry via videoconferencing and their potential to improve patient care and satisfaction, and reduce emergency department overcrowding. Frantzidis et al. [28] developed a remote monitoring system for the elderly and chronically ill. Tang et al. [63] used a multimedia system to improve medication adherence in elderly care. The growing number of aged population indicates that this form of telemedicine will become an important research area for many developed countries.

Almost all technologies we review here could be used in conjunction with telemental health technology. For instance, it will be possible to use automated speech analysis methods (e.g., [24, 40, 59, 65]) while the patients are being interviewed by psychiatrists to provide objective analysis of speech and language disorder or to monitor improvements in mental health conditions.

Much needed research is now being devoted to the development of more sophisticated tele-mental health technologies that integrate various technologies. This chapter reviews some of these technologies, with the aid of quantitative evaluation, rather than anecdotal qualitative evaluations [68]. Chapters 2, 3, and 4 of this book examine the use of modern communication technologies for tele-mental health and contemporary issues in mental health, such as how technology is changing the way health care services are delivered and how the relationship between patients and health care providers is changing.

1.3 Automated Assessment Systems

Many mental health assessment methods are time consuming and highly subjective. To improve efficiency as well as to provide more objective assessments, various automated mental health assessment methods have been developed. The methods can be broadly classified based on what type of data are collected and analyzed.

1.3.1 Image and Behaviour Analysis

Cowie et al. [13] reviewed the use of image analysis techniques in detecting emotional cues from facial expressions (still face images) and gestures (movements of facial features). According to [13], two emotion detection paradigms are one detecting (seven) archetypal expressions and another one detecting nonarchetypal expressions (e.g., modulated, falsified, or mixed expressions). The majority of existing literature and available data clearly focus on the method of detecting archetypal expressions (e.g., [48, 51, 67]). Much work needs to be done on the detection of richer nonarchetypal emotional expressions and gestures. These approaches now focus on the detection of action units (AU) defined by Ekman et al. [21]. For instance, Valstar and Pantic [66] used a facial point detector based on Gabor-feature-based boosted classifiers, achieving AU recognition rate of 95.3 %. On the application of facial expression detection method on the diagnosis of mental health problems, Stone and Wei [61] used a facial expression detector to measure cognitive load, which is conventionally assessed using EEG or EMG measurements. However, there is little research on the use of facial emotional detection methods for clinical diagnosis of mental health problems. This may be due to the fact that image processing techniques are more difficult than other techniques, such as sound processing, and large variations on emotional expressions make it difficult to develop reliable measurements that are correlated with underlying psychological problems.

Instead of relying on face detection methods, Nambu et al. [45] developed a simple image processing technique for monitoring behaviours and diagnosing poor health in the elderly. The researchers developed an automatic diagnosis system that can assess physical conditions as well as mental conditions from behaviours of elderly watching TV. They used only the recordings of the start time of watching TV obtained from a running monitor of the television. Initially, they tried to utilize various other sensors, such as a running monitor of electric appliances or door switches, but found the resulting data to be difficult to objectively analyze them, as their data appear to be not correlated to each other. The start times of watching TV are recorded by dividing each day into 15 min intervals. An interval is given a certain value, say 1, when an elderly participant starts the TV in the interval and another value, say 0, otherwise. This way, a 30×96 pixel image could be constructed for visualizing behaviours of elderly watching TV. Their hypothesis was that the subjects watched the television at roughly fixed times if they were healthy. To measure productiveness of their TV watching behaviour, the researchers measured non-randomness of the patterns on the visualized behaviour using the maximum entropy method (MEM). The image compression rate was measured as an indication of the health condition. The lower compression rate (larger size of compressed image) was used as an indication of unhealthy condition.

1.3.2 Biosignals

Biosignals, such as skin conductance, EEG, EMG, and EGA measurements, have been used to monitor various physiological and psychological conditions. Since the introduction of affective computing [53], applications of bio-signals have attracted a lot of research interest, but mainly on detection of emotion for their application to human computer interactions. However, there are a few studies that tried to combine HCI and biosignals in medical applications (e.g., [5, 39, 41]). Here we review some examples.

Tarvainen et al. [64] used derived features from galvanic skin responses (GSR) to detect emotional responses to external stimulus (surprising sounds). GSR responses are produced by changes in the electrical properties of the skin in response to sweat gland functions responding to different kinds of stimuli. In a sense, GSR are similar to skin conductance responses (SCR). Tarvainen et al. [64] derived the features using principal component analysis (PCA), and clustering technique was applied to build a classifier that can distinguishing whether a response pattern belongs to a control or psychotic patient. Their method was tested using measurements from 33 participants: 20 healthy controls and 13 psychotic patients. It was observed that healthy controls showed clearer response patterns to external stimulus. The system achieved the overall correct ratings of 82 %. As GSR measures are much easier to obtain than EEG signals, it has been used on wearable computers. For instance, Lisetti and Nasoz [39] used GSR in conjunction with heart rate and temperature monitors mounted on wearable computers to monitor certain emotions (sadness, anger, fear, surprise, frustration, and amusement) noninvasively.

Electrodermal activity (EDA) is another term for GSR. It also results from sympathetic neuronal activity. Critchley [14] provides a detailed review of the relationship between the central nervous system, periperi, and EDA measures, indicating that a vast amount of information on mental and physiological conditions can be extracted from EDA measurements.

Frantzidis et al. [28] developed a method of detecting early psychological disorders by means of detecting frequent mood changes using EEG and EDA signals. Their research was based on the assumption that affective states of depression, anxiety, and chronic anger negatively influence the human immune system [32]. This is a neurophysiology-oriented approach that monitors the subjects' biosignals, providing a more objective mental health assessment. In their approach, EEG and EDA signals are recorded and features are computed. ERP, ERS, and ERD features are computed from EEG data, and SCR features are computed from EDA. Attribute selection is applied to EEG features using Best-First search. The C4.5 data mining algorithm is applied to the selected EEG features to generate valence discrimination function. The subjects' gender and the valence information extracted from the decision tree are then used to select one of four Mahalanobis distance functions (positive/negative pictures male, pos/neg pictures female) for arousal discrimination. The Mahalanobis distance of the vector of selected features from the centre of the selected Mahalanobis distance functions are then used to estimate the arousal level. The result of the detection is one of four classes: LL (Lower valence-Low arousal), LH (Lower valence-High arousal), HL (High valence-Low arousal), and HH (High valence-High arousal). Their average reported accuracy rate was 77.68 % for the discrimination of the four emotional states, differing both in their arousal and valence dimension.

1.3.3 Language Use in Patients with Schizophrenia

Speech and language disorders (SLD), such as incoherent discourse, occur in various mental disorders, such as mania, depression, and schizophrenia [1, 19, 36]. SLD is often termed thought disorder by schizophrenia researchers. Disorganized speech, such as incoherent discourse, has been considered one of the important aspects in diagnosing schizophrenia [1]. Indeed, incoherent discourse is considered an important symptom in diagnosing many psychiatric and neurological conditions [24]. DSM-IV [20] also uses disorganized speech as one of the diagnostic criteria for schizophrenia. Therefore, various formal methods have been proposed in an attempt to characterize disordered discourse related to mental disorders. The followings are some of the well validated rating scales of thought disorder: the assessment of Thought, Language and Communication (TLC) [3], the Clinical Language Disorders Rating Scale (CLANG) [9], the Communication Disturbances Index [17] and the Thought Disorder Index (TDI) [58].

SLDs occur in various mental disorders and provide critical information for assessing mental disorders. However, these formal methods are subjective, time consuming, and costly. Therefore, various automated SLD assessment methods for diagnosing mental disorders have been developed. Examples include statistical analysis of letter and category fluency [8], Latent Semantic Analysis (LSA) based speech incoherence analysis [24, 25], Ex-Ray [16], and Discriminant-Words [59].

SLD is also considered to be associated with cognitive impairments [15, 24] and as an early vulnerability indicator for schizophrenia [6, 42, 49, 52]. This is because schizophrenia is considered a neurodevelopmental disorder rather than a neurodegenerative disorder that occurs early in development, long before observable symptoms appear [18]. This suggests that deficits in brain function may present early in life [24]. This indicates that SLD analysis can provide early diagnosis of schizophrenia.

We can broadly classify automated SDL analysis tools into three categories:

1. Statistical analysis of letter and category fluency.
2. Latent Semantic Analysis (LSA) Based Analysis of Speech Disorder.
3. Machine Learning Approaches.

Statistical analysis of letter and category fluency is an earlier approach that measures word statistics of spoken or written content. LSA-based analysis approaches go further into word-to-word, word-to-sentence, or sentence-to-sentence semantic relations. Machine learning approaches use derived features from both word statistics and semantic relations to build models of underlying mental health conditions. Recent advances include generation of rules for explaining diagnosis results in terms of the input features.

1.3.3.1 Statistical Analysis of Letter and Category Fluency

The statistical analysis of letter and category fluency is one of the earliest SLD approaches in diagnosing schizophrenic patients. It measures performance on verbal fluency and semantic fluency tasks. These are measured by counting the number of words generated to letter cues or category cues within a certain time period [8]. Bokat and Goldberg [8] reported that patients with schizophrenia underperformed on both category and letter fluency tasks. In addition, they reported that schizophrenic patients demonstrated greater impairments on semantic fluency than letter fluency. However, these approaches may provide very limited information on disordered discourse, as they rely mostly on linguistic features, such as vocabulary size of patients [24]. Some researchers (e.g., [24]) suggested that communicative features, such as tangentiality (e.g., semantic similarity between questions and answers), provide more relevant information as to the underlying conditions [24].

1.3.3.2 Latent Semantic Analysis (LSA) Based Analysis of Speech Disorder

Elvevag et al. [25] used Latent Semantic Analysis (LSA) [38] to measure coherence of speech, and reported its performance in discriminating speech generated from schizophrenia patients and controls. They compared their research participants' performance and correlation with a standard clinical measure of ThD (the Scale for the Assessment of Thought, Language and Communication; and TLC [3]).

The authors defined "coherence" of speech as the semantic similarity of words or sentences to words or sentences. The researchers measured discourse coherence in schizophrenics to assess abnormalities in the use of language to provide objective and reliable assessment of coherence in discourses of schizophrenia patients. Their method could be able to discriminate schizophrenia patients with both low and high ThD from controls. In particular, they showed that LSA could be used to identify which part of speech production is incoherent and estimate the levels of incoherence.

In their approach, four language tasks were designed: a word coherence test, a verbal fluency test, a two-way dialog coherence test (between utterances), and a similarity test between participants (for identical questions compare semantic similarity of responses between participants). The first two tests were compared with blind human ratings on the global ThD assessment. The third test was compared with the average scores for tangentiality, content, and organizational structure ratings of TLC. The last test was compared with the average scores on tangentiality, coherence, and content ratings of TLC. These tests were designed to test choice of words, expression of meaning, relatedness of discourse, and coherence.

The problem with these instruments lies in the choice of questions and what measures (words, sentences, window size) are best in increasing sensitivity to group differences. LSA was trained on a corpus of written texts which are somewhat different from spoken discourse [38]. However, LAS was able to discriminate the groups in spoken discourse [24, 25, 37].

In their follow up study [24], they showed that a similar method can be used to assess relatives of patients with schizophrenia, as schizophrenia is considered to be heritable. Transcribed free-speech samples were obtained from four groups of participants: schizophrenia patient, schizophrenia patients' family, normal, and normal family. Although it is not exactly clear how features were represented, three types of features were claimed to be used: surface features, statistical language features, and semantic features. Linear Discriminant Analysis (LDA) was used for feature selection and classification. The overall classification accuracy over not-well vs. well was 77.1 %. The overall classification accuracy of well family participants versus control non-family participants was 90.0 %.

1.3.3.3 Ex-Ray on Schizophrenia

Ex-Ray [16] and Discriminant-Words [59] apply machine learning techniques, such as support vector machines, to a text classification task to diagnose mental health problems using transcribed speech samples from ''structured-narrative tasks''. The task of Ex-Ray is to determine whether the speech belongs to a schizophrenia patient or not. Ex-Ray uses the bag-of-words feature representation where a fixed size vocabulary (e.g., 1,100 words in [16] is used to compute feature values, and each feature value is the frequency of each word in the vocabulary appearing in each speech sample. The feature values are also normalized to the length of documents. Ex-Ray and Discriminant-Words use Support Vector Machines (SVMs) [11] for the classification task. Ex-Ray achieved 80 % accuracy on a schizophrenia-versus-control classification task. Discriminant-Words achieved 75 % accuracy for an autism-versus-control similarity-measure task.

In Tilaka et al. [65], the performance of Ex-Ray was compared with two SLD scales: the Thought, Language and Communication Scale (TLC) [2] and the Clinical Language Disorder Rating Scale (CLANG) [9]. The same bag-of-words feature representation was used. Tilaka et al.'s SVM classifier achieved 98 % accuracy for a schizophrenia versus control task. This was comparable to the SLD scales on the same samples: TLC (98 % accuracy) and CLANG (97 % accuracy).

In a similar study by Felin et al. [26], it was also shown that a language model can be built from only one group of participants (schizophrenia) and used for discriminating them from others groups (e.g., normal). In this study, a one-class SVM classifier was built using 27 transcribed speech samples and tested against a total of 66 speech samples comprising speech samples from 27 patients and 39 controls. The SVM classifier achieved 81 % accuracy, whereas the two-class classifier trained on the entire database achieved 98 % accuracy. These findings suggest that machine learning approaches may be very practical, as there are often times when an appropriate control group is difficult to obtain. This one-class SVMs was compared to TLC and CLANG in diagnosing disorganized speech as well and shown to perform better.

Goh et al. [31] used Ex-Ray technology for the classification of autism assessment reports into positive and negative autism cases, using the term frequency features. The empirical evaluation was done on two sets of autism assessment reports: assessments that were confirmed to be autism or normal. The autism diagnosis reports were obtained from mental health clinics and comprised a total of 236 reports: 217 positive cases and 19 negative cases.. The autism text documents are represented as attribute-value vectors ("bag of words" representations) where each distinct word corresponds to a feature whose value is the frequency of the word in the text sample. The Ex-Ray method has been evaluated against well established validation tools: Gillian Autism Rating Scale (GARS-2) [29], Social Communication Questionnaire (SCQ) [7, 55], and Social Responsiveness Scale (SRS) [10]. In this study SVM-2C achieved ROC areas of 0.938, whereas GARS-2, SCQ, and SRS achieved ROC areas of 0.750, 0.810, and 0.810, respectively.

1.3.4 Acoustic Analysis of Speech

Speech provides nonlinguistic information, such as voice quality and prosody, that provide information on emotional states of speakers, and, therefore, acoustic analysis of the human voice can be used for the detection of various mental health problems affecting emotional states of affected individuals [57]. For instance, Ellgring and Scherer [23] have shown that simple acoustic properties of speech, such as increased speech rate and decreased pause duration, are effective indicators of the level improvements of depression. Automated voice analysis for the diagnosis of mental health dates back to 1930, when a German psychiatrist, Zwirne, developed a fundamental frequency (F0) tracking device to measure voice changes in depressed patients [47]. Since then, automated acoustic feature analysis of speech has regained interest only recently, due to the increasing number of mental health patients [27], the limitations of subjective approaches to diagnosing mental health conditions and the effects of treatments [23, 44], and the amount of resources required for clinical assessments [27].

Earlier research focused on prosodic features: fundamental frequencies (F0) [23, 47, 54], pause duration [23], and speech rates [23, 47]. Later studies utilized more complicated features: power spectral density measures [27], voice quality [12], vocal tracking [44], glottal features [40, 44], and TEO-based features [40]. Almost all approaches combine more than one category of features and report on the best combinations of features for the diagnosis of each mental health conditions. However, almost all approaches include prosodic features as part of their feature sets. This indicates that prosodic features can be effective indicators in the detection of emotion, stress, and depression. Table 1.1 summarizes developments in features and their uses. We now describe previous and current approaches in more detail.

Pope et al. [54] investigated the association of acoustic features of speech with anxiety and depression in 10 min monologues. Anxiety was positively related to rate of verbal productivity and speech disturbance, and negatively related to silent pauses. Depression was negatively related to rate of productivity and filled pauses and positively to silent pauses. A positive relationship was found between anxiety and resistiveness in speech and a negative relationship between depression and superficiality.

Nilsonne [46] and Nilsonne et al. [47] used the rate of change of fundamental frequencies (F0) to measure the level of clinical improvements in depression. Based on their study involving 16 depressed patients, they found that the standard deviation of F0 (SDF0), the standard deviation of the rate of change of F0 (SDF0RC), and the average speed of change of F0 (AF0S) were significantly greater after recovery from depression.

Ellgring and Scherer [23], and Low et al. [40] have shown that there are large gender differences in depressive speech behaviour. For instance, Ellgring and Scherer [23] study showed that the minimum fundamental frequency (F0) of speech in female was a good predictor of mood improvement.

Table 1.1 Summary of acoustic speech analysis methods for mental conditions

Authors	Features	Mental conditions
Pope et al. [54]	Speech rate Speech disturbance	Anxiety, depression (evaluated on 6 patients: 4 females and 2 males)
Nilsonne [46], Nilsonne et al. [47]	Rate of change of F0 Pause time Total reading time	Depression (evaluated on 16 depressed patients before and after recovery)
Ellgring and Scherer [23]	Speech rate Pause duration F0	Depression (evaluated on 16 de-pressed patients (11 female and 5 male) be-fore and after recovery)
France and Shiavi [27]	Formant Power spectral density measurements	Depression, suicide Evaluated on 48 female participants (10 control, 17 dysthymic patients, and 21 major depressed patients) and 67 male subjects (24 control, 21 major depressed patients, and 22 high-risk suicidal patients)
Cowie and Douglas-Cowie [12] Cowie et al. [13]	Prosodic features (pitch, voice quality)	Emotion, stress
Moore Ii et al. [44]	Combination of glottal and prosodic features	Depression
Low et al. [40]	TEO-based features Glottal features	Depression in adolescence

France and Shiavi [27] analyzed prosodic features (F0, formant measures, amplitude modulation) and spectral features (power spectral density measurements) in discriminating depressed individuals. To generate features, [27] segmented speech samples into frames and calculated the feature sets (range, variance, mean skewness, kurtosis, and coefficient of variation) for each frame slot. Based on their study involving a sample of participants comprising of 48 female participants (10 control, 17 dysthymic patients, and 21 major depressed patients) and 67 male participants (24 control, 21 major depressed patients, and 22 high-risk suicidal patients), formant (features derived from F1, F2, and F3) and power spectral density (the percentage of total power in four 500 Hz sub-bands) measurements were found to be the best discriminators in both the male and female participants. For male subjects, amplitude modulation (AM) features were found to be a strong class discriminators. Features describing F0 were generally ineffective discriminators in both sexes.

Cowie et al. [13] reviewed relationships between prosodic features (pitch, intensity, speech rate, voice quality) and emotion for use in their human computer interaction framework (the PHYSTA project), which is a hybrid system capable of using information from faces and voices to recognize people's emotions. Their review consolidated relevant knowledge from both psychology and linguistics.

Moore Ii et al. [44] provided detailed statistical analysis on the use of a combination of glottal, prosodic, and vocal track features for clinical analysis of emotional disorders, in particular for discriminating depressed speech. Base on their study involving 15 males (9 controls, 6 patients) and 18 females (9 controls, 9 patients), Moore Ii et al. [44] reported that the combination of glottal and prosodic features produced better discrimination overall than the combination of prosodic and vocal tract features.

Low et al. [40] used acoustic correlates of depression in adolescents (aged 13–20 years) for early detection of depression. It was argued that emotional disturbances caused by depression affect acoustic properties of people with depression. They applied various time-series signal processing techniques, such as TEO-based features, Mel-frequency cepstral coefficients (MFCCs), and prosodic, spectral, and glottal features to extract acoustic properties of people with depression and to distinguish the speech of nondepressed from the speech of clinically depressed adolescents. They achieved classification accuracies of 87 % for males and 79 % for females using only TEO-based features, suggesting that TEO-based features most closely correlate with depression in adolescents among other combinations of those features. The combinations of glottal features with prosodic and spectral features was also found to be closely correlated with depression, achieving accuracies of 69 % for males and 75 % for females.

1.3.5 Knowledge Based Approaches

Panagiotakopoulos et al. [50] developed an integrated medical record management system that provides a series of applications and personalized services for patients with anxiety disorder by managing patient data collection and automatically assessing stress level based on user modelling to assist personalized treatments. Their experiment data were collected using a stress monitoring test comprising survey questions (e.g., "where were you at this time?", "what were you doing at this time?"). Panagiotakopoulos et al. [50] used Bayesian modelling to build association rules for the prediction of stress levels of participants. The classifier were built and evaluated on 10 anxiety patients over 30 days. The classifier achieved Receiver Operating Curve (ROC) areas (AUC) of 0.841.

1.4 Online Support and Information Management

Other relevant technologies for mental health informatics are newly-emerging online support and care technologies, such as online health systems [43], health social networks (e.g., PatientsLikeMePatientsLikeMe[1] and the IBM Patient Empowerment System[2]), and online forums.

---

[1] http://www.patientslikeme.com/all/patients

[2] http://www-03.ibm.com/press/us/en/pressrelease/33944.wss

A health social network is an online information service which facilitates information sharing between closely related members of a community. Also known as social media on the Internet, or Health 2.0, a health social network empowers patients and health service providers by promoting collaboration between patients, their caregivers, and clinicians [56]. At its basic level, a health social network provides emotional support by allowing patients to find others in similar health situations. They can also share information about conditions, symptoms, and treatments [62]. Other services include physician Q&A and self-tracking of conditions, symptoms, treatments, and other biological information [62]. The self-supporting community is particularly important for future sustainability in the case of lifelong conditions, such as autism.

Other forms of online support systems are being integrated into general support systems, such as web sites for supporting student services. For instance, McKay and Martin [44] discuss the use of information and communications technologies (ICT) in higher education as effective interventions for people with mental health issues, such as Web-mediated courseware design to meet the specific needs of people recovering from mental illness. As ICT tools have been successfully used for providing distance education, the same approach could be used to provide non-interrupted education for students with chronic mental health conditions as well as providing assessment and support services [44].

More traditional forms of health informatics are the uses of information systems to solve the data management problems arising from different forms and data requirements involving various stakeholders including patients. One of the challenges of mental health informatics is the data privacy issue, as the perceived lack of privacy is the main barrier to the growth of tele-mental health [69].

1.5 Conclusion

Mental health informatics is a multi-disciplinary endeavour incorporating many areas of research in information technology, communication, computer science, neuroscience, physiology, psychiatry, and psychology. Telepsychiatry and health social networks seem to be relatively well established with a great deal of industry and government support. In the recent years, many web-based online psychology counselling services have also been observed. Still, there remains much to be done, in particular more extensive and structured trials of the proposed methods seem warranted. However, many studies indicate the potential power of each of the approaches in solving current mental health care problems.

References

1. Allen, H.A., Liddle, P.F., Frith, C.D.: Negative features, retrieval processes and verbal fluency in schizophrenia. British J. Psych. **163**((DEC)), 769–775 (1993)
2. Andreasen, N.C.: Thought, language, and communication disorders: i. clinical assessment, definition of terms, and evaluation of their reliability. Arch. Gen. Psychiatry **36**(12), 1315–1321 (1979). doi:10.1001/archpsyc.1979.01780120045006
3. Andreasen, N.C.: Scale for the assessment of thought, language, and communication (TLC). Schizophr. Bull. **12**(3), 473–482 (1986)
4. Angaran, D.M.: Telemedicine and telepharmacy: Current status and future implications. Am J Health-Syst Pharm **56**(14), 1405–1426 (1999)
5. Bamidis, P.D., Papadelis, C., Kourtidou-Papadeli, C., Pappas, C., Vivas, A.B.: Affective computing in the era of contemporary neurophysiology and health informatics. Interact. Comput. **16**(4), 715–721 (2004)
6. Bearden, C.E., Rosso, I.M., Hollister, J.M., Sanchez, L.E., Hadley, T., Cannon, T.D.: A prospective cohort study of childhood behavioural deviance and language abnormalities as predictors of adult schizophrenia. Schizophr. Bull. **26**(2), 395–410 (2000)
7. Berument, S.K.R., Rutter, M., Lord, C., Pickles, A., Bailey, A.: Autism screening questionnaire: Diagnostic validity. British J. Psychiatry **175**, 444–451 (1999)
8. Bokat, C.E., Goldberg, T.E.: Letter and category fluency in schizophrenic patients: A meta-analysis. Schizophr. Res. **64**(1), 73–78 (2003)
9. Chen, E.Y.H., Lam, L.C.W., Kan, C.S., Chan, C.K.Y., Kwok, C.L., Nguyen, D.G.H., Chen, R.Y.L.: Language disorganisation in schizophrenia: Validation and assessment with a new clinical rating instrument. Hong Kong J. Psychiatry **6**(1), 4–13 (1996)
10. Constantino, J.N., Gruber, C.P.: Social Responsiveness Scale (SRS). Western Psychological Services, Los Angeles, CA (2005)
11. Cortes, Corinna, Vapnik, V.: Support-vector networks. Machine Learn. **20**(3), 273–297 (1995)
12. Cowie, R., Douglas-Cowie, E.: Automatic statistical analysis of the signal and prosodic signs of emotion in speech. Proc. ICSLP **1996**, 1989–1992 (1996)
13. Cowie, R., Douglas-Cowie, E., Tsapatsoulis, N., Votsis, G., Kollias, S., Fellenz, W., Taylor, J.G.: Emotion recognition in human-computer interaction. IEEE Signal Process. Mag. **18**(1), 32–80 (2001)
14. Critchley, H.D.: Electrodermal responses: What happens in the brain? Neuroscientist **8**(2), 132–142 (2002)
15. DeLisi, L.E.: Speech disorder in Schizophrenia: Review of the literature and exploration of its relation to the uniquely human capacity for language. Bulletin **27**(3), 4 (2001)
16. Diederich, J., Al-Ajmi, A., Yellowlees, P.: Ex-ray: Data mining and mental health. Appl. Soft Comput. J. **7**(3), 923–928 (2007)
17. Docherty, N.M.: Cognitive impairments and disordered speech in Schizophrenia: Thought disorder, disorganization and communication failure perspectives. J. Abnorm. Psychol. **114**(2), 269–278 (2005)
18. Dr, W.: Implications of normal brain development for the pathogenesis of Schizophrenia. Arch. Gen. Psychiatry **44**(7), 660–669 (1987)
19. DSM-IV-TR: Diagnostic and Statistical Manual of Mental Disorders, Text Revision, 4th edn. American Psychiatric Association, USA (2000)
20. DSM-IV: Diagnostic and Statistical Manual of Mental Disorders. American Psychiatric Association, USA (1994)
21. Ekman, P., Rosenberg, E.L., Heller, M.: What the face reveals. Basic and applied studies of spontaneous expression using the facial action coding system (FACS). Psychotherapies **18**(3), 179–180 (1998)
22. Elkin, N.: How America searches: Health and wellness (2008)

23. Ellgring, H., Scherer, K.R.: Vocal indicators of mood change in depression. J. Nonverbal Behav. **20**(2), 83–110 (1996)
24. Elvevag, B., Foltz, P.W., Rosenstein, M., DeLisi, L.E.: An automated method to analyze language use in patients with schizophrenia and their first-degree relatives. J. Neurolinguist. **23**(3), 270–284 (2009)
25. Elvevag, B., Foltz, P.W., Weinberger, D.R., Goldberg, T.E.: Quantifying incoherence in speech: An automated methodology and novel application to Schizophrenia. Schizophr. Res. **93**(1–3), 304–316 (2007)
26. Felin, Joachim, D., Song, I.: An alternative method of analysis in the absence of control group. In: Diederich, J., Song, I., Yellowlees, P. (eds.) Mental Health Informatics. Springer (2011)
27. France, D.J., Shiavi, R.G.: Acoustical properties of speech as indicators of depression and suicidal risk. IEEE Trans. Biomed. Eng. **47**(7), 829–837 (2000)
28. Frantzidis, C.A., Bratsas, C., Klados, M.A., Konstantinidis, E., Lithari, C.D., Vivas, A.B., Papadelis, C.L., Kaldoudi, E., Pappas, C., Bamidis, P.D.: On the classification of emotional biosignals evoked while viewing affective pictures: An integrated data-mining-based approach for healthcare applications. IEEE Trans. Inf. Technol. Biomed. **14**(2), 309–318 (2010)
29. Gilliam, J.E.: Gilliam Autism Rating Scale, 2nd edn. PRO-ED, Austin, TX (2006)
30. Glover, G.: Mental health informatics and the rhythm of community care. Information systems in psychiatry must be released from the asylums and updated. Br. Med. J. **311**(7012), 1038–1039 (1995)
31. Goh, T.J., Diederich, J., Song, I., Sung, M.: Using diagnostic information to develop a machine learning application for the effective screening of autism spectrum disorders. In: Diederich, J., Song, I., Yellowlees, P. (eds.) Mental Health Informatics. Springer, NY (2011)
32. Goleman, D.: Emotional Intelligence. Bantam Books, New York (1995)
33. Harrison, R., Clayton, W., Wallace, P.: Can telemedicine be used to improve communication between primary and secondary care? Br. Med. J. **313**(7069), 1377–1381 (1996)
34. Hilty, D.M., Luo, J.S., Morache, C., Marcelo, D.A., Nesbitt, T.S.: Telepsychiatry: An overview for psychiatrists. CNS Drugs **16**(8), 527–548 (2002). doi:10.2165/00023210-200216080-00003
35. Hilty, D.M., Marks, S.L., Urness, D., Yellowlees, P.M., Nesbitt, T.S.: Clinical and educational telepsychiatry applications: A review. Can. J. Psychiat. Rev. Can. Psychiat. **49**(1), 12–23 (2004)
36. Kuperberg, G.R.: Language in Schizophrenia. Part I. An introduction. Lang. Linguist. Compass **4**(8), 576–589 (2010)
37. Landauer, T., Foltz, P., Laham, D.: An introduction to latent semantic analysis. Discourse Process. **25**, 259–284 (1998). doi:citeulike-article-id:2243850
38. Landauer, T.K., Dumais, S.T.: A solution to Plato's problem: The latent semantic analysis theory of acquisition, induction, and representation of knowledge. Psychol. Rev. **104**(2), 211–240 (1997)
39. Lisetti, C.L., Nasoz, F.: Using noninvasive wearable computers to recognize human emotions from physiological signals. Eurasip J. Appl. Signal Process. **11**, 1672–1687 (2004)
40. Low, L.S.A., Maddage, N.C., Lech, M., Sheeber, L.B., Allen, N.B.: Detection of clinical depression in adolescents' speech during family interactions. IEEE Trans Biomed Eng **58**(3 PART 1), 574–586 (2011)
41. Luneski, A., Bamidis, P.D., Hitoglou-Antoniadou, M.: Affective computing and medical informatics: State of the art in emotion-aware medical applications. Stud. Health Technol. Inform. **136**, 517–522 (2008)
42. Makowski, D., Waternaux, C., Lajonchere, C.M., Dicker, R., Smoke, N., Koplewicz, H., Min, D., Mendell, N.R., Levy, D.L.: Thought disorder in ado-escent-onset Schizophrenia. Schizophr. Res. **23**(2), 147–165 (1997)
43. McKay, E., Martin, J.: Mental health and wellbeing: Converging HCI with human informatics in higher education. Issues Inf. Sci. Inf. Technol. **7**(3), 339–351 (2010)

44. Moore Ii, E., Clements, M.A., Peifer, J.W., Weisser, L.: Critical analysis of the impact of glottal features in the classification of clinical depression in speech. IEEE Trans. Biomed. Eng. **55**(1), 96–107 (2008)
45. Nambu, M., Nakajima, K., Noshiro, M., Tamura, T.: An algorithm for the automatic detection of health conditions. IEEE Eng. Med. Biol. Mag. **24**(4), 38–42 (2005)
46. Nilsonne, A.: Acoustic analysis of speech variables during depression and after improvement. Acta Psychiatr. Scand. **76**(3), 235–245 (1987)
47. Nilsonne, A., Sundberg, J., Ternstrom, S., Askenfelt, A.: Measuring the rate of change of voice fundamental frequency in fluent speech during mental depression. J. Acoust. Soc. Am. **83**(2), 716–728 (1988)
48. Otsuka, T., Ohya, J.: Recognition of facial expressions using HMM with continuous output probabilities. Proc. IEEE Int. Workshop Robot Human Commun. **2**, 323–328 (1996)
49. Ott, S.L., Roberts, S., Rock, D., Allen, J., Erlenmeyer-Kimling, L.: Positive and negative thought disorder and psychopathology in childhood among subjects with adulthood schizophrenia. Schizophr. Res. **58**(2), 231–239 (2002)
50. Panagiotakopoulos, T.C., Lyras, D.P., Livaditis, M., Sgarbas, K.N., Anastassopoulos, G.C., Lymberopoulos, D.K.: A contextual data mining approach toward assisting the treatment of anxiety disorders. IEEE Trans. Inf. Technol. Biomed. **14**(3), 567–581 (2010)
51. Pantic, M., Rothkrantz, L.Ü.M.: Automatic analysis of facial expressions: The state of the art. IEEE Trans. Pattern Anal. Mach. Intell. **22**(12), 1424–1445 (2000)
52. Parnas, J., Schulsinger, F., Schulsinger, H., Mednick, S.A., Teasdale, T.W.: Behavioral precursors of schizophrenia spectrum: A prospective study. First published doi:10.1001/archpsyc.1982.04290060020005 (1982)
53. Picard, R.W., Vyzas, E., Healey, J.: Toward machine emotional intelligence: Analysis of affective physiological state. IEEE Trans. Pattern Anal. Mach. Intell. **23**(10), 1175–1191 (2001)
54. Pope, B., Blass, T., Siegman, A.W., Raher, J.: Anxiety and depression in speech. J. Consul. Clinical Psychol. **35**(11), 128–133 (1970)
55. Rutter, M., Bailey, A., Lord, C.: Social Communication Questionnaire. Western Psychological Services, Los Angeles, CA (2003)
56. Sarasohn-Kahn J (2008) The wisdom of patients: Health care meets online social media. California HealthCare Foundation iHealth Reports
57. Scherer, K.R., Zei, B.: Vocal indicators of affective disorders. Psychother. Psychosom. **49**(3–4), 179–186 (1988)
58. Solovay, M.R., Shenton, M.E., Gasperetti, C., Coleman, M., Kestnbaum, E., Carpenter, I.X., Holzman, P.S.: Scoring manual for the Though Disorder Index (rev. version). Schizophr. Bull. **12**, 483–496 (1986)
59. Song, I., Marsh, N.V.: Anonymous indexing of health conditions for a similarity measure. IEEE Trans. Inf. Technol. Biomed. **16**(4), 737–744 (2012)
60. Soni, A,: The five most costly conditions, 1996 and 2006: Estimates for the U.S. civilian noninstitutionalized population medical expenditure panel survey. Agency for Healthcare Research and Quality (2009)
61. Stone, R.T., Wei, C.S.: Exploring the linkage between facial expression and mental workload for arithmetic tasks, pp. 616–619 (2011)
62. Swan, M.: Emerging patient-driven health care models: an examination of health social networks, consumer personalized medicine and quantified self-tracking. Int. J. Environ. Res. Public Health **6**(2), 492–525 (2009)
63. Tang, L., Zhou, X., Yu, Z., Liang, Y., Zhang, D., Ni, H.: MHS: A multimedia system for improving medication adherence in elderly care. IEEE Syst. J. **5**(4), 506–517 (2011)
64. Tarvainen, M.P., Koistinen, A.S., Valkonen-Korhonen, M., Partanen, J., Karjalainen, P.A.: Analysis of galvanic skin responses with principal components and clustering techniques. IEEE Trans. Biomed. Eng. **48**(10), 1071–1079 (2001)

65. Tilaka, A.D., Diederich, J., Song, I., Teoh, A.: Automated method for diagnosing speech and language dysfunction in schizophrenia. In: Peter, Y., Joachim, D., Margaret, L.I.S. (eds.) Mental Health Informatics. Studies in Computational Intelligence Springer, NY (2013)
66. Valstar, M.F., Pantic, M.: Fully automatic recognition of the temporal phases of facial actions. IEEE Trans. Syst. Man Cybern. B Cybern. (2011)
67. Yacoob, Y., Devis, L.S.: Recognizing human facial expressions from long image sequences using optical flow. IEEE Trans. Pattern Anal. Mach. Intell. **18**(6), 636–642 (1996)
68. Yellowlees, P., Burke, M.M., Marks, S.L., Hilty, D.M., Shore, J.H.: Emergency telepsychiatry. J. Telemed. Telecare **14**(6), 277–281 (2008). doi:10.1258/jtt.2008.080419
69. Young, K.S.: An empirical examination of client attitudes towards online counseling. Cyberpsychol. Behavior **8**(2), 172–177 (2005)

Chapter 2
The Rise of Person-Centered Healthcare and the Influence of Health Informatics and Social Network Applications on Mental Health Care

Michelle Burke Parish and Peter Yellowlees

2.1 Introduction

Social networks are rapidly becoming the new frontier of healthcare. The use of social networking in healthcare has been spurred by a shift to person-centered healthcare models and a patient driven movement towards greater transparency and communication with providers. Connecting with patients over social networks could allow providers to be more fully informed about patients' day-to-day issues, symptoms and lifestyle choices. The click of a mouse could open a window into patients' daily lives and give patients access to their providers in the convenience of their own home. Social media could foster a revival of the house-call or rather become the digital house-call of the future. Such an approach may find no better home than in the field of mental health where relationships and communication are paramount to treatment success. However, one might ask, what would this picture of mental healthcare look like? Might mental health care soon involve clinicians logging onto online social networks: checking patients' online activity, evaluating patients' moods, administering surveys and determining if additional appointments are needed, adjusting medications, reviewing video of a significant event or issue uploaded by a patient, or even running software algorithms or other diagnostic tools to evaluate a patients mental state though the language and information shared over social networking? Although this picture of mental health treatment may seem a bit farfetched, the technology to support these methods exists and research to examine these approaches is already underway. As patient-provider interaction online increases and the popularity of social networks booms to an all-time high, clinicians having direct links to their patients through web-based and mobile applications is just around the corner from becoming common place. Yet,

M. B. Parish · P. Yellowlees (✉)
Department of Psychiatry and Behavioral Sciences, University of California, Davis, U.S.A

M. Lech et al. (eds.), *Mental Health Informatics*,
Studies in Computational Intelligence 491, DOI: 10.1007/978-3-642-38550-6_2,

research in this area is new and limited, and important ethical issues as well as patient privacy, security and confidentiality must be considered as this "new frontier" in healthcare merges into the mainstream.

2.2 Person-Centered Healthcare and the Influence of Health Informatics in Mental Healthcare

2.2.1 Rise of Person-Centered Healthcare

The use of information technology in healthcare has long been driven by the need to expand services to those less reachable and to increase the convenience of health care delivery. We have recently seen a paradigm shift in healthcare from provider-driven models to more person-centered approaches. Person-centered healthcare is a patient driven movement towards greater transparency and communication between health care providers and patients that has become a standard model of care throughout the medical and mental health fields. Patient centered healthcare centralizes care with the patient, and encourages patient-provider communication and patient input in treatment, where patient needs are considered more closely. Providers strive to tailor patient care to each individuals' unique care needs, focus on the importance of caring for the whole person [1] and to know the person behind the patient [2].

Patient demand for more accessible health care information and greater communication with providers has spurned the now widespread use of the internet to facilitate care and patient knowledge [3] and has been the catalyst for the use of social networking applications in healthcare. Health IT applications are now widely accessible to patients to support patient care, and many researchers and healthcare providers are beginning to realize the potential of these tools to improve healthcare, market services, conduct research and reach at risk and difficult to access populations [4]. Email communications and appointment reminders, websites providing general health care and provider information and scheduling, and more recently, social networks to encourage more direct patient-provider contact, administer convenient health and illness information, and allow for convenient patient support groups are beginning to become common place. Technology such as online forums or blogs, instant messaging platforms, video-chat, and social networks are reengineering the way doctors and patients interact. Social networking applications in healthcare have the potential to facilitate the person-centered care model far beyond current practice standards by providing clinicians with a window into patients' daily lives, informing a more holistic patient approach.

2.2.2 *Influence of Health IT and Popularity of Social Networks*

Telemedicine is the practice of providing health consultations via video conferencing or other electronic formats. Telemedicine has a long history in healthcare dating back to the 1950s and is routinely used nationwide [5]. Over the last three decades, an infrastructure has been established to support the use of telemedicine in most major healthcare facilities, and it is used across multiple disciplines including radiology, dermatology, ophthalmology, cardiology and pathology [6–14] and psychiatry [15–17]. The advent of telemedicine and other forms of online communication between patient and provider (i.e. email, secure chat) marked a paradigm shift in healthcare that has developed into mass integration of health IT applications within the field.

Many individuals already seek medical advice and services online and thorough social networks from expert and community sources. While there is wide variation in reports, studies suggest that at least 40 % and up to 80 % of adults with internet access use the internet for health purposes such as to research health related issues, communicate with providers, or receive treatment [18]. As technology based convenience tools have become a part of everyday life for providers and patients alike, providers are utilizing tools ranging from email to specialized social network sites and smart phone applications (apps) to connect with patients and even to provide health services.

Social networking has been defined as "web-based services that allow individuals to (1) construct a public or semi-public profile within a bounded system, (2) articulate a list of other users with whom they share a connection, and (3) view and traverse their list of connections and those made by others within the system" [19]. Social networks have become a fast growing phenomenon across the globe. Sites such as Facebook (https://www.facebook.com/), Myspace and Google+ have revolutionized the way many people connect socially. According to Facebook, one of the most popular social networking sites worldwide, over 600 million people are members of this site, or rather it is used by 1 in every 13 people worldwide (https://www.facebook.com/). For a more extensive history of social networking sites see [19].

The mass popularity of these sites among consumers has driven social networks into the healthcare arena. Most healthcare institutions offer online tools for patients such as access to their electronic chart, lab results and appointment scheduling, and many are now connecting with and engaging patients over social networks like facebook and twitter. Social networking is becoming an important element in providing patient-centered care. Providers are discovery that social networks allow for the development of closer relationships and increased communication with patients which can lead to greater patient engagement in treatment.

2.2.3 Applications of Social Networks in Healthcare

Social networking applications are now being considered as a research tool for social scientists and other researchers to access patient data and as platforms for administering surveys and other data collection devices (Snee 2008; Mahapatra, 2010; Procter et al. 2010). Some medical social networking sites are now aggregating patient data to show trends in treatment success and disease progression. The site PatientsLikeMe (http://www.patientslikeme.com/) is a consumer driven site where individuals log-on to connect with others in the community who are experiencing similar medical issues. Users can look up symptoms, treatments and medications related them, and enter their own medical information to share with others on the site. This data is aggregated by the site and patients and researchers can look up an array of aggregate reports on a large number of medical issues and drugs including reported side-effects, effective dosages of drugs and even warning signs of specific illnesses. This aggregated data can also be purchased by researchers and has been used successfully in studies evaluating patient perceptions of medical treatments and illnesses such as treatment perceptions in individuals with amyotrophic lateral sclerosis (ALS) [20] and for developing and validating illness specific rating scales [21]. While social networking sites such as PatientsLikeMe may be valuable and useful tools for aggregating and disseminating large cross sections of patient reported data, concerns have been raised about the validity of this form of data collection. Brubaker et al. (2010) note that researchers must take heed when evaluating and interpreting patient driven self-report data from such sites. On these sites, users select the data that they report based on the symptoms or issues most salient to them and such data may not provide a full picture of disease progression or side-effects for everyone. Further, such platforms for patient data collection may not be equitable as data generated from social networking sites would only be representative of a subset of the population that is sufficiently educated and financially secure to consistently access the Internet to participate on social networking sites (Brubaker et al. 2010).

2.3 Mental Health Care and Social Media

2.3.1 Social Networking Applications and Mental Health Care: Research and Current Trends

Over the past 50 years, the mental health field has seen a great shift to community based, person-centered, patient-facilitated treatment [17], and has been at the forefront of advancing patient care onto more convenient and accessible health IT platforms such as telepsychiatry, eTherapy and now social networks.

Mental health care consumers are increasingly interested in health IT platforms for mental health treatment and resources [22, 23]. Many different social networks for patient groups are already largely available online. One such social network is Mental Health Social Network supported by Psych Central (http://www.mentalhealthsocial.com/index.php?ref=index.html.var). Mental Health Social Network allows users to log on and interact with others in the community who are experiencing similar issues and symptoms. Illness-specific information is available, some informational questionaries and access to local mental health referrals are also accessible within the site.

Social networks may be a useful tool for providing social support to those with mental health issues, and may even be utilized for identifying those at risk for mental illness. This tool may prove to become a valuable source of information for mental health providers about patient's state of mind, mood, social support and coping resources. However, in many ways our understanding of the impact of social networking tools in mental health is still in its infancy, and research on the effective use of this health IT tool is only beginning to be undertaken.

Studies have been conducted evaluating the use of social networks to support the mental health needs of those in select populations. Social networking sites may provide a stress buffering resource for those serving in the military who experience adverse life events [24]. In military populations the fear of stigma among other concern reduces treatment seeking for mental health issues [25, 26]. Technology-based approaches may increase mental health care access for this population. One study found that 33 % of Soldiers who reported that they were not willing to talk to a counselor in person, were willing to utilize at least one technology based platform for mental health care [27]. Social networks have also been found to be a useful social support tool for some groups such as cancer survivors who have limited social support [28]. Accessing social networks may be particularly beneficial for individuals with limited social support resources or those who have limited social interaction or are experiencing significant life transitions. For example, blogging and social networking was found to improve new mothers' well-being through increasing feelings of connectedness to the world outside their home through the Internet [29]. Further, social networking may provide additional or adjunct support to patients in crisis [30], for individuals with mental illness in rural areas [31] and strengthen social support for adults over 50 [32, 33]. Adolescents and young adults, or digital natives, may be the most accessible population via social networks as they are the most likely to regularly access the Internet and to utilize it as a health care and mental health care resource.

Adolescents and young adults make up the largest population of Internet and social network users and many in this age range are using the internet to access information about mental health. One study found that 76.9 % of the young people sampled (aged 12–25) use the internet to connect with others and 38.8 % reported seeking information about mental health problems for themselves or others online [34]. In a small sample of adolescents (n = 75) over half surveyed reported having turned to the internet for mental health support. Online social networking sites were found to be used regularly by 82 % of those surveyed and 47 % of student in this study believed these sites could help with mental health problems [31]. Thus, social networking applications may have a unique advantage for accessing adolescent and youth populations for mental health intervention and education [35].

Individuals in this age range may face barriers to care in addition to fear of social stigma such as lack of financial and other support resources or over all lack of access [36]. Thus social networks may become a key tool in more effectively reaching this population through a resource that a large majority already accessed frequently, and may be particularly useful for communicating with some at risk and difficult to access adolescent populations. For example, social networks could be used to keep in contact with homeless youth and children who are wards of the state or in foster care who may frequently relocate. Homeless youth may be able to regularly access free internet at public libraries, schools, and shelters and could potentially keep in contact with mental health providers, or even receive treatment and support over these channels. Social networking use may provide mental health benefits for this population as well. Rice et al. [37] found that social networking provided a buffer against anxiety and depression, acting as a useful coping recourse for teens faced with homelessness. In-person interactions with other homeless peers presented a risk factor for anxiety and depression. However, when teens interacted with home-based friends through social networks, it was found to be protective for depression and to reduce substance abuse in this population [37].

Social networking approaches to mental health treatment or treatment support may reduce barriers such as fear of stigmatization which is considered a key component in underutilization of metal health services for adolescents and young adults [38]. Adolescence is often a tumultuous developmental period marked by peer pressure, self-image concerns, relationship difficulties among other difficulties. Many mental health issues including schizophrenia, depression, and bipolar disorder first become apparent during adolescence and young adulthood [39] and early intervention may reduce the severity of the primary illness and reduce the likelihood of developing secondary mental health issues such substance abuse.

2.3.2 The Application of Social Networks in Mental Health Treatment: Assessment and Intervention

Social media applications may be useful tools to evaluate for mental illness. In a recent study, researchers reviewed the public social networking accounts of college students to assess for symptoms of depression, finding that 25 % of college students, whose social networking communications were evaluated, exhibited depressive symptoms, based upon the Diagnostic and Statistical Manual of Mental Disorders (DSM) criteria, and 2.5 % met the DSM criteria for major depressive disorder. Researchers noted that those who received online reinforcement from their friends were more likely to discuss their depressive symptoms publicly via social networking sites [44]. Such studies indicate that social networks could provide useful insight into patient wellbeing and even be used as an instrument for mental illness assessment. Many cutting-edge technologies are now being utilized for mental health evaluation and treatment support including mobile applications (apps.). Mobile apps can be used to map symptoms and even support specific interventions or function as a coping tool for patients. A recently developed app, Live OCD Free (http://www.liveocdfree.com/), utilizes exposure and response prevention techniques though the app to assist users with managing and coping with obsessive compulsive disorder (OCD) related symptoms. Exposure based therapy techniques to treat disorders such as OCD find success by simulating the anxiety provoking situation and implementing techniques to reduce anxiety and facilitate coping. Mobile based interventions act in real-time; no simulation needed. Such technology has the power to provide exposure based therapy in the context of real-life situations, an achievement that can take months or years to reach in the therapeutic setting. Other apps have been developed to map mood (MoodyMe https://itunes.apple.com/us/app/moody-me-mood-diary-tracker/id411567371?mt=8), and behavior patterns across time, including triggers, diet, sleep and other related factors. This technological approach to treatment support and intervention has the potential to provide patients and providers a much broader and holistic picture of individual mental health. Triggers can be tracked more precisely and thus, may be more effectively addressed in treatment. The classic "homework" utilized in cognitive behavioral therapy (CBT) can now be taken off paper and put into a device that most patients carry with them everywhere they go. One issue that may be particularly receptive to mobile tracking is Posttraumatic Stress Disorder (PTSD). The National Center for PTSD and the National Center for Telehealth and Technology have created an app called PTSD Coach (http://www.ptsd.va.gov/public/pages/PTSDCoach.asp) designed to help veterans learn about and manage symptoms that commonly occur after trauma. The app features information on PTSD and treatments, tools for screening and tracking symptoms, tools to manage stress and direct links to support and help. While such apps are not designed to act as a substitute for treatment, this technology may become an important tool for managing and even initially detecting PTSD symptoms. Apps are beginning to be used in many useful ways to support behavioral health intervention including: symptom assessment, illness-specific education, treatment resource location, and tracking of treatment progress [45]. These platforms are also now allowing for live two-way communication between patient and provider which may begin to take the place of more traditional telemental health approaches.

Technology engineers are currently developing computer software programs to assess and evaluate mental health. Software programs have been developed to accurately detect mood in the voice of the user or "Artificial intuition" which is the use of technology to evaluate human emotions. Researchers at the University of Rochester have developed an algorithm that can detect human emotions through speech analysis which can correctly identify human emotions with roughly 80 % accuracy [46]. This technology could be imbedded in a myriad of health IT platforms including smartphones and social networking platforms to allow clinicians to evaluate patients mood and to track changes in mood over time. This technology could be utilized to detect the onset of illness-specific episodes such as a major depressive or manic episode, to track mood for the purposes of titrating medication (i.e. antidepressant, mood-stabilizing and anxiolytic medications) or to evaluate treatment effectiveness and medication compliance. Further, similar technologies may be adapted to detect specific symptom patterns to evaluate for mental illness via speech and language analysis that could be placed within health IT resources.

Mobile mental health applications are an exciting and interesting new platform for mental health and the possibilities for these tools are vast. These techniques and applications could be utilized via mobile and other, more universally accessible, health IT platforms such as secure social networking sites. Symptom tracking applications can be easily imbedded within social networks and information could be stored for patient and clinician access. Online social networks have the potential to encompass many aspects of patient care. In addition to providing symptom tracking and implementing therapeutic techniques in real-time, online social networks could provide a "one-stop" portal for contact between patients and providers, assessment, intervention and community mental health support with other users dealing with the similar issues. As the use of social networking applications boom amongst patients and providers alike, clinicians may be faced with new ethical dilemmas, and unique clinical and ethical guidelines associated with patient contact via social networks are needed.

2.3.3 *Ethical and considerations for Social Networking Use in Mental Health Care: Privacy, Confidentiality and Security*

2.3.3.1 Social Media Presence and Advertisement—Privacy and Security on Social Networks for Non-treatment Use

Developing a presence on social media has become a highly effective marketing tool and can be very useful for engaging patients in treatment and disseminating general educational and organizational information. However, privacy and security issues still arise even when using social networking sites strictly for non-treatment purposes. Providers or organizations intending to access patients over non-secured public social networking sites should ensure that secure data is not stored or transferred, treatment is not be provided, staff are adequately trained in secure social network use and security and that patients are adequately notified of the risks of sharing private information on the site.

Considering the complexity of this issue and the evolving security controls of social networking sites, it is advisable that providers or health care entities utilizing social media seek legal advice early and often to assist with the development of a social media policy. Policies should describe the limits to privacy and confidentiality when sharing information over social networking sites and should be clearly posted and easily accessible to patients logging onto the site. The social media policy should be detailed in patient consent forms and privacy notices used in standard practice. Policies should: "explain appropriate use of social media platforms, clearly define how information posted there will be used, specify what degree of privacy can be expected, state clearly that these forums are not to be used for personal medical advice, state clearly that the site is NOT monitored 24 h a day, seven days a week [47]". One issue of concern that should be considered is ability for the provider to respond in the case of a threat posted on the social networking site i.e. a patient posts threats of self-harm or violence towards others on the providers or organizations site. Providers are legally and ethically bound to respond in a timely manner to emergent situations where patients may be at risk for harming themselves or others. Policies posted on these sites and provided to patients should include limits to confidentiality in such cases and document how providers will respond to threats of self-harm or harm to others that are publically posted on the site. Risk of unforeseen disclosure of information on a provider's page due to a computer virus or "hacking" should also be included and posted in social media policies [48].

2.3.3.2 Social Media in Mental Health Practice and Treatment: Legal Considerations—Privacy, Security, and HIPAA Compliance

Ethics codes such as the American Psychological Association, American Counseling Association and American Psychiatric Association, provide guidelines for how mental health professionals must manage ethical concerns and avoid ethical violations. Yet, while more recent professional guidelines such as the APA Ethics Codes, call for an extension of these codes to technological transactions, limited guidelines exist to guide clinicians in ethical interactions via social networking sites. Before the use of social networking sites can be introduced into mainstream in mental health practice, many legal and ethical questions regarding privacy, security and confidentiality must be fully considered. Moreover, the ability to maintain communication practices that are compliant with the Health Insurance Portability and Accountability Act (HIPAA) is a legal concern of the utmost importance.

Practice laws and ethical guidelines have fallen behind rapid and ever evolving technological advances. Mental health treatment or treatment adjunctive support via social networking sites has the potential to encompass many different platforms of patient-provider contact or treatment including online counseling, email communication, telepsychiatry, asynchronous telepsychiatry, and guidelines for each form of interaction should be considered before contact is made or treatment is established. Above and beyond these guidelines that apply universally across all online treatment, privacy and security are paramount to any treatment based interaction over social networking as much of the communication occurs on a public or semi-public forum. Batchelor et al. [49] note that, with regard to providing therapy via online social networking, capacity to give informed consent to contracts, protection of online privacy including sharing and controlling data, data leaks between different digital platforms, and management of digital identities and footprints are important ethical and security issues to take into consideration [49].

With the widespread use of social networking sites among patients and providers alike, it is reasonable to assume that providers may begin to be approached over social networking sites for advice from patients. While specific practice guidelines have not been developed, precedent exists for provider-patent interactions on online social networking sites. For example, many medical social networking sites are designed so that users can log-on and receive medical advice from experts without having to make an appointment. Providers participating on "ask-a-doctor" type sites can respond to direct queries from individuals soliciting advice online who are not already established patients. Providers must be cautious to protect the privacy of the individuals soliciting advice and are bound by the laws and ethical codes that govern their license and the rules of the site. However, in this role, a treatment relationship has not been established. Thus, it may be very difficult for the individuals soliciting advice to be sure that they are communicating with an actual licensed physician and providers must be careful not to engage in treatment provision over these sites. Treatment and diagnosis over the internet is considered to be unethical in the absence of a previously established treatment relationship [50].

Once providers begin engaging patients on social networks designed for treatment, education, community support and quick advice for established patients, they have entered into an entirely new legal and ethical territory. Providers must be aware that they are legally accountable for advice given to established patients over social networking sites and should use caution in providing treatment [51]. Providers must be vigilant to fully establish patient care and treatment planning and to request in-person evaluations when warranted. Further, when providers are engaging with clients over social networking sites where other patients are participating, they must determine how to respond to clients' in a manner that provides useful information while still protecting the client's privacy. It is not safe for the provider to assume that he or she has the freedom to answer a patient's query openly online, particularly if the patient's condition or issues are rare and may make them unwittingly identifiable to others online.

Bishop et al. (2011) discuss the privacy implications of the use of social media in the provision of healthcare. They note that the possibility of eavesdropping, delay, and provider verification, are potentially complicating factors in the communication between provider and patient online. Further, Bishop et al. illustrate guidelines for communicating with patients online such as that general advice may be given on more open forums but that more detailed personal information should be discussed on HIPAA compliant channels that are private and secure. However, it may be difficult for providers to determine which social networking sites are secure enough as most public sites are not set up to be HIPAA compliant. How is a provider to know if a site is secure enough for communication with patients and what information can be shared, if any at all, over social networking sites?

2.3.3.3 HIPAA Compliance of Social Networking Sites

The Health Insurance Portability and Accountability Act, or HIPAA [52], provides "federal protections for personal health information held by covered entities and gives patients an array of rights with respect to that information" [52]. HIPPA laws allow for the exchange of protected health information (PHI) electronically as long appropriate measures are taken to ensure the security of the transaction (e.g. provider-to-provider email consultation on their secure email accounts that are protected by a medical centers firewall and internet security systems). HIPAA address both privacy and security of patients' information that is transmitted or store electronically. The Privacy Rule addresses the saving, accessing and sharing of medical and personal information of any individual. The Security Rule more specifically outlines national security standards to protect health data created, received, maintained or transmitted electronically. Providers who "host" or store any protected patient data with a hosting provider must have administrative, physical and technical safeguards in place to be HIPAA compliant. A supplemental act was passed in 2009 called The Health Information Technology for Economic and Clinical Health (HITECH) Act which supports the enforcement of HIPAA requirements by raising the penalties of health organizations that violate HIPAA Privacy and Security Rules (2009). HIPAA rules apply to all covered entities which include health plans, health care providers and their business partners that transmit health information electronically. This applies to: doctors, clinics, psychologists and therapists, dentists, chiropractors, nursing homes and pharmacies [52].

The basic requirements for a covered entity or business associate to be compliant are as follows:

1. **Physical safeguards**—include limited facility access and control, with authorized access in place. Policies must be in place about use and access to workstations and electronic media, including transferring, removing, disposing and re-using electronic media and electronic protected health information. These requirements apply to the physical location and equipment that the provider uses to connect to patients, interact and store protected patient information (i.e. electronic consent forms, treatment recommendations, logs of treatment sessions or interactions with patients would all be considered PHI). Providers business or the organization that they are employed under must meet these requirements to store and transmit patient data and should develop policies for providers interacting with patients on social networking sites. These policies should specify who is and isn't allowed physical access to your facilities and equipment and how the policy is enforced (i.e. security badges, key-codes, access logs and the like.)
2. **Technical safeguards**—require access control to allow only those who are authorized to access electronic protected health data such as using unique user IDs, an emergency access procedure, automatic log off and encryption and decryption. There should be specific policies and procedures on how users are

granted access to programs, sensitive data, or equipment. This includes how access is requested and authorized, how administrators are notified to disable accounts when appropriate, frequency of account audits, and how records of all this activity are maintained. Audit reports, or tracking logs, must be implemented to keep records of activity on hardware and software in order to investigate the source or cause of any security violations.

3. **Technical policies**—should also cover measures put in place to confirm that PHI hasn't been altered or destroyed. Disaster recovery plans must be in place in case of an emergency, security breach or prolonged power outage and offsite backup are important to ensure that any electronic media errors or failures can be quickly remedied and patient health information can be recovered accurately and intact.
4. **Network/data transmission security**—is required of HIPAA compliant hosts to protect against unauthorized public access of PHI over all channels for transmitting data (i.e. email, Internet, or even over a private network, such as a "private cloud" or a social networking site).

Source "What is HIPAA compliance?" [53].

HIPAA compliance is a complicated issue and requires technical and legal expertise to design systems, policies, prepare reports and respond to audits and emergencies. Social networking platforms must comply with HIPAA security standards to allow for the exchange of protected information in this space. Most popular social networking sites such as facebook, twitter and myspace do not comply with HIPAA security standards. Thus, providers who access patients and store or exchange patient information via a non-HIPAA compliant social networking site using unsecured computer equipment are surely in violation of HIPAA regulations. Providers and health organizations may protect themselves from liability by avoiding violating HIPAA laws, and being vigilant about developing and communicating social media polices. However, providing care or transmitting protected information over unsecured channels is clearly not advisable. Providers and health care organizations are bound to keep abreast of the legal and ethical requirements of communicating over social networking sites and guidelines should be developed for utilizing social networks for intervention, assessment and treatment.

2.4 Guideline Considerations for Mental Health Care via Social Networks

Ethical guidelines specific to distance and other health IT approaches to mental healthcare provision such as telepsychiatry or more relevantly, the provision of treatment in virtual social networking environments, have been reported and provide a useful starting point for the development of guidelines specific to patient-provider communication or care provision via social networking. Yellowlees et al. [54] provide the following guidelines for conducting therapy in online virtual environments such as Second Life (http://secondlife.com/) where providers and patients (represented by electronic virtual figures or avatars) can logon and meet on virtual "islands" or "clouds"("private" virtual locations within the site that can depict a variety of scenes including a virtual therapy office). The virtual reality therapy guidelines presented are largely applicable to treatment communications over social networking sites [54]:

1. Patients who are only receiving generic educational information on an open virtual reality environment can be anonymous, and should not be tracked in any way. Any providers on that island should be fully identified, and should have named or numbered avatars that clearly identify who they are, and that link to biographies published on a defined public website so that any patients or users of the island may obtain accurate information about the providers expertise and interests as would be expected on any health information website.
2. Patients who wish to move to a secure virtual reality environment for some form of virtual therapy, whether this is individual counseling or cognitive behavioral therapy should be treated in accordance with the following protocols to ensure high practice standards, and legal and ethical processes:
    a. All patients should undergo a face-to-face or telemedicine assessment to: evaluate patient safety and appropriateness for treatment with this modality, establish care, confirm their diagnosis, create a treatment plan and discuss consent. This is particularly important in a potential emergency situation where therapists have to know the physical location of a patient, as per telemedicine guidelines, in order to call for help.
    b. All patients should then sign a written consent form if required in the state in which they reside (which can be done electronically), be trained in how to use the virtual environment, be given a tour of the private island, and receive a copy of their diagnostic assessment and treatment plan.
    c. HIPAA compliance of the virtual environment must be documented, verifiable and ensured prior to patient contact.
    d. If patients and providers are federal employees, then patients can be treated in the virtual environment from any state, by any provider. If the patient or the provider is not a federal employee, the treating provider must be licensed to practice in the state from which the patient logs in.
    e. All providers will have fully authenticated avatars using their real names, and will have biographies published that link their professional identities to their avatars for patients to read.
    f. Patients and providers will then schedule sessions on the private island for either counseling or cognitive behavioral therapy, or a combination of both.
    g. Any major changes to the treatment plan, such as altered medications, should require a face-to-face or telemedicine consultation.
    h. Either the provider or patient may at any time either cease therapy, or request a telemedicine or face to face consultation to review progress.

The virtual therapy guidelines and other similar online therapy guidelines [55] are a useful starting point for developing guidelines for mental health treatment via social networking platforms. Many of the basic principles apply to patient contact or treatment over any online platform. The primary guidelines to take into consideration before interacting with patients over social networks for treatment or treatment-adjunctive purposes are:

1. **Establishing care**—patients must be an identifiable established patient (in accord with the state that the provider is licensed). This typically evolves having undergone an initial in-person or telemedicine evaluation where informed consent has been established.
2. **Verification**—the patient's physical location is established so that the provider can respond in the case of an emergency and an emergency contact plan is established. The provider is clearly identified in the online forum with all relevant professional credentials and contact information clearly posted and accessible to the patient. As in telemedicine consultations, the provider must be licensed in the state that the patient is located in or must have verifiable permission to practice in that state.
3. **Informed consent**—informed consent should take account of continued follow-up online or any online communication used as an adjunct to therapy. Providers should develop a social media policy and take account of this policy in the consent form, detail the appropriate avenues for contact in case of an emergency in the consent form and give clients a copy for their records. Detail the social media policy and emergency procedure and contact information on the social networking profile.
4. **Ensuring security**—Treatment and any interactions involving the exchange or storage of protected health information must be conducted over secure HIPAA compliant channels. The provider is responsible for verifying and documenting compliance.
5. **Provider education**—Providers should consult with other professionals and legal contacts, take continuing education in HIPAA security, liability and clinical practice which, if not locally accessible, are frequently available online for mental health professionals.

Uniform guidelines are needed for patient provider interaction over online platforms such as social networking sites [56] and ethics codes should take online communication and treatment into account as it is rapidly becoming a fixture in mental health practice. In the absence of clear guidelines, providers must be aware of the potential legal pitfalls and ethical dilemmas when patient contact occurs online. Providers must uphold the laws and ethical codes that govern their licenses and remain aware of evolutions in technology and privacy restrictions online. Providers must be vigilant in using their clinical and ethical judgment in these situations to determine the level of privacy required for the information that is shared and be sure that any exchange of protected information is secure and confidential.

2.4.1 Special Considerations: Ethical Guidelines for Personal Social Network Use Amongst Mental Health Providers

In light of the ethical pitfalls that may await unprepared providers extending their mental health practice onto social networking sites, some providers may opt out- at least as long as possible—of social networking site use in their professional arena. However, the vast majority of young professionals are connected to social networking sites for private use [57, 58]. Are there ethical dilemmas associated with personal use of social networking sites for mental health providers? Might some providers inadvertently violate patient privacy by discussing patient issues on private social networks with colleagues? How should mental health providers respond if a client or former client attempts to initiate a relationship on the provider's personal social networking site by sending a message or "friend" request? What is a provider's responsibility if a client messages them about information that he or she would be mandated to report in a professional capacity? The primary ethical issues that arise with personal use of social networking sites for mental health providers concern: boundary violations, self-disclosure, privacy concerns and nonmaleficence [48].

2.4.2 Establishing Boundaries on Social Networking Sites: Privacy Settings, Self-Disclosure and "Friend" Requests

With the surge in networking via online social media applications, personal information is more public than ever before, and personal and professional boundaries are becoming more difficult to define (Behnke 2008). Online social networks have become a platform for individuals to share very personal and intimate aspects of their lives electronically. The appeal of these applications is immense; individuals can log on from nearly anywhere in the world and communicate with loved ones and friends, maintaining and expanding these relationships through text, video and picture archives of their lives. Online social networks are now expanding to include colleagues and other professional contacts and personal information may easily become available patients, colleagues, students, former patients and the like. In the face of such occurrences, the question arises: what are the risks for mental health providers who communicate personal information online?

Ultimately it is within a patient's rights to research a healthcare provider, and even though this may feel like a violation of privacy to a provider, patients can and often do seek out information about their providers online. Professional boundaries can become quite blurry if private information posted on a social networking site becomes available to patients with the click of a mouse. What are the risks for patients who might access, intentionally or unintentionally, providers' personal information online? Can personal information, if shared with clients' online, blur the professional boundaries and impact the therapeutic relationship?

One study conducted across a sample of psychology graduate students reported that their social network sites contained personal information that they would not want their colleagues (6 %), professors (13 %), or particularly their clients (37 %) to access. When asked about experiences of client contact on personal social networks, a small percent (7 %) of the student sample reported that clients had directly reported to them that they had researched them online. A surprisingly large portion of the students (27 %) reported seeking out information about their clients online [58]. Evidence suggests that there have been high occurrences of medical and graduate students displaying unprofessional conduct online [59] and that young providers may not use very stringent privacy settings on their personal social networking sites [60]. Even for providers who are cautions about privacy setting or information shared on social networking sites, online exposure of providers' private information may still occur as most popular social networking sites are not secure and may be subject to hacking, and providers may not be fully aware of the limits of social networking privacy controls. Privacy on social networks varies by site and the privacy settings within the same site may change periodically as the site upgrades and evolves.

Further, clinicians should be aware of the amount and scope of information about themselves that can be made available to clients on online search engines. Another issue to consider is the existence of old social networking site accounts that are no longer used, but may still contain personal information, and may be accessible to patients, colleagues. Students and social networking accounts can be difficult to delete on some sites, and changes in the ever-evolving privacy controls for these sites may inadvertently allow for private information to become public [48].

Managing patient "friend" requests may be another issue of concerns for providers utilizing social networks for personal use. What should a clinician do if he or she logs onto a personal social networking site only to discover a friend request form a patient or former patient? Is it appropriate to for clinicians to accept such "friend" requests on personal social networking sites? In most cases the answer to this question is no. The American Medical Association (AMA) recently developed a new policy on physician use of social media that warns against physicians engaging in personal relationships online. The report states that physicians should protect their professional relationship with patients, colleagues, and others by not engaging in social relationships or connections online and keeping personal social networking accounts, blogs, and other web content private and separate from professional content online. The report advises against searches of patients or allowing patients access to personal information online by either accepting a patient's request to connect, extending a request to connect to a patient, or keeping privacy settings such that others may view personal content without making a formal connection as physicians may risk a variety of repercussions if patients view this information, including loss of trust or respect [61].

Tunick et al. [62] present the following guidelines for managing patient contact over personal social networking sites:

- Develop a social medial policy—be transparent with clients about your social media policy and discuss ethical issues with social networks with trainees and colleges.
- Maintain awareness of the ethical dilemmas that may arise on social networks. Providers may be sought out by clients on their personal social networks and sent a friend request by a patient. Consider what the boundary implications are for "friending" a client online? How might online "friendships" influence treatment and what other dilemmas might arise from such contact—for instance, what is a clinician's responsibility if a client posts concerning information on their personal social network page? What is the clinician's ethical obligation in this situation and how would one address this issue with a client or even the authorities if necessary?
- Remain aware and diligent about privacy settings—Privacy settings are ever evolving on social networking sites and information that is presumed to be private may become public to clients and colleagues. To avoid requests, clinicians can set privacy setting to be very restrictive, preventing other users from searching for them by name or messaging them [62].

2.4.3 Protecting Patient Privacy, Unintentional Disclosures and Nonmaleficence

Social networking sites provide a potential avenue for clinicians to intentionally and unintentionally violate patient privacy. One study evaluating medical residents social network sites found that patient privacy violations did occur over social networking sites [63]. Instances of medical professionals sharing patient information over social networking sites have been documented. The Federation of State Medical Boards recently published a report describing inappropriate online behaviors on personal and professional social networks which they recommended should lead to investigation by state medical boards. However, it may be difficult for some mental health professionals to differentiate between appropriate and inappropriate disclosure of patient information. Tunick et al. [62] investigated how psychologists view their own social media use as well as how they approach interacting with clients online. While many respondents indicated participating in social networks and even accessing patient information online, there was no clear consensus amongst those surveyed about how psychologists should handle matters of Internet safety and privacy with their clients.

Another emerging issue is that of clinicians reviewing clients' social profiles, often without client permission. One can imagine the potential allure of accessing clients social networking profiles as the sites provide rich and potentially valuable personal data that would likely be an asset to therapy if utilized properly and ethically. However, researchers caution against accessing client's information online without permission [61]. According to the Australian Psychological Society, internet searches of client information should be limited to very specific circumstances where it is considered to be in the best interests of a client such as if a client's safety is at risk and his or her social networking profile may provide information about his or her whereabouts or may be accessed for signs of suicidal ideation or intent [61]. Some caution against the review of client information online even in emergent situations, but it is ultimately the clinician's decision if the patient's safety is sufficiently at risk to warrant such a violation of privacy without permission. In non-emergent situations, clinicians should strongly consider the risks and benefits of accessing clients' information online and should obtain permission from the client first. If a clinician feels it might be beneficial to the therapeutic process to evaluate a patients social networking site, such as to evaluate the clients perception of a particular interaction or relationship, challenge the clients self-perception or obtain a more objective view of the clients interactions with others, it is advisable that the clinician obtain permission and only review the information with the client [62]. The information should only be considered for use if the process would be beneficial to the client. Private client information should never be researched online simply to satisfy the clinician's curiosity or to determine if the client is providing accurate information in therapy, such queries should be directly addressed with the client in the context of therapy.

It is imperative for clinicians to be aware that public social networking sites are simply not set up for secure communication. Privacy is limited here and patient communication over such channels risks violating patient privacy and confidentiality. Even if providers are not communicating patient specific mental health information over public social networks, it is not ethically advisable to discuss patient information or consult with colleagues over social networking sites. In addition to the ubiquitous privacy and security risks with mental health information shared online, there are important quality of care issues and population-specific risk factors to consider for online mental health care resources and treatment.

2.5 Special Considerations for Social Media in Mental Health: Quality and Equity of Care and at Risk Populations

2.5.1 Quality and Equity of Care

Social media may provide may benefits in mental health care such as: increasing communication between patients and providers, greater patient empowerment, facilitating a sense of self-control and choice in mental health treatment for patients, increasing understanding and enhancement of self-management skills, making successful prevention or treatment of future episodes more likely, increasing access to major international experts, and increasing access to exciting new treatment and assessment tools that are now being developed for use over social media. However, as mental health care adapts to the demand for health IT, inequities develop as this is not a universally accessible resource. Individuals who have low socioeconomic status have limited access to the internet and mobile smartphones or may have their access frequently suspended because of difficulty making payments for Internet and phone services [64]. Thus, those with low socioeconomic status may not be able to fully benefit from the ever increasing mental health resources available online. Further, the newer technologies may be more expensive or only be supported by more expensive, less universally available, platforms such as smartphones. In addition to access to technology, technological aptitude and the ability to utilize technology effectively to access health care information, also known as e-health literacy, is a significant issue that may impede patent access and treatment success with social media platforms. Those with poor e-health literacy may have great difficulty successfully utilizing online health service which may increase inequities in mental health care access. Level of e-health literacy has been shown to impact the benefit of online health information [65], and those with mental illness may be particularly vulnerable to poor e-health literacy due to lower levels of general literacy and education [66] or illness-specific deficits such as attention deficit [64]. Clinicians must take each patient's eHealth literacy into consideration before engaging with them on social media for evaluation, education or treatment support and consider ways to grant access to technological services for patients who have limited access due to financial constraints or poor e-health literacy.

While the convenience of the internet may be greatly appealing to health consumers, particularly adolescents and young adults, ensuring the accuracy of information transmitted online is challenging and there may be some general risks for patients utilizing online sources for primary mental health treatment. It may be difficult for clinicians and patients alike to evaluate the quality or the source of information online. Clinicians must be able to verify patients' identity and location to effectively establish treatment and respond in the case of an emergency. Patients may be at risk for fraud or misrepresentation with clinicians who they access solely on online forums. If patients are not able to accurately evaluate clinicians credentials they may be at risk of receiving receive poor advice or even damaging "treatment" from unverifiable sources. They may also fall victim to fraud and may incur financial loss through poor choices of doctors or products.

2.5.2 At Risk Patient Populations and Mental Health Care on Social Networks

Certain at-risk populations may not be appropriate for receiving mental health care online including those who are actively in crisis (i.e. at risk for self-harm or harm to others), experiencing extreme psychosis or severe mental health symptoms (e.g.

severe depression, hopelessness, mania or severe anxiety) or at risk for becoming unstable. Individuals experiencing such symptoms should be closely monitored and provided inpatient hospitalization until stabilized. It may be difficult for clinicians to monitor such patients in an online format and to respond effectively in the case of an emergency if proper emergency procedures are not in place. It is possible that social media applications could be utilized to keep in close contact with such patients and even used to locate a patient in crisis; however clinicians should carefully consider any potential risks of utilizing social media with such patients.

2.6 Conclusion

Social media is now an important fixture in health care. Social networks are becoming a new and exciting resource for disseminating mental health information and may soon provide a valuable platform for providing cutting-edge treatment, connecting with patients and reaching at-risk populations. However, many legal and ethical issues abound concerning patient privacy and information security online. Guidelines must be established before this novel treatment platform can be fully realized in mental health care. Recommendations to consider in guideline development include: understanding and ensuring HIPAA compliance, developing a social media policy, establishing a treatment relationship and consent before making treatment related contact online, and developing procedures to respond to emergency situations.

References

1. Miles, A., Mezzich, J.: The care of the patient and the soul of the clinic: Person-centered medicine as an emergent model of modern clinical practice. Int. J. Pers. Centered Med. **1**(2), 207–222 (2011)
2. Ekman, I., Swedberg, K., Taft, C., Lindseth, A., Norberg, A., Brink, E., et al.: Person-centered care—ready for prime time. Eur J. Cardiovasc. Nurs. **10**(4), 248–251 (2011)
3. Zurhellen, W.M., Kim, G. R.: Building a medical home. AAP News **32**(5), 28 (2011)
4. Hawn, C.: Take two aspirin and tweet me in the morning: How twitter, facebook, and other social media are reshaping health care. Health Aff. **28**(2), 361–368 (2009)
5. Brown, F.W.: Rural telepsychiatry. Psychiatr. Serv. **49**(7), 963–964 (1998)
6. Giansanti, D., Castrichella, L., Giovagnoli, M.R.: Telepathology requires specific training for the technician in the biomedical laboratory. Telemed J E Health **14**(8), 801–807 (2008)
7. High, W.A., Houston, M.S., Calobrisi, S.D., Drage, L.A., McEvoy, M.T.: Assessment of the accuracy of low-cost store-and-forward teledermatology consultation. J. Am. Acad. Dermatol. **42**(5 Pt 1), 776–783 (2000)
8. Hooper, G.S., Yellowlees, P., Marwick, T.H., Currie, P.J., Bidstrup, B.P.: Telehealth and the diagnosis and management of cardiac disease. J Telemed. Telecare **7**(5), 249–256 (2001)
9. Mahnke, C.B., Mulreany, M.P., Inafuku, J., Abbas, M., Feingold, B., Paolillo, J.A.: Utility of store-and-forward pediatric telecardiology evaluation in distinguishing normal from pathologic pediatric heart sounds. Clin. Pediatr. (Phila) **47**(9), 919–925 (2008)

10. Marcin, J.P., Nesbitt, T.S., Cole, S.L., Knuttel, R.M., Hilty, D.M., Prescott, P.T., et al.: Changes in diagnosis, treatment, and clinical improvement among patients receiving telemedicine consultations. Telemed J E Health **11**(1), 36–43 (2005)
11. Rashid, E., Ishtiaq, O., Gilani, S., Zafar, A.: Comparison of store and forward method of teledermatology with face-to-face consultation. J. Ayub. Med. Coll. Abbottabad **15**(2), 34–36 (2003)
12. Rotvold, G.H., Knarvik, U., Johansen, M.A., Fossen, K.: Telemedicine screening for diabetic retinopathy: Staff and patient satisfaction. J. Telemed. Telecare **9**(2), 109–113 (2003)
13. Thrall, J.H.: Teleradiology. Part I. History and clinical applications. Radiology **243**(3), 613–617 (2007)
14. Williams, S., Henricks, W.H., Becich, M.J., Toscano, M., Carter, A.B.: Telepathology for patient care: What am i getting myself into? Adv. Anat. Pathol. **17**(2), 130–149 (2010)
15. Neufeld, J.D., Yellowlees, P.M., Hilty, D.M., Cobb, H., Bourgeois, J.A.: The e-mental health consultation service: Providing enhanced primary-care mental health services through telemedicine. Psychosomatics **48**(2), 135–141 (2007)
16. Ruskin, P.E., Silver-Aylaian, M., Kling, M.A., Reed, S.A., Bradham, D.D., Hebel, J.R., et al.: Treatment outcomes in depression: Comparison of remote treatment through telepsychiatry to in-person treatment. Am. J. Psychiatry **161**(8), 1471–1476 (2004)
17. Wootton, R., Yellowlees, P., McLaren, P.: Telepsychiatry and e-mental health. Royal Society of Medicine Press Ltd, Road Lake (2003)
18. Baker, L., Wagner, T.H., Singer, S., Bundorf, M.K.: Use of the internet and e-mail for health care information: Results from a national survey. JAMA **289**(18), 2400–2406 (2003)
19. Boyd, D.M., Ellison, N.B.: Social network sites: Definition, history, and scholarship. J. Comput-Mediated Commun. **13**(1), 210–230 (2007)
20. Nakamura, C., Bromberg, M., Bhargava, S., Wicks, P., Zeng-Treitler, Q.: Mining online social network data for biomedical research: A comparison of clinicians' and patients' perceptions about amyotrophic lateral sclerosis treatments. J. Med. Internet Res. **14**(3), (2012)
21. Wicks, P., Vaughan, T.E., Massagli, M.P.: The multiple sclerosis rating scale, revised (msrs-r): Development, refinement, and psychometric validation using an online community. Health Qual. Life Outcomes **10**(1), 70 (2012)
22. Horgan, A., Sweeney, J.: Young students' use of the internet for mental health information and support. J. Psychiatr. Ment. Health Nurs. **17**(2), 117–123 (2010)
23. Gowen, K., Deschaine, M., Gruttadara, D., Markey, D.: Young adults with mental health conditions and social networking websites: Seeking tools to build community. Psychiatr. Rehabil. J. **35**(3), 245–250 (2012)
24. Lewandowski, J., Rosenberg, B.D., Jordan Parks, M., Siegel, J.T.: The effect of informal social support: Face-to-face versus computer-mediated communication. Comput. Hum. Behav. **27**(5), 1806–1814 (2011)
25. Ben-Zeev, D., Corrigan, P.W., Britt, T.W., Langford, L.: Stigma of mental illness and service use in the military. J. Ment. Health **21**(3), 264–273 (2012)
26. Pietrzak, R., Johnson, D., Goldstein, M., Malley, J., Southwick, S.: Perceived stigma and barriers to mental health care utilization among oef-oif veterans. Psychiatr. Serv. **60**(8), 1118–1122 (2009)
27. Wilson, J.A., Onorati, K., Mishkind, M., Reger, M.A., Gahm, G.A.: Soldier attitudes about technology-based approaches to mental health care. CyberPsychology Behav. **11**(6), 767–769 (2008)
28. McLaughlin, M., Nam, Y., Gould, J., Pade, C., Meeske, K.A., Ruccione, K.S., et al.: A videosharing social networking intervention for young adult cancer survivors. Comput. Hum. Behav. **28**(2), 631–641 (2011)
29. McDaniel, B., Coyne, S., Holmes, E. : New mothers and media use: Associations between blogging, social networking, and maternal well-being. Matern. Child Health J., 1–9 (2011)

30. Good, A., Sambhanthan, A., Panjganj, V., Spettigue, S.: Computer interaction and the benefits of social networking for people with borderline personality disorder: Enlightening mental health professionals (2011)
31. O'Dea, B., Campbell, A.: Healthy connections: Online social networks and their potential for peer support. Stud. Health Tech. Inform. **168**, 133 (2011)
32. Hogeboom, D.L., McDermott, R.J., Perrin, K.M., Osman, H., Bell-Ellison, B.A.: Internet use and social networking among middle aged and older adults. Educ. Gerontol. **36**(2), 93–111 (2010)
33. Sundar, S.S., Oeldorf-Hirsch, A., Nussbaum, J., Behr, R.: Retirees on facebook: Can online social networking enhance their health and wellness? Paper presented at the Proceedings of the 2011 annual conference extended abstracts on Human factors in computing systems (2011)
34. Burns, J.M., Davenport, T.A., Durkin, L.A., Luscombe, G.M., Hickie, I.B.: The internet as a setting for mental health service utilisation by young people. Med. J. Aust. **192**(11 Suppl), S22–S26 (2010)
35. Shandley, K., Austin, D., Klein, B., Kyrios, M.: An evaluation of 'reach out central': An online gaming program for supporting the mental health of young people. Health Educ. Res. **25**(4), 563–574 (2010)
36. Burns, J.M., Durkin, L.A., Nicholas, J.: Mental health of young people in the united states: What role can the internet play in reducing stigma and promoting help seeking? J. Adolesc. Health **45**(1), 95–97 (2009)
37. Rice, E., Milburn, N.G., Monro, W.: Social networking technology, social network composition, and reductions in substance use among homeless adolescents. Prev. Sci. **12**(1), 80–88 (2011)
38. Schomerus, G., Angermeyer, M.C.: Stigma and its impact on help-seeking for mental disorders: What do we know? Epidemiologia e psichiatria sociale **17**(01), 31–37 (2008)
39. Kessler, R.C., Amminger, G.P., Aguilar-Gaxiola, S., Alonso, J., Lee, S., Ustun, T.B.: Age of onset of mental disorders: A review of recent literature. Curr. Opin. Psychiatry **20**(4), 359 (2007)
40. Ybarra, M.L., Mitchell, K.J.: How risky are social networking sites? A comparison of places online where youth sexual solicitation and harassment occurs. Pediatrics **121**(2), e350–e357 (2008)
41. O'Keeffe, G.S., Clarke-Pearson, K.: The impact of social media on children, adolescents, and families. Pediatrics **127**(4), 800–804 (2011)
42. Borzekowski, D., Schenk, S., Wilson, J., Peebles, R.: E-ana and e-mia: A content analysis of pro-eating disorder web sites. Am. J. Public Health **100**(Suppl 8), 1526–1534 (2010)
43. Lewis, S., Heath, N., Michal, N., Duggan, J.: Non-suicidal self-injury, youth, and the internet: What mental health professionals need to know. Child Adolesc. Psychiatry Ment. Health **6**(1), 13 (2012)
44. Moreno, M.A., Jelenchick, L.A., Egan, K.G., Cox, E., Young, H., Gannon, K.E., et al.: Feeling bad on facebook: Depression disclosures by college students on a social networking site. Depression Anxiety **28**(6), 447–455 (2011)
45. Luxton, D.D., McCann, R.A., Bush, N.E., Mishkind, M.C., Reger, G.M.: Mhealth for mental health: Integrating smartphone technology in behavioral healthcare. Prof. Psychol.: Res. Practice **42**(6), 505–512 (2011)
46. Bosker, B.: Your next phone will know what you're feeling The Huffington Post. Retrieved from http://www.huffingtonpost.com/2012/12/04/phone-emotional-intelligence_n_2239657.html (2012)
47. Hinmon, D.: Step #4 understand the rules for a hipaa-compliant social media strategy. Social Media Strategy Blog, vol. 2013. February 15, 2011
48. Hidy, B., Porch, E., Reed, S., Parish, M. B., Yellowlees, P.: Social networking and mental health. Telemental Health: Clinical, Technical, and Administrative Foundations for Evidence-Based Practice, 367 (2012)

49. Batchelor, R., Bobrowicz, A., Mackenzie, R., Milne, A.: Challenges of ethical and legal responsibilities when technologies' uses and users change: Social networking sites, decision-making capacity and dementia. Ethics Inf. Technol. **14**(2), 99–108 (2012)
50. Eysenbach, G.: Towards ethical guidelines for e-health: Jmir theme issue on ehealth ethics. J. Med. Internet Res. **2**(1), (2000)
51. Deady, K.E.: Cyberadvice: The ethical implications of giving professional advice over the internet. Geo. J. Legal Ethics **14**, 891 (2000)
52. Health insurance portability and accountability act, 110 Stat. 1936 (1996)
53. What is hipaa compliance? Online Tech. HIPAA Compliant Hosting. Retrieved from http://www.onlinetech.com/compliant-hosting/hipaa-compliant-hosting/resources/what-is-hipaa-compliance
54. Yellowlees, P.M., Holloway, K.M., Parish, M.B.: Therapy in virtual environments—clinical and ethical issues. Telemedicine and e-Health, (2012)
55. Grady, B., Myers, K.M., Nelson, E.-L., Belz, N., Bennett, L., Carnahan, L., et al.: Evidence-based practice for telemental health. Telemedicine e-Health **17**(2), 131–148 (2011)
56. Finn, J., Barak, A.: A descriptive study of e-counsellor attitudes, ethics, and practice. Counselling Psychother. Res. **10**(4), 268–277 (2010)
57. Lehavot, K.: "Myspace" or yours? The ethical dilemma of graduate students' personal lives on the internet. Ethics Behav. **19**, 129–141 (2009)
58. Lehavot, K., Barnett, J., Powers, D.: Psychotherapy, professional relationships, and ethical considerations in the myspace generation. Prof. Psychol: Res. Pract. (2010)
59. Chretien, K.C., Greysen, S.R., Chretien, J.-P., Kind, T.: Online posting of unprofessional content by medical students. JAMA, J. Am. Med. Assoc. **302**(12), 1309–1315 (2009)
60. MacDonald, J., Sohn, S., Ellis, P.: Privacy, professionalism and facebook: A dilemma for young doctors, vol. 44. Oxford, ROYAUME-UNI: Wiley (2010)
61. Devi, S.: Facebook friend request from a patient? Lancet **377**(9772), 1141–1142 (2011)
62. Tunick, R.A., Mednick, L., Conroy, C.: A snapshot of child psychologists' social media activity: Professional and ethical practice implications and recommendations. Prof. Psychol.: Res. Pract. **42**(6), 440 (2011)
63. Thompson, L.A., Black, E., Duff, W.P., Paradise Black, N., Saliba, H., Dawson, K.: Protected health information on social networking sites: Ethical and legal considerations. J. Med. Internet Res. **13**(1), (2011)
64. Richardson, A.: Online public health interventions: A good strategy for those with mental illness. J. Mass. Commun. Journalism **2**, e126 (2012)
65. Norman, C.D., Skinner, H.A.: Ehealth literacy: Essential skills for consumer health in a networked world. J. Med. Internet Res. **8**(2), (2006)
66. Breslau, J., Lane, M., Sampson, N., Kessler, R.C.: Mental disorders and subsequent educational attainment in a US national sample. J. Psychiatr. Res. **42**(9), 708–716 (2008)

Chapter 3
The Changing Doctor-Patient Relationship: A Move to Anytime, Anywhere

Najia Nafiz and Peter Yellowlees

3.1 Introduction

The advent of the Internet has undoubtedly changed the way the world communicates and is already dramatically changing the doctor-patient relationship.

With the move towards Web 2.0, a term used to refer to a new era of Web-enabled applications built around user-generated content such as blogs, podcasts, wikis, and social networking sites (such as Facebook) finding information and staying in contact with friends, family, and now healthcare providers has dramatically changed [32]. The advent of telemedicine has revolutionized healthcare in areas such as dermatology and pathology [22, 41] and it has great potential for uses in other fields such as mental healthcare as well.

Here is an example of how Internet based telemedicine works everyday. Imagine you have a sore throat and visit your healthcare provider, who could be a nurse practitioner, general physician, or depending on where you live, an unlicensed healthcare worker in your village. Upon examination your healthcare provider recommends a referral to see a specialist for a follow up diagnosis and treatment plan. Whereas traditionally you would have to see this specialist in person, which could require anywhere from a 50 min drive to a full day traveling by boat, your provider can now connect you directly to the specialist via telemedicine.

http://www.telemedicine.com/whatis.html

The example above would not have been possible a few decades ago. The Internet has not only revolutionized daily communication, with rapid exchanges of information via Instant Messaging and E-mail, but also the way healthcare is

N. Nafiz
California State University, Sacramento. 6000J Street, Sacramento, CA 95819, USA

P. Yellowlees (✉)
Department of Psychiatry and Behavioral Sciences, University of California-Davis, Sacramento, CA, USA
e-mail: pmyellowlees@ucdavis.edu

M. Lech et al. (eds.), *Mental Health Informatics*,
Studies in Computational Intelligence 491, DOI: 10.1007/978-3-642-38550-6_3,

accessed and delivered. If medical consultation is needed from a specialist we can now get that consultation from any specialist around the world online, we can also read reviews on physicians, research our symptoms and treatment options, find support groups and even schedule our appointment online.

E-revolution, a phenomenon that includes everyday use of the Internet by the general public, has the potential to reshape the trillion-dollar health care industry in the USA by improving patient self-management and health outcomes [13]. Patients use the Internet not only to gather information (with Web sites such as WebMD providing symptoms, possible diagnoses, and treatments) but also to share their experiences and become advocates. As consumers are spending more of their own income on health care, with an estimated increase of 2.5–3.5 % per year of increasing age [42], they are also taking more responsibility for their health [43]. In this chapter we explore how the Internet has influenced the doctor-patient relationship by examining the following five questions:

1. How are patient expectations and behaviors changing?
2. Who is using the Internet for Mental Health Care?
3. What online Mental Health Services are currently being offered?
4. How are current and past models of the doctor-patient relationship being affected?
5. What are benefits and possible downfalls of using the Internet in the doctor-patient relationship?

3.2 How are Patient Expectations and Behaviors Changing?

The The Internet is now used so commonly by patients that it has literally become part of the doctor-patient relationship [43]. Gardiner has recently described a transition from the informed patient to patient informed care [20], reflecting what is now being called participatory medicine and participative patients. Participatory medicine is defined as "a movement in which networked patients shift from being mere passengers to responsible drivers of their health, and in which providers encourage and value them as full partners" [19].

Organizations such as The Society for Participatory Medicine have developed to equip and empower patients to take control of their health care needs. The Society helps promote the e-patient movement (the term e-patient, also known as Internet Patient or Internet Savvy-Patients, refers to those who seek online guidance for not only themselves but also family and friends). If you type in e-patient in a Google search one of the first websites you are likely to see is e-patient Dave:

> Dave deBronkart, known online as "e-Patient Dave" is the leading spokesperson for the e-patient movement–Empowered, Engaged, Equipped, Enabled. A high tech executive and

online community leader for many years, he was diagnosed in 2007 with Stage IV kidney cancer, with median survival 24 weeks. He used the Internet in every way possible to partner with his care team; today he is well. In 2008 he discovered the e-patient movement, and began studying, blogging, and speaking at conferences, and in 2009 was elected founding co-chair of the new Society for Participatory Medicine [11].

The Internet has empowered patients by offering extraordinary choice of self-help ranging from information about disease and treatment to group discussions and support from those affected with the same disorder to survivors of the disorder. Patient-driven research (PDR) centers online offer those with rare diseases a place to connect with others and exchange treatment options as well as provide and receive support. PDR is considered a radical shift from the classical research model due to the cost effectiveness and increased speed at which results are disseminated. PDR is especially important for those with orphan diseases where the speed of exchanging information can be the difference between life and death [18]. Norman Scherzer, considered the George Washington of e-patients, compares the speed at which information can be distributed about a disease and its treatments using PDR rather than the traditional scholarly journals:

One of the great benefits of PDR is its speed. We can get lifesaving information out to the people who need it right away, much faster than professional researchers, who must go through many time-consuming steps. First you design your study. Then you arrange for funding. Then you must get everything approved—sometimes by several different committees. Then you recruit your subjects. So at last you can begin. Then you must wait for your results to trickle in. But that's only the beginning.

Next you must analyze and interpret your data. You must write everything up. After all that, you'll need to find a peer-reviewed journal to publish your work. And if you're lucky enough to find one, you must go through even more long rounds of reviews, revisions, corrections, and proofing—as well as possible editorial or production delays. This can take several years. So professional research has a built-in lethal lag time—a period of delay between the time some people know about an important medical breakthrough and the time everybody knows. As a result of this delay, many patients who could have been saved by the latest treatments die unnecessarily. In my experience, this lethal lag time is rarely less than two to three years. And it can sometimes be four to five years, or even more. Physicians are subject to this delay just like everyone else [12].

One One example of PDR is the Association of Online Cancer Resources (ACOR) which is an information and support network with over 600,000 patients and caregivers using its 163 public online communities [18]. ACOR provides its users with information on different types of cancers, treatment options, support, research publications and ongoing clinical trials.

Web sites such as PatientsLikeMe.com (Fig. 3.1) offer a health data-sharing platform that allows patients to share and learn from real-world, outcome-based health data. PatientsLikeMe was co-founded in 2004 by three MIT engineers: brothers Benjamin and James Heywood and longtime friend Jeff Cole. Five years earlier, their brother and friend Stephen Heywood was diagnosed with Lou Gehrig's disease at the age of 29 (Lou Gehrigs, named after the famous New York Yankees player Ludwig Heinrich Gehrig, is an incurable fatal neuromuscular

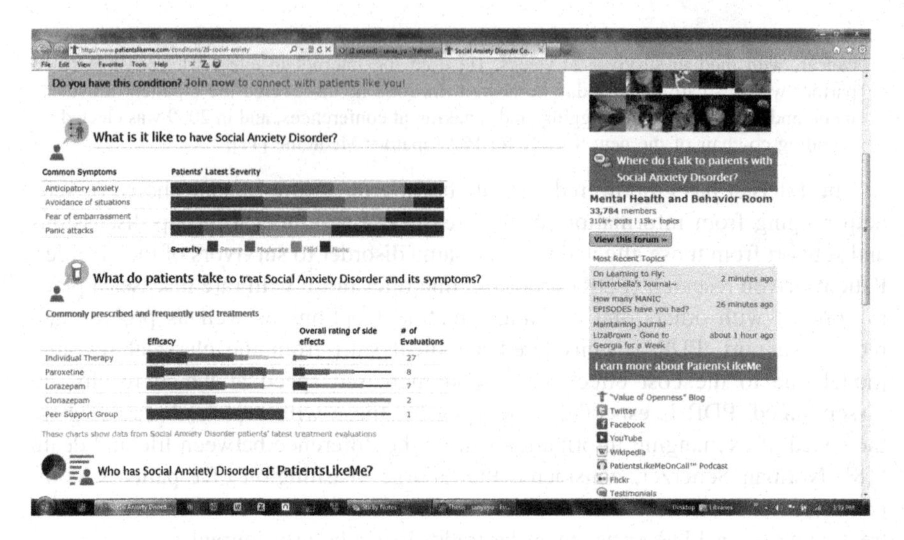

Fig. 3.1 A screenshot of PatientsLikeMe (Accessed 03-10-2012, http://www.patientslikeme.com/conditions/26-social-anxiety)

disease which attacks nerve cells in the brain and spinal cord that control voluntary muscle movement, 25 % of patients survive more than 5 years after diagnosis). The Heywood family soon began searching the world over for ideas that would extend and improve Stephen's life (he died at the age of 37). Inspired by Stephen's experiences, the co-founders and team conceptualized and built a health data-sharing platform that could transform the way patients manage their own conditions, change the way industry conducts research and improve patient care.

Although the company was started as a result of Stephen Heywood's struggles with Lou Gehrig's disease the Web site has hundreds of different disorders that users can get information on and blog about. The following screen shot is from a page about social anxiety disorder in which one can see statistics about symptoms and treatments available from people who have the disorder, there are also forums in which patients can share their experiences and get in touch with others:

Patients report that the information they find online helps them manage their overall health and comply with prescribed treatments, and those who use the Internet frequently are two to three times more likely than infrequent users to take action that affects their diagnosis and treatment [21].

3.3 Who is Using the Internet for Mental Health Care?

Globally Africa, the Middle East, and Latin America are the fastest growing populations in terms of Internet usage [36]. In the United States, Internet use has grown dramatically over the past decade, with a jump from 44 % of the population using the Internet in 2000 to 77 % in 2010 [37]. It is estimated that 80 % of Internet users look online for health care information with the most commonly researched topics being specific diseases, treatments, and health care providers [16]. According to a recent Pew Internet report people searching for health care information online are most likely:

- Female (86 % of women versus 73 % of men);
- Females significantly outpace males online in their pursuit of information about specific diseases or medical problems, certain treatments or procedures, doctors or other health professionals, hospitals or other medical facilities, food safety or recalls, drug safety or recalls, and pregnancy and childbirth;
- Seventy-nine percent of caregivers (a term used for adults who provide unpaid care to a parent, child, friend or other loved ones) have access to the Internet. Of those, 88 % look online for health information;
- Differences among adults with various levels of education are echoed in health information gathering online: 89 % of Internet users with a college degree do so, compared with 70 % of Internet users with a high school degree. The numbers drop even further when looking at adults who have less than a high school education—just 38 % go online and, of those, 62 % say they gather health information online;
- Income is another strong predictor of Internet access: 95 % of adults who live in households with $75,000 or more in annual income go online, compared with 57 % of adults who live in household with $30,000 or less in annual income. Again, the disparity is repeated in the two groups' likelihood to look online for health information: once online, 87 % of upper-income Internet users do so, compared with 72 % of Internet users living in lower-income households [14];
- It is estimated that 1 in 5 Internet users have gone online to find others who may have similar health concerns. This peer-to-peer consultation is especially seen in patients with a chronic condition such as high blood pressure, diabetes, heart condition or cancer where 1 in 4 Internet users have used the Internet to find others like them. Other groups that go online to find people who share their health concerns include: Internet users caring for a loved one; those who have experienced a medical crisis in the past year; and those who have experienced a significant change in their health such as pregnancy, weight loss or gain and quitting smoking [15]. A recent Harris Interactive poll shows:
  - The proportion of people who are online who report that they "often" look for information about health topics on the Internet has increased to 39 %, up from 22 % in 2009, and 32 % in 2010;
  - The majority of individuals use search engines (69 %) and medical websites (62 %) to look for health information online (sometimes called "cyber-chondriacs" if they search too much—an Internet term similar to hypochondria);
  - The proportion of individuals who say that their searches were very or somewhat successful has increased to 90 % this year, up from 83 % in 2009 and 86 % in 2010;

- Individuals who say that they believe the information they obtained was reliable has risen to 90 % this year from 87 % and 85 % in the two previous years; Fully 57 % of such people report that they discussed information obtained online with their doctors, up from 44 % and 53 % in the last two years;
- Those who report that they searched online for medical information based on discussions with their doctors has increased to 57 % from 49 % in 2009 and 51 % in 2010 [40].

According to the Pew Research Center, mental health research online is also on the rise with the percentage of Internet users looking up mental health issues jumping from 22 to 28 % between 2002 and 2008, a statistically significant increase. It is estimated that 1 in 5 Internet users have looked online for mental health information (such as depression, anxiety or stress) [31].

Research again shows that women are more likely to seek mental health information online compared to men (35 % women versus 22 % males). Over the past 6 years women have accounted for much of the growth in online research of mental health whereas males have shown no difference. Those with higher levels of education are significantly more likely to seek mental health information online (32 % of college graduates versus 24 % who have a high school education). Age also plays a factor with those under the age of 65 being twice as likely as wired seniors to use the Internet for mental health information [17].

For practitioners, eighty-six percent of U.S. doctors currently report that the Internet is essential to their clinical practices:

- 65 % search the Internet more than once a day;
- The majority of doctors access the Internet from their offices (92 %), or with a patient in the examination room (21 %);
- Most commonly these physicians are searching specific drug information (77 %), general condition information (75 %), treatment side effects (68 %), drug safety information (66 %) and information for patients (61 %). Actions taken as a result of these searches include conducting further research (48 %), printing out information for a patient or directing a patient to a Web site (45 %) and recommending further testing based on symptomology (32 %).

Nearly one-third of the physicians make changes to a patient's medication as a result of a search. The above statistics refer to practitioners in general, specific information on the use of the Internet for psychiatrists and other mental health care professionals is sparse and hard to find unfortunately.

At the 2009 annual meeting of the American Association of Technology in Psychiatry it was estimated that only about 2 % of the approximately 46,000 U.S. psychiatrists have used telepsychiatry for clinical purposes even though research shows that telepsychiatric appointments are cancelled significantly less frequently by patients than traditional face-to-face appointments [25]. The American Psychiatric Association (APA) states "telepsychiatry has been shown to improve collaborative services between professionals. Studies indicate that healthcare professionals feel telepsychiatry has given them an opportunity to work more effectively as a team. Patients surveyed say they felt that the communication between their physicians had improved their outcomes" [3].

Although there are no specific data for psychiatrists, judging from other specialties it can be estimated that 20–30 % of psychiatrists probably use email with patients and that about 10 % use electronic medical records (it is estimated that 17 % of physicians in general use electronic health records).

3.4 What Online Mental Health Services are Currently Being Offered?

Telemedicine consultations are now so common that they are undertaken on broadband Internet systems and professionals from all areas in mental health (from psychiatrists, psychologists, marriage and family therapists to career counselors) now deliver e-therapy. According to Yellowlees and Nafiz [43] the mental health resources and services available to patients at home or in the community are provided through a multitude of Internet devises, ranging from computers to iPhones, including:

- Online/video/telephone-based patient support groups and Web sites for health information
- Telepsychiatry consultations and email/phone/instant messaging with physicians and other providers from fixed and mobile locations
- Multimedia educational materials developed by patients and providers for both patient and provider education
- Scheduling systems, personal electronic health records, and tools for self-directed decision support and chronic disease management

Web sites such as http://Healthlinknow.com and http://Acesspsych.com not only offer information for both professionals and clients on how telepsychiatry works, but also services such as any variety of mental health consultations for clients in larger cities to smaller remote communities, prisons and clinics. Online cognitive behavior therapy (CBT) programs, such as fearfighter.com and "beating the blues" offer computer aided cognitive behavior therapy (CCBT) for a fraction of the cost of a traditional face-to-face therapy. Fearfighter is a Web site designed to treat panic and phobia with multi step interventions, full outcome measurement tracking and patient support in the forms of email, telephone or even face-to-face (http://fearfighter.com).

It is estimated that 46 % of Americans own smartphones and 17 % of cell phone owners, or 15 % of adults, have used their phone to look up health or medical information. There are numerous mood-tracking applications for cell phones now. The apps are generally either free or cost a few dollars (generally $2–$4). These apps allow users to track their quality and amount of sleep, triggers, general health and most important their mood (ranging from depression, anxiety, stress, post-traumatic stress, brain injury and many more). There are reminder alarms if you forget to check in and notepad features that allow users to journal each day. The following are screen shots of T2 Mood Tracker (developed by the National Center for Telehealth and Technology). The T2 Mood Tracker in Fig. 3.2 allows users to pick and choose which symptoms apply them and tracks their symptoms.

The following are comments by users of the T2 Mood Tracker application:

> I have Adult ADD, depression and GAD. The reminder feature is very helpful or I wouldn't remember to use it consistently. I like that I can track each of my issues separately, which helps me to notice which issues are giving me more trouble. This makes me feel a lot less anxious in itself, since part of the problem with managing mental issues is knowing which ones are the root symptoms, and which are symptoms of the root cause not being addressed.

> This tool (T2 Mood Tracker) provides the tracking and journaling that so many psychologists and other mental health providers encourage clients to use in order to really monitor a person's functioning. If used regularly, this app could be phenomenal with a person's control over their own mind and body! And this is great for anyone- not just those in treatment. (Accessed from ITunes Preview, http://itunes.apple.com/us/app/t2-mood-tracker/id428373825?mt=8.

Developed by universities and experts in the field there are also free self-help Web sites for those seeking alleviation from symptoms of mental disorders. MoodGYM is an innovative, interactive Web program designed by researchers at

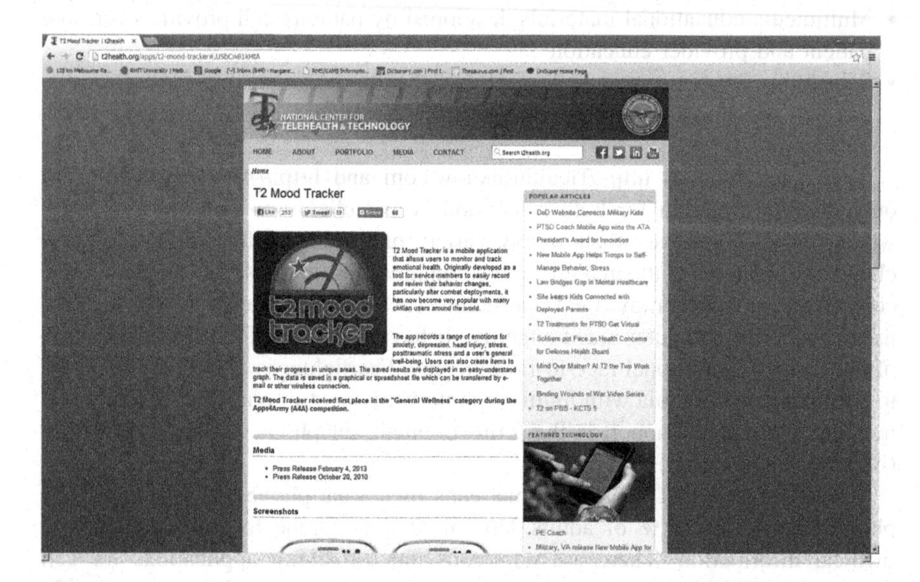

Fig. 3.2 A screenshot of the T2 Mood Tracker (Accessed from http://t2health.org/apps/t2-mood-tracker#.USbDih1kMtB)

the Centre for Mental Health Research at the Australian National University for the treatment of depression and anxiety. Using flash diagrams and online exercises MoodGYM teaches its users (400,000 plus registered users) cognitive behavior therapy—a proven treatment for depression, as well as relaxation and meditation techniques. Research trials have shown that MoodGYM significantly reduces depression symptoms for its users, and the benefits have been shown to last after 12 months when compared to control groups [9, 26].

Research shows that online mental health interventions are as effective as traditional face-to-face therapy for disorders such as depression and anxiety [1, 7, 23]. For example, treatment outcomes are comparable with both face-to-face and online cognitive behavioral therapy in alleviating symptoms of panic disorder and agoraphobia [23]. Based on a 30 month follow up study for treatment of social phobia research showed that the long-term effects of face-to-face delivered cognitive behavior therapy (CBT) was comparable to Internet based treatment [8]. In regards to depression, research shows that both CBT and psychoeducation obtained online can reduce symptoms of depression [42].

Telepsychiatry consultations are now well established with guidelines existing for both adult and child psychiatry [American Telemedicine Association [4] and have been demonstrated to be diagnostically valid and show substantial patient satisfaction [27, 29].

3.5 How are Current and Past Models of the Doctor-Patient Relationship Being Affected?

On a typical day, military psychologist Ray Folen, PhD, might provide an hour of therapy to a patient struggling with anxiety in Guam, another hour to a client in Japan experiencing post-traumatic stress disorder and a third hour to a soldier in his home state of Hawaii who might be dealing with depression. All of this therapy is provided from Folen's office at Tripler Army Medical Center in Honolulu, but only one of the sessions is done face-to-face [28].

The doctor-patient relationship is central to the general practice of medicine but it is especially important in psychiatry and other mental health care fields because it plays a prominent role in the therapeutic process. In his book The doctor, his patient and the illness, Balint described the doctor-patient relationship as a process involving three stages: the collection of symptoms from the patient (including the physical and mental state exams), a diagnostic evaluation, and seeking mutual agreement on a management plan [6].

Psychiatrists have been described as having three potential roles in the doctor-patient relationship-that of authority, facilitator, or partner [6]. In the authority role the psychiatrist makes all the decisions for the patient, this is becoming less common. In the facilitator role the psychiatrist guides his or her patients to appropriate information that will help the patient make informed treatment choices. Finally, in the partner role the psychiatrist assists with research into therapeutic options and information analysis but the patient is often the primary researcher [43].

With the advent of videoconferencing, E-mail and Instant Messaging the relationship of the doctor-patient has undoubtedly changed, however, as Andersson [5] writes, "Emerging evidence across trials clearly suggests that the computer cannot totally replace human contact". Face-to-face consultations will remain the core of most psychiatrist-patient relationships but the Internet is becoming a major component of most health consultations and will continue to change the way that psychiatrists work. Initially patients may have a traditional face-to-face visit but this might be followed with video visits such as online therapy and psychoeducation with in-person visits occurring as needed [43].

Psychiatrists can now videoconference with their patients, this requires that both the psychiatrist and patient have access to web cam technology. In videoconferencing both psychiatrist and patient can see one another as they chat. This form of e-therapy has been labeled as more similar to the traditional face-to-face therapy since the psychiatrist and patient can see one another. The downfall to videoconferencing could be the disruption in service should the server crash [2].

E-mail is another versatile tool for fast, easy communication between the psychiatrist and his or her patients. However, the psychiatrist should be aware of the emerging laws concerning the Internet and medicine with respect to HIPAA regulations [2].

Instant messaging is similar to e-mail with the added benefit of real-time response. This has been compared to a conversation via the telephone but typed instead of spoken. Voice-over-Internet-protocol (VOIP) technology enables voice communications via the Internet and is gaining popularity. Live chat rooms could be used for group therapy since it allows for multiple people to communicate simultaneously [2].

With the use of e-therapy it is vital that both practitioners and clients understand and appreciate the limited nature of this medium and practitioners need to:

- Assess if the client is suitable for online treatment, taking into consideration if the client is in immediate crisis, is engaged in active suicidal ideation or if there are other serious concerns such as domestic violence or severe drug use;
- Have back-up resources in place to address urgent issues;
- Educate clients and provide informed consent;
- Assess the suitability of clients and work within ethical parameters.

3.6 What are Benefits and Possible Downfalls of Using the Internet in the Doctor-Patient Relationship?

E-therapy has numerous benefits, such as the convenience of getting treatment in the privacy of your home versus having to drive to see a mental healthcare provider. It allows patients and practitioners to bypass time and geographical boundaries, allowing access to mental health care for those with limited mobility or for people who live in remote locations. And although face-to-face therapy is considered the gold standard researchers are discovering that online treatments can be as effective and therapeutic, but, this is not to say that there aren't opposing opinions and certain issues that still need addressing.

3.6.1 Distance

One issue with online therapy is the artificial distance created between the doctor and the client and researchers have argued that this can have both positive and negative consequences. The clinical limitations of distance involve lack of visual and auditory cues, body language, and spontaneous clarification (if communication is via Email or Text), which can be very important in some instances in therapy [38].

However, with treatments of disorders that have a potential element of shame, stigma or embarrassment, such as post-traumatic stress disorder, eating disorders, or for those struggling with social anxiety, the prospect of receiving treatment from a distance can be appealing [5, 24]. Researchers have hypothesized that online counseling may create a sense of disinhibition where clients feel more comfortable discussing sensitive topics online versus in a traditional face-to-face setting [39]. Dr. Fishkind, a psychiatrist based out of Texas writes:

> We've had over 60,000 patient encounters…only six have been refused to be seen via teleconferencing…when it comes to mental health issues and the difficult things you need to talk about in a crisis, a lot of patients feel it's less threatening and easier to be open and communicative via telemedicine.

In the treatment of children and adolescents Pakyurek et al., argue that in certain cases telepsychiatry might be a superior method of psychiatric assessment than face-to-face consultations. They discuss five case studies, one of which is the following:

> A 15-year old girl was referred for a consultation by her primary care provider, and she agreed to individual face-to-face therapy for the first time after her first telepsychiatry consultation. Despite multiple attempts in the past, she had declined to do so. The girl stated that she felt more comfortable in front of a monitor than with "a real psychiatrist." Both the girl and her mother reported that in the past she had refused to open up. After the telepsychiatry session, an appointment with a local psychologist was secured for individual therapy. At 2-month follow up, the girl reported improvement with her energy level, sleep, and social motivation. She had been meeting with her therapist consistently every week since the initial consultation with us [30].

In another example Dr. Chandran, who treats adolescents based out of Virginia notes:

> [patients] feel great about seeing me on the television and they actually become more animated when they see me that way, especially kids with anxiety issues. They do very well with telemedicine.

Distance (when E-mail is utilized as a medium) also allows for a 'zone of reflection', which [38] describes as a slowing down of the therapy process and allowing both parties to pay close attention to their own thoughts and feelings while still engaged in a dialogue. Some clients might also be more comfortable expressing themselves in writing and the process of writing itself can be therapeutic and encourage insight.

3.6.2 Cost

Traditional therapy visits can range anywhere from $50 to $150 for a 50 min session (depending on where you live and what type of services you need) plus the cost of travel to and from the visit. With e-therapy, depending on which online services you choose, an email question can cost about $25–$60 and a chat or videoconferencing session can range between $50–$120 for 60 min (http://asktheinternettherapist.com; National Directory of Online Counselors). If your computer does not have a webcam one can be purchased for roughly $80.

Although e-therapy can be cheaper than face-to-face therapy, there is still an issue with insurance companies reimbursing practitioners. Practitioners also need to consider the cost of expenses incurred in conducting e-therapy, such as website hosting fees, website development, computer expenses and Internet service fees.

3.6.3 Ethics

Numerous ethical and legal questions are being raised as the healthcare field advances towards the use of the Internet, including:

- The use of E-mail in the doctor-patient relationship.
- State licensing concerns if therapist and client are in different states.
- Confidentiality.

The use of E-mail has created a slew of legal concerns with respect to the ethics of the doctor-patient relationship. Mental health care professionals may be faced with difficult ethics-related decisions regarding answering unsolicited e-mails from their patients, the patient's family or the general public [33], and, at what point does an E-mail exchange between a psychiatrist and his/her patient turn into e-therapy? Recupero [33] argues that while E-mail may be incidental, e-therapy can constitute the practice of medicine online (such as prescribing medicine, conducting psychotherapy or psychiatric examinations).

Although one benefit of e-therapy is that it has no geographical boundaries, and this can be beneficial for both the practitioner and client, licensing issues arise. License and certifications to practice counseling are state issued, therefore with each state having its own licensing requirements issues arise if the therapist and client are in different states [34].

In order to ensure confidentiality the practitioners needs to utilize safeguards such as firewalls and password protection, but even with these precautions a misdirected e-mail to an unintended recipient increases liability exposure for the psychiatrist. A possible solution to this could be the use of encryption technology. An encrypted e-mail has unintelligible sequence of characters that can be unscrambled with a decryption key from the sender (the psychiatrist in this example) [33].

Although many of the same APA ethics code apply to online therapy such as informed consent, doing no harm, and competence to practice, Deborah Baker, JD, director for prescriptive authority and regulatory affairs in APA's Practice Directorate states, "...technology is pushing ahead at a rapid pace, psychology licensing laws have not yet caught up. All health and mental health-care professions are wrestling with many of the same issues" [10].

3.7 Summary

The locus of power in health care is shifting. Instead of the doctor having full control of the patients' needs a consumerist model has emerged in which patients and their doctors are partners in managing the patients' care [13]. The age of the "Industrial Age Medicine" has been replaced by the new model of the "Information Age Care" as envisioned by Ferguson [12] and Smith [35]. In this new information age the relationship of healthcare practitioner and patients are increasingly becoming collaborative partnerships as patients have more control over their healthcare needs than ever before:

- In general medical care we see a trend towards e-monitoring with e-devices such as e-scale (which sends alerts to healthcare professionals when a patient's weight exceeds the desired range) e-shirt (which can be worn to transmit heart rate and respiratory rate over the Internet) to the ability of diabetic patients testing their blood glucose with the click of a computer mouse [13];
- The use of the Internet for mental healthcare is catching up with applications for smartphones for tracking mood, anxiety and general health to online treatments for most mental health ailments;
- E-therapy has been demonstrated to not only be time and cost effective but research also shows that the treatment outcome is comparable to that of the gold standard (face-to-face) therapy. And for some individuals the artificial distance of e-therapy can be more therapeutic than the gold standard;

- Relatively few psychiatrists and other mental health care providers are currently using the Internet to aid with their practice. The main barriers to use telepsychiatry have been reported as scheduling, reimbursement, and organizational issues, rather than technical problems. However, the mental healthcare field will need to catch up as demand for this type of therapy is bound to increase in the near future;
- Face-to-face therapy will still remain the gold standard in therapy, and there will always be cases that require the physical presence of both the therapist and client for the best treatment outcome, however, online therapy is a novel tool that therapists and clients can use to supplement the traditional form of therapy.

Telemedicine has had a tremendous impact on the way health care is accessed and delivered in fields such as optometry, radiology, pathology and cardiology. The use of telemedicine in the mental health field is still a new concept but from the preliminary uses and research it has great potential to reshape the way mental health care is accessed and delivered. It has the potential to make mental health care far more accessible and affordable and perhaps less stigmatizing due to the privacy of getting care from home. The Industry Council Chairman for the American Telemedicine Association predicts that telemedicine will continue to grow as demands for real-time remote delivery systems grow across the healthcare spectrum. The mental health care field needs to seize this opportunity, as this is clearly where the future of healthcare is headed.

References

1. Amstadter, A.B., Broman-Fulks, J., Zinzow, H., Ruggiero, K.J., Cercone, J.: Internet-based interventions for traumatic stress-related mental health problems: A review and suggestion for future research. Clin. Psychol. Rev. **29**(5), 410–420 (2009). doi:10.1016/j.cpr.2009.04.001
2. American Psychiatric Association.: The Internet in clinical psychiatry. Retrieved from http://www.psych.org/Departments/EDU/Library/APAOfficialDocumentsandRelated/ResourcesDocuments/200920.aspx
3. American Psychiatric Association.: Telepsychiatry. Retrieved from http://www.psychiatry.org/practice/professional-interests/underserved-communities/telepsychiatry (2011)
4. American Telemedicine Association.: Telemedicine standards & guidelines. Retrieved from http://www.americantelemed.org/i4a/pages/index.cfm?pageID=3311 (2012)
5. Andersson, G.: Using the Internet to provide cognitive behaviour therapy. Behav. Res. Ther. **47**(3), 175–180 (2009). doi:10.1016/j.brat.2009.01.010
6. Balint, M.: The doctor, his patient and the illness. International Universities Press, New York (1957)
7. Carlbring, P., Ekselius, L., Andersson, G.: Treatment of panic disorder via the Internet: a randomized trial of CBT vs. applied relaxation. J. Behav. Ther. Exp. Psychiatry **34**(2), 129–140 (2003). doi:10.1016/S0005-7916(03)00026-0
8. Carlbring, P., Nordgren, L.B., Furmark, T., Andersson, G.: Long-term outcome of Internet-delivered cognitive-behavioural therapy for social phobia: a 30-month follow-up. Behav. Res. Ther. **47**(10), 848–850 (2009). doi:10.1016/j.brat.2009.06.012

9. Christensen, H., Griffiths, K.M., Jorm, A.F.: Delivering interventions for depression by using the internet: Randomised controlled trial. Br. Med. J. **328**, (2004). doi:10.1136/bmj.37945.566632.EE
10. DeAngelis, T.: Practicing distance therapy, legally and ethically. Retrieved from American Psychological Association website http://www.apa.org/monitor/2012/03/virtual.aspx (2012, March)
11. E-Patient Dave.: Retrieved from http://epatientdave.com/about-dave/#.UNz3QZgqNFQ (2012)
12. Ferguson, T.: E-patients: How they can help us heal healthcare? Retrieved from http://www.nationalehealth.org/sites/default/files/e-patients_white_paper_0.pdf (2007)
13. Forkner-Dunn, J.: Internet-based patient self-care: the next generation of health care delivery. J. Med. Int. Res. **5**(2), e8 (2003). doi:10.2196/jmir.5.2.e8
14. Fox, S.: Health topics: 80 % of Internet users look for health information online. Retrieved from Pew Internet & American Life Project website: http://www.pewinternet.org/~/media//Files/Reports/2011/PIP_Health_Topics.pdf (2011a)
15. Fox, S.: Peer-to-peer healthcare: Many people-especially those living with chronic or rare diseases-use online connections to supplement professional medical adive. Retrieved from Pew Internet & American Life Project website: http://www.pewinternet.org/~/media//Files/Reports/2011/Pew_P2PHealthcare_2011.pdf (2011b)
16. Fox, S.: Pew Internet: Health. Retrieved from Pew Internet & American Life Project website: http://www.pewinternet.org/Commentary/2011/November/Pew-Internet-Health.aspx (2012)
17. Fox, S., Jones, S.: The social life of health information: Americans' pursuit of health takes place within a widening network of both online and offline sources. Retrieved from Pew Internet & American Life Project website: http://www.pewinternet.org/~/media//Files/Reports/2011/PIP_Health_Topics.pdf (2009)
18. Frydman, G.: Patient-driven research: Rich opportunities and real risk. J. Participatory Med. **1**(1). Retrieved from http://ojs.jopm.org/index.php/jpm/article/view/28/18
19. Frydman, G.: A patient-centric definition of participatory medicine. Retrieved from e-Patients.net website http://e-patients.net/archives/2010/04/a-patient-centric-definition-of-participatory-medicine.html (2010)
20. Gardiner, R.: The transition from 'informed patient' care to 'patient informed' care. Studis in Health Technology and Informatics, pp. 137, 241–256. Retrieved from http://www.ncbi.nlm.nih.gov/pubmed/18560085 (2008)
21. HarrisInteractive.: The increasing impact of e-Health on consumer behavior. Retrieved from http://www.ehealthstrategies.com/files/hi_v1_21.pdf (2001)
22. Kayser, K.: Interdisciplinary telecommunication and expert teleconsultation in diagnostic pathology: present status and future prospects. J. Telemed. Telecare **8**(6), 325–330 (2002). doi:10.1258/135763302320939202
23. Kiropoulos, L.A., Klein, B., Austin, D.W., Gilson, K., Pier, C., Mitchell, J., Ciechomski, L.: Is internet-based CBT for panic disorder and agoraphobia as effective as face-to-face CBT? J. Anxiety Disord. **22**(8), 1273–1284 (2008). doi:10.1016/j.janxdis.2008.01.008
24. Leibert, T., Archer, J., Munson, J., York, G.: An exploratory study of client perceptions of Internet counseling and the therapeutic alliance. Journal of Mental Health Counseling, **28**(1), 69–83. Retrieved from http://search.proquest.com.proxy.lib.csus.edu/cv_775533/docview/198720837/13B1B57FC335A9D31DE/6?accountid=10358 (2006)
25. Leigh, H., Cruz, H., Mallios, R.: Telepsychiatry appointments in a continuing care setting: kept, cancelled and no-shows. J. Telemed. Telecare **15**(6), 286–289 (2009). doi:10.1258/jtt.2009.090305
26. Mackinnon, A., Griffiths, K.M., Christensen, H.: Comparative randomised trial of online cognitive-behavioural therapy and an information website for depression: 12 month outcomes. Brit. J. Psychiatry **192**, 130–134 (2008). doi:10.1192/bjp.bp.106.032078
27. Neufeld, J.D., Yellowlees, P.M., Hilty, D.M., Cobb, H., Bourgeois, J.A.: The e-Mental Health Consultation Service: Providing enhanced primary-care mental health services through telemedicine. Psychosomatics **48**(2), 135–141 (2007). doi:10.1176/appi.psy.48.2.135

28. Novotney, A.: How can psychologists stay ahead of the curve—and keep patients safe? Monitor Psychol. **42**(6), Retrieved 03-10-2012, from http://www.apa.org/monitor/2011/06/telehealth.aspx (2011, June)
29. O'Reilly, R., Bishop, J., Maddox, K., Hutchinson, L., Fisman, M., Takhar, J.: Is Telepsychiatry equivalent to face-to-face psychiatry? Results from a randomized controlled equivalence trial. Psychiatr. Serv. **58**(6), 836–843 (2007). doi:10.1176/appi.ps.58.6.836
30. Pakyurek, M., Yellowlees, P., Hilty, D.: The child and adolescent Telepsychiatry consultation: Can it be a more effective clinical process for certain patients than conventional practice? Telemed. e-Health **16**(3), 289–292 (2010). doi:10.1089/tmj.2009.0130
31. Pew Internet.: American search online for mental health, insurance, and drug information. Retrieved from http://www.pewinternet.org/Press-Releases/2003/Americans-Search-Online-for-Mental-Health-Insurance-and-Drug-Information.aspx (2003)
32. Pew Internet.: Web 2.0. Retrieved from http://www.pewinternet.org/topics/Web-20.aspx?typeFilter=5 (2012)
33. Recupero, P.R.: E-mail and the psychiatrist-patient relationship. J. Am. Acad. Psychiat. Law **33**(4), 465475. Retrieved from http://jaapl.org/content/33/4/465.full (2005)
34. Ross, W.: Ethical issues involved in online counseling. J. Psychol. Issues Organ. Culture **2**(1), 54–66 (2011). doi:10.1002/jpoc.20047
35. Smith, R.: The future of healthcare systems. Brit. Med. J. **314**(7093), 1495–1496. Retrieved from http://www.jstor.org.proxy.lib.csus.edu/stable/25174647 (1997)
36. Internet World Stats.: Internet users in the world-Distribution by world regions-2011. Retrieved from http://www.internetworldstats.com/stats.htm (2011a)
37. Internet World Stats.: United States of America: Internet usage and broadband usage report. Retrieved from http://www.internetworldstats.com/am/us.htm (2011b)
38. Suler, J.: Psychotherapy in cyberspace: A 5-dimensional model of online and computer-mediated psychotherapy. CyberPsychology & Behavior **3**(2), 151–159 (2000). doi:10.1089/109493100315996
39. Suler, J.: Assessing a person's suitability for online therapy: The ISMHO clinical case study group. Cyberpsychol. Behav. **4**(6), 675–679 (2001). doi:10.1089/109493101753376614
40. Taylor, H.: The growing influence and use of health care information obtained online. Retrieved from Harris Interactive website http://www.harrisinteractive.com/NewsRoom/HarrisPolls/tabid/447/ctl/ReadCustom%20Default/mid/1508/ArticleId/863/Default.aspx (2011)
41. Whited, J.D.: Teledermatology: Current status and future directions. Am. J. Clinical Dermatol. **2**(2), 59–64. Retrieved from http://www.ingentaconnect.com/content/adis/derm/2001/00000002/00000002/art00001 (2001)
42. Yellowlees, P.: Your Health in the Information Age: How You and Your Doctor can Use the Internet to Work Together. iUniverse, Bloomington (2008)
43. Yellowlees, P., Nafiz, N.: The psychiatrist-patient relationship of the future: anytime, anywhere? Harvard Rev. Psychiat. **18**(2), 96–102 (2010). doi:10.3109/10673221003683952

Chapter 4
Novel Approaches to Clinical Care in Mental Health: From Asynchronous Telepsychiatry to Virtual Reality

Abdullah Maghazil and Peter Yellowlees

This chapter is divided into 5 main sections. The first part is an introduction to the process of patient consultations, and how the process of these consultations can be redesigned to make it work more effectively with a range of technologies and devices. We provide some guidelines for providers to enable them to focus their direct services on more important tasks than routine work, which can often be done using a range of technologies. The second part reviews a number of technologies that are changing the way we communicate whether in our daily lives or in our healthcare practices, particularly smartphones, tablets and a range of medical devices intended for use at home. The third part is designed to focus on synchronous or real-time Telepsychiatry, which encompasses live and interactive communication between the patient and the provider for diagnosis, analysis, and data collection. The fourth part reviews Asynchronous or Store & Forward Telepsychiatry, a clinical process that we have pioneered and which we believe will become very common in future. Asynchronous medicine is the transmission of medical information from the patient to the provider, or vice versa, over a distance, with a review of the information later on. The information is literally "stored and forwarded" and viewed asynchronously. This is similar to sending a lab test result or an x-ray image to the doctor who then reviews the results whenever they have time available to provide suggestions or treatment. The final section will focus on the future, and in particular on the use of virtual reality in mental health.

A. Maghazil
Health Informatics Graduate Program, UC Davis Medical Center, Sacramento, USA

P. Yellowlees (✉)
Department of Psychiatry and Behavioral Sciences, University of California-Davis, Sacramento, CA, USA

M. Lech et al. (eds.), *Mental Health Informatics*,
Studies in Computational Intelligence 491, DOI: 10.1007/978-3-642-38550-6_4,

4.1 New Approaches to Care: The Underlying Principals

In any actual doctor/patient consultation, we know that across multiple different specialties about 80 % of all consultations that any doctor has with any patient about any type of problem are generally straightforward. The patient has got a fairly clear set of symptoms. The doctor is able to make the diagnosis fairly easily. There is no need for specialist referral or multiple lab or radiology tests. The consultation tends to be short and the patient does not need to return for substantial follow up. The whole interaction is reasonably straightforward, and the patient's symptoms or signs do not deviate from what is often called a "classical presentation".

The 80/20 rule is a concept that essentially means about 20 % of the patients that doctors see take up about 80 % of resources. These are the people who have chronic illnesses, who need multiple admissions, who see a lot of different specialists, and who have multiple different tests. Meanwhile, the other 80 % of the patients that doctors see only take up about 20 % of resources. They are the patients who are relatively younger, relatively fitter, don't have chronic illnesses, and have shorter-term disorders that can be treated effectively. These 80 % of patients who take up 20 % of resources are the ones most likely to benefit from automated systems such as are in tele-health and m-health, although increasingly the 20 % who have chronic illnesses are being helped by technology focused on improving their long term disease management with home monitors and similar devices and support tools.

If we look at banking systems, as a parallel example to healthcare, most transactions, as high as 80 %, are made at the ATM machine and the rest of the 20 % of transactions are made inside the banking facility by specialists. If ATM machines did not take most of the load work of simple transactions from the banking facility, the quality of service would be poor and transactions would be slower leading to dissatisfied customers.

This 80/20 phenomenon means that in healthcare we really need to concentrate on the simple transactions and make the whole system of care work more efficiently; especially to be able to free up people to undertake the more complicated transactions that involve more specialized interference. In healthcare, we essentially have the equivalent to the actual bank's records in our EMRs which typically involve data, along with lab results, different types of electronic documents, digital images, and even photographs or video digital images. This is the healthcare equivalent of the bank ATM. We have already moved into a world where electronic records are multimedia and this multimedia data should be accessible almost anywhere using the equivalent of an ATM for health which includes computers, monitoring devices, smartphones, tablets and medical devices in general. These data sources are already collected and should be able to be delivered through a single portal, to either patients or doctors whenever or wherever they want.

There are two very important informatics and computer science principles that we need to remember that underlie the use of technology in medicine and mental health care.

The first is what is called the complementarity principle. This is a really simple concept that states that computers do well what humans do badly, and vice versa. If you think about it, computers are basically fairly unintelligent. They are machines that have to be programmed and they will only do what they are told to do; but they never forget and they are really good at scheduling, remembering, and reminding. So they can do a lot of the essential mechanical transactions that humans often forget to do. We forget phone numbers, dates and impossible to remember large data sets but computers don't forget any of these things.

On the other hand, humans are creative, are very good at analyzing data, and are much better at decision-making than computers. Look how long it has taken for a computer to beat a human at chess—and how big a computer it took. So when we are designing a new system, we need to think about the skills computers have versus the skills humans have, and not mix up what humans can do that computers can do better, and vice versa. This is what ATM healthcare entitles us to do. We should be able to use computers to do many of the simple health transactions, particularly remembering and ordering prescriptions and lab tests, scheduling appointments, providing all sorts of preventative individualized health information and the like.

Humans, on the other hand, can look at large numbers of data streams, can analyze them and work out diagnoses. But once the diagnosis is completed, we can often move back into tasks that computers do better than humans. These tasks can be; ordering the whole series of tests (often called an "order set"), coordinating the requirements of a treatment protocol, sending out reminders, making sure the right investigations are done at the right time, and ensuring that all results get back to humans at the right time so that they can analyze them.

The second principle concerns the importance of redesigning, or reengineering, a system before putting in a new technology or software solution, rather than trying to match a technology to a currently inefficient system. This is an essential principle held high in companies like Toyota who learned very early that there was no point in just introducing new technologies if a bad workflow process existed. They learned that it was essential to redesign the whole workflow before introducing any technology. The lack of recognition of this issue that has been really significant problem in the health industry, where, unfortunately, a lot of electronic medical records from early, and even current years, were designed to support bad business practices. We need to remember, and acknowledge, that a lot of what we do in healthcare is very inefficient. It is based essentially on a sort of 19th Century mentorship model of healthcare at which time it was essential for the doctor and the patient to physically be together to undertake a consultation. And, of course, increasingly, that is just not the case anymore.

So we need to redesign the workflows and redesign the work processes in healthcare prior to introducing any new technology so that we can use information technology more effectively and efficiently. That is exactly what has happened in the banking system where nowadays, if you want to withdraw money out of a bank, you don't have to stick to certain opening hours, or if it is busy time or not. All what you have to do is just go to a machine in the wall and get your money—fast and convenient.

So what could ATM healthcare look like? The initial target is the 80 % of straightforward clinical interactions, not the 20 % of consultations where you really need a high-level practitioner to analyze and undertake a particularly difficult consultation. We are not suggesting that the process of Internet healthcare or ATM healthcare should supersede what is essentially still the gold standard in healthcare—when a physician is talking to and examining a patient in person to derive their conclusions and plan their treatments. ATM healthcare should manage the simple routine consultations we absolutely can undertake electronically either synchronously or asynchronously.

This brings us up to telemedicine, whether it is video consulting in real times, which is called synchronous telemedicine, or whether it is delayed time store and forward telemedicine, also called asynchronous telemedicine. These are now proven technologies that are getting widely implemented and used, and which will ultimately increasingly be used as part of ATM healthcare. This is happening with the "minute clinics" now springing up in pharmacies and major retailers where mid-level providers are typically beamed into the store from afar to deal with a specific range of simple consultations. These technologies and clinical processes are rapidly becoming the equivalent of teller machines. The area of mobile health, or m-health, is moving beyond this with email, messaging and wireless video chatting that we increasingly do from our mobile phones giving us better communication between the providers and patients. Now how is all this going to happen? Well, clearly, there are a lot of forces that are moving forward to introduce ATM healthcare more widely. Look at the way smartphone applications, for example, are changing the way people use and interact with their mobile devices. Patients are the most important force to move us all towards a healthcare ATM world. We are confident that this is going to happen, as patients demand that their doctors use technology to improve healthcare quality in general.

4.2 New Medical Devices for Mental Health Provisions: Smart Phones & Tablets

Consumer focused devices and applications are the target of many researchers and manufacturers nowadays since they have great value and huge potential in improving personal healthcare. They allow patients to collect their own data and involve themselves and their families in the treatment progress of their health. When the patient is personally involved in their own treatment the increased convenience and confidence leads to better health outcomes for patients and their family members. It also gives providers more collected data to analyze and test [1].

80 million Americans own a smartphone. 20 million iPads, or their tablet equivalents, were sold in 2011. 70 % of doctors own these devices. We now have generations of children who are "digital natives" and have been brought up surrounded by electronic devices. Video recordings are everywhere—captured on a sea of smartphones—youtube and social networking sites have terabytes of video uploads per day and "skype" has entered our language as a verb. Online healthcare is becoming more accepted by both patients and doctors and new clinical practices that support patient focused and individualized care that simply haven't been possible in the past are rapidly appearing [13, 14, 15].

In the field of telemedicine several companies have created mobile health IT platforms for smartphones that enable video medical consultations, both synchronously and asynchronously, secure instant messaging and email, as well as telephony. These mobile consults from virtual networks of clinicians available anytime, anywhere, can be direct to patients or primary care providers, to clinics, emergency departments and homes. Such mobile systems will increasingly enable not only patient and provider communication, but also web-based care coordination, e-Prescribing, practice management, health education and wellness promotion, online scheduling, billing and electronic health record interoperability and health information exchange all in one app.

As part of this revolution in healthcare we also need to let patients use the power of their phones and mobile devices to capture clinically significant events on video and transmit these direct to their providers. CNN has promoted the concept of "iReports"—videos taken by news observers on the ground. Maybe we should be promoting "hReports"—videos taken of clinically significant "health" events which are transmitted to treating physicians. Think of the opportunities—the ability to watch a seizure, observe the evolution of a stroke, see a dozen different people with infectious disease symptoms in different locations, review an autistic child's behavior, examine a compound fracture or watch the football accident that led to a neck injury. Mobile platforms offer so many possibilities for assessment, treatment and prevention in healthcare. So let us celebrate the fact that, in the field of telemedicine, there is an already an app for that. And let's promote and integrate these apps into our daily healthcare environment.

Mobile Health or sometimes referred to as M-Health is a concept that is being adopted by many companies including the healthcare industry that are benefiting from interfaced applications in smartphone devices to promote their products. Mobile phones have been in development for many years prior to the concept of the "Smartphone". They are derived from a combination of a personal digital assistant (PDA) and a telephone, both of which have been in use for decades. A Smartphone is simply a regular mobile phone combined with a PDA or a palm device to provide greater convenience for the user. In the past ten years, manufacturers have been competing to provide the best smartphones to the public with maximum functionality [7].

In most cases to create an "app", only software is needed since the mobile device's operating system is available as a base for programming, whether it be apple, android, or others. This has opened the door for many vendors to build and use smartphones for their products [19, 20]. We will now go over some interesting examples of applications in health care for mobile devices.

In Apple's App Store there are currently over 20,000 applications categorized under medical and healthcare, and these are only targeted at the iPhone and iPad. Many other applications are targeted at Android users and other smartphone operating systems. Some of these applications are targeted at clinicians but the vast majority are targeted at consumers. Certain applications are intended to gather health related data to allow monitoring of the patient often connecting it to a personal health record (PHR), with instant access. This is potentially a great aid to physicians if used properly although personal health records have yet to be taken up ubiquitously by consumers.

Tablets or tablet computers, are simply a mobile computer that has the functions of a smartphone, usually without cell phone capabilities and larger than a mobile phone. Tablets come in different types; some have a multi-touch screen while others use a stylus pen to navigate through the applications on the device's screen. Many tablets have no physical keyboard but provide an alternative usually referred to as virtual keyboard. A lot of tablet prototypes and products were launched prior to about 2010 but none achieved widespread adoption due to their limited functionality, short battery life, and high price. In 2010, Apple Inc. launched the iPad with many features as well as long battery life, a high resolution touch screen, relatively light weight, simplicity, and low cost [5] and the market for tablets changed overnight. Many other companies adopted the same features and the use of tablets has since increased exponentially.

Some advantages of tablets include:

- Easier to use in certain environments than the typical keyboard and mouse, such as while standing or lying on bed.
- Lighter weight than regular computers and can be used in many locations.
- Multi-touch and relatively large screen that allows using the finger tips which can help with drawing, painting and faster navigation.
- Connects easily to the high speed internet either through Wi-Fi or a cellular data signal.

Some disadvantages of tablets include:

- Slower input speed on virtual keyboard compared to a physical keyboard.
- May not be comfortable for the wrist especially when typing on the tablet while looking into the screen.
- Weaker video processing since tablets usually do not have an integrated video card due to space restrictions.
- Might be at higher risk of being dropped and misused which might damage the screen and many delicate materials inside the tablet.

After the introduction of the iPad in 2010, the use of tablets has been relatively widely used in many hospitals either by physicians on their own or being adopted by the hospital administration to be used by clinicians. At UC Davis, for example, in a 2012 survey of 1200 faculty physicians, almost all owned a smartphone, and over 700 also owned an iPad or tablet computer.

Some of the usages and features of tablets in hospital settings include:

- As a display unit during surgery
- View X-rays and EKG
- Ordering labs and viewing results
- Accessing patient records and entering data when needed prescribing medication
- Clinical decision support
- Educational tool for providers through online resources and alternative surgical or clinical techniques
- Educational tool for patients through videos or presentations
- An entertainment and distraction tool/toy for pediatric patients
- Remote monitoring
- A tool for relaxation and anxiety reduction
- A tool for instructing patients before and after an operation
- An instrument for easily taking notes at point of care.

A wide range of mental health applications are available from the iTunes store for both smartphones and tablets and a lot are for free. Here are some interesting ones [8].

- *Depression check*: after answering certain questions, the application gives you results concerning depression, anxiety, bipolar disorder, and post-traumatic stress.
- *Psych Terms*: a simple tool for mental health professionals that includes over 1,000 frequently used terms, phrases and definitions.
- *Symptom Checker*: search for any mental or non-mental health symptom and the application will find you information about possible illnesses and injuries and a list of local doctors that can treat your condition with their contact information.
- *Inspiring Quotes 5,000*: quotes on success, perseverance, courage, inspiration and hope.
- *Pharmacist's Letter*: find unbiased advices and recommendations by subscribing to the popular Pharmacist's Letter.
- *Medicinal Herbs*: search and find information about traditional herbs and botanicals used for mental health treatments.
- *Drugs and Medications*: research medications by name or shape and color of the pill.
- *Health tips1000*: nutrition and exercise tips to help boost mood and health in general.
- *Power of Positivity*: powerful, positive quotes and information to enhance wellbeing.
- *Bible Promises*: more than 500 popular verses on meaningful topics.

Many other long used applications that were previously only available via PC's have now become available as useful smartphone and tablet apps. Examples here include Micromedex, ePocrates and Medscape.

Relaxation and Stress Reduction Apps

Relaxation and stress reduction techniques are very helpful in maintaining good mental health and preventing relapses from depression, anxiety, stress and eating disorders. Here are some examples of interesting and simple applications that intend to relax and reduce stress:

- *Deep Relaxation*: scientifically proven brain technology that gives you relaxation and meditation through specific tracks.
- *Pure Sleep Ambiscience^{TM}*: help you sleep deeply and peacefully by using binaural and isochronic entertainment techniques that send specific sounds to each ear.
- *Relax Waterfall*: natural sounds that will help with relaxation and feeling rejuvenated.
- *Relax Completely*: hypnosis session for deep relaxation.
- *Silent Island Relaxation*: sleep, meditation and relaxation tool through videos, slideshows and sound tones.
- *Yoga Free*: over 250 yoga poses and video yoga classes. You can also create your own yoga program by using different sets of poses within the application.
- *Relax Dream*: offers rejuvenating, authentic sounds to de-stress.

4.2.1 Stop Smoking Apps

This application is called "My Last Cigarette" and is an interesting and helpful Smartphone application that encourages the user to stop and keep away from smoking. After the user enters some personal information into the phone, the application will provide a lot of variant and useful information including:

- A readout of the Nicotine level estimated
- The Carbon Monoxide level in the blood
- Statistical facts on deaths out of smoking since the user quit smoking
- Time since the user have been a non-smoker
- The increase of life expectancy readout
- Number of cigarettes NOT smoked
- The risk of a heart attack compared to the risk before stopping to smoke
- The risk of lung cancer compared to the risk before
- How much money saved after stopping smoking
- Expected circulatory improvement
- Expected lung function improvement
- Daily picture and diagram.
- Daily motivational quote or a medical fact.

All calculations used to generate this data are based upon the latest medical knowledge and statistics. Hopefully after going through these readouts, the user will be more motivated to keep away from smoking.

4.2.2 Medical Devices and the Medical Home

According to the definition by the US Food and Drug Administration [23], a device is:

> An instrument, apparatus, implement, machine, contrivance, implant, in vitro reagent, or other similar or related article, including any component, part, or accessory, which is:
>
> (1) Recognized in the official National Formulary, or the United States Pharmacopeia, or any supplement to them,
> (2) Intended for use in the diagnosis of disease or other conditions, or in the cure, mitigation, treatment, or prevention of disease, in man or other animals, or
> (3) Intended to affect the structure or any function of the body of man or other animals, and which does not achieve its primary intended purposes through chemical action within or on the body of man or other animals and which is not dependent upon being metabolized for the achievement of its primary intended purposes.

Medical devices have been in use for many years and there are literally thousands of them. The FDA has a large section of its organization devoted to the auditing and registration of a myriad of these devices. Try putting the term "medical device" into google to see the range. It is not possible to attempt to cover the whole field in this piece, however we have chosen a few examples of interesting "devices" that we think will evolve and take their place in mainstream mental healthcare over time.

4.3 Mobile Therapy Watch

This simple but effective medical device watch is capable of helping in the treatment of one of the most difficult mental disorders, Schizophrenia [24]. This illness affects around 1 % of the U.S. population and may lead to severe disability for the patient and their families. One of the symptoms of this disorder is auditory hallucinations whereby they hear voices threatening them, for example, and making them afraid to go outside.

One of the ways to treat this type of disorder is by a technique called "look, point, and name technique". This treatment technique is applied by the patient anytime they hear voices to overcome them. By looking at as many objects in the room, pointing and naming it, the patient is distracted from the voices in their head which will help with overcoming the hallucination. The mobile therapy watch's goal is to remind the patient at different times of the day to start using the technique. The watch can also be preprogrammed to show certain messages and alerts so the patients will be able to follow the treatment and not get caught up with their hallucinations. This technique will not only temporarily relieve the patient from the distressing symptom but also may give the patient the confidence in themselves to overcome these symptoms by gaining some control over the voices they hear [22].

4.3.1 Health Monitoring Mirror

This mirror concept reflects a persons' image like normal mirrors, but also monitors the health of the user on a day-to-day basis. The mirror has an encyclopedic medical database that is embedded in it and uses facial recognition technology to show results in the interactive mirror. The facial recognition software can determine if the patient is ill or not. The "Health Monitoring Mirror" can in theory not only assess users personal health but will be able to tell them that they require urgent medical attention by giving immediate alerts.

4.3.2 LifeShirt Wearable Mental Illness Monitor

The LifeShirt allows continuous monitoring of mentally disordered patients' movements. The device has so far been developed for patients with bipolar affective disorder and schizophrenia. Both disorders lead to abnormal movements of some patients, where hyperactivity is associated with bipolar patients and restricted movement is associated with patients who have schizophrenia. Patients wear the vest that is embedded with sensors to monitor hyperactive and repetitive movements while collecting data on respiration, heart rate and other physiological measurements. By collecting these data, psychiatrists are able to monitor and treat patients with the appropriate treatment. Precise measurements are a key role in achieving the best treatment outcome, which is accomplished by this device since it allows patients to move freely in different environments and settings [6].

4.3.3 Global Positioning Shoes for Alzheimers Patients

Many patients with Alzheimer disease might easily get lost or wander away from their families due to the disease. A simple integration between GPS technology and shoes can be very helpful in saving lives. Shoes embedded with a GPS device are easier than putting on a necklace or a bracelet embedded with GPS device. Shoes are highly unlikely to be lost or misplaced. The shoes can be tracked through Google maps on a web browser or through smartphones and can alert families by sending an SMS or an email if the patient went out of a pre-set set of geographic parameters, or if their movements suddenly reduced, suggesting a possible fall [18].

4.3.4 The Patient Centered Medical Home

The "Medical Home" is a new and evolving concept that is also called the "Patient-Centered Medical Home (PCMH)". This concept gives the patient access to a personal healthcare provider who manages all the patient's needs. This increases the patient's satisfaction and improves personal health in general. The relationship between the patient and their provider, and sometimes the family, will improve which will lead to better healthcare. The approach should provide the patient with the right care, in the right setting, and at the right time. This includes offering health care after being discharged from a hospital; therefore, reducing the risk of being readmitted to the hospital or a another visit to the emergency room [3].

In 2002, a project called *The Future of Family Medicine* was created through the collaboration of seven U.S. national family medicine organizations. The main goal was to revolutionize and renovate the specialty of family medicine to target more patients and enhance the quality of care. The project was proposed that services should be "accessible, accountable, comprehensive, integrated, patient-centered, safe, scientifically valid, and satisfying to both patients and their physicians [11]. In a literature review published by Starfield and Shi [21], it was determined that medical homes are associated positively with a patient's good health. Medical homes also offer an overall lower cost while maintaining a very good standard of health for patients.

The model of care for the patient centered medical home is as described in the seminal guide produced by the Agency for Health Care Research and Quality (AHRQ), *Integrating Mental Health Treatment into the Patient Centered Medical Home (PCMH)* [1], which cites the importance of Health IT tools in this process.

The guide was a response to a critical public mental health problem: the need to improve access to high quality, patient centered mental health services in underserved populations, supporting the PCMH. The PCMH is an important component to improving mental health care, particularly for underserved individuals. Mental health needs are inadequately met for underserved individuals (racial minorities, immigrants/undocumented workers, low-income, uninsured, those living in rural areas and the elderly). Mental health care is most often provided in the primary care setting by PCPs, who typically have poor access to specialty consultation. The provision of mental health care solely by primary care providers is rapidly growing. However, 2/3 of U.S. providers report poor access to mental health services and support, and mental health care needs are not adequately met in primary care, particularly for underserved groups. Though some mental health issues can be effectively managed in primary care, primary care is best utilized as a "pathway to care". The PCMH is a patient centered approach that aims to improve patient health across specialty referral and other services and the model, utilized in many Western Countries, allows centralization of health care in primary care with specialty providers consulting with and supporting the PCP which has been shown to improve patient care and health in many groups. Significant patient improvement has been found when specialist consultation is available to PCPs for managing mental health issues. One study found that patent's treated by PCP with access to psychiatric consultation improved 35 % more than patients who were treated by a PCP alone. Coordination of care among specialty mental health services and primary care is a cornerstone of the PCMH and an essential step in improving patient care. However, approaches to incorporate mental health treatment into the PCMH are limited. Health information technology has been noted as an essential component to developing and maintaining an effective medical home.

Telepsychiatry is being increasingly used throughout the USA. It is estimated by the American Telemedicine Association (www.atmeda.org) that about 2 % of US psychiatrists currently perform about 80,000–160,000 telepsychiatrist consults per year, with this number is expanding rapidly. Most telepsychiatry is synchronous, which typically relies on live, two-way interactive videoconferencing to facilitate a "real-time" consultation between a specialist and a PCP and patient, who are located in different areas, and multiple studies have demonstrated the diagnostic reliability, patient satisfaction and positive clinical outcomes associated with this modality. Asynchronous telemedicine makes use of the transmission of clinical information via email or web applications for review by a specialist at a later time and is now commonly used in radiology, dermatology, ophthalmology, cardiology and pathology.

The traditional psychiatric consultation model throughout the world is for a primary care physician to refer a patient to go and physically see a psychiatrist for an opinion. This is often a very inefficient, slow, and costly process, and as a result it is common for referring doctors to phone specialist colleagues for a "curbside consultation" where a brief discussion will frequently lead to the implementation of specialist recommendations often made on the basis of very cursory information. Many studies have examined ways of improving the process of primary care psychiatry referral and standard or synchronous telepsychiatry in some settings has either augmented or replaced this in-person and the "curbside" models. Our view is that packaged multi-approach telepsychiatry services offer a much more rapid, efficient, and patient-centered process for consultation than the traditional in-person, or unsupported phone/"curbside" models. Hence in the future we expect to see multiple technological approaches to providing mental healthcare in the PCMH, synchronous and asynchronous telepsychiatry, email, telephony and social networking and online education.

Home-Health monitoring allows the collection of data from patients in the convenience of their homes, or wherever they may be, for further diagnosis and analysis. Some monitoring devices save the data collected into a personal health records (PHR) and some others transmit the data to the healthcare provider [16].

Home-Health monitoring can also benefit patients when connected to physicians, for:

- Patient education
- Medication supervision
- Wound care
- Heart and blood pressure monitoring
- Nutritional counseling
- Oncology services
- Cardiac care
- Post-surgical care
- Behavioral health
- Asthma programs.

4.3.5 Mobile Health Clinics

Mobile health clinics reach medically disenfranchised individuals who do not normally have access to primary healthcare in urban and rural settings. A mobile health clinic is a large RV-like trailer that has a mini functional clinic. These mobile health clinics provide screenings, preventive care services and sometimes minor procedures. This takes a huge load off emergency rooms and sometimes can be the only accessible healthcare provided to some patients.

These mobile clinics can travel too hard to reach areas where a permanent clinic is difficult to provide and are conveniently available for use in national disaster situations.

4.4 Asynchronous Telepsychiatry: A Novel Model of Care and a Disruptive Innovation?

Most X-rays are no longer physically taken by radiologists. Instead the images are usually taken by a radiology technician, who is highly trained in this process, and then sent to radiologists who writes diagnostic reports which are returned to the referring doctors, often with advice on treatment or the need for other investigations. This process of asynchronous medical reporting and decision making (sometimes called "store and forward telemedicine") has become common in a number of specialties such as radiology, pathology, cardiology, dermatology and ophthalmology [4, 10].

We believe, with digital video recordings of patients now so easy to create and upload, that the time has come for such recordings made in primary care clinics, or potentially in patient's homes or other environments, to be used as clinical data that is the equivalent of an X-ray, and sent to experts, such as psychiatrists, neurologists, pediatricians and geriatricians for asynchronous opinions and reporting. This approach is an improved version of the traditional "curbside consultation" that many specialist physicians are accustomed to providing for colleagues, whereby a video of the patient can be reviewed instead of a description of symptoms as given in a phone call or a hallway conversation. This asynchronous approach to reporting has the potential to markedly improve access to experts, such as psychiatrists, for primary care providers. Video data can then be combined with other electronic data such as patient history or clinical notes and passed from provider to provider through an electronic medical record.

We have conducted the first published study of asynchronous telepsychiatry (ATP) in a sample of 127 English and Spanish speaking patients. Our study also involved the first demonstration of ATP across languages [2, 17, 25, 27, 28, 29]. We developed our own novel ATP technical platform to evaluate the feasibility and diagnostic reliability of ATP. The ATP datasets were reviewed by a psychiatrist who wrote a report containing a diagnostic assessment and treatment plan for the referring doctor to implement if they wished. We demonstrated the feasibility of this process in 60 English language consultations and then in 24 Spanish speaking patients, interviewed and recorded in Spanish, and assessed by both Spanish speaking psychiatrists, and after translation of the interviews by medical interpreters, by English speaking psychiatrists. Inter-rater reliability among the English and Spanish speaking psychiatrists was acceptable. We concluded that ATP has a unique advantage over real-time care in that patient data can be improved en-route by adding to, or altering, the information before sending it to a consulting specialist, thereby broadening the scope of providers who can evaluate it, and making the data presented to the reporting provider either more focused or more appropriate. The final part of this first study of ATP was a cost-benefit analysis, where we demonstrated that ATP, using our model, was indeed what Christensen has called a "disruptive innovation" where we changed the process of care in a way that was more cost-effective than either in-person psychiatric consultations or traditional real-time (synchronous) telepsychiatry consultations.

Further studies are needed to replicate these results and fully examine the reliability and validity of this process in larger samples and in non-research clinical settings. Clinical outcomes studies are also necessary. The language translation approach we used, involving the creation of real-time interpreted audio files, was not ideal, and we believe that an approach using sub-titles, with automated voice-to-text and digital translation, would be better. Replication is necessary with larger and more diverse diagnostic groups, as well as with other languages. Despite these methodological issues ATP does appear to be a feasible way of conducting distant psychiatric consultations, and to do this across languages. We believe ATP could be useful in many areas where access to psychiatrists is currently difficult, including correctional services, military environments, and other difficult to access groups either by reason of geography, economics or culture and ethnicity. Future iterations of the ATP platform could add other data enhancements such as facial and language analytic tools to improve diagnostic screening capacity.

The ATP consultation platform and process is ripe for research initiatives. Apart from the developments above, it is important to know whether subtitles instead of an audio file, could be beneficial for multiple types of language translations, including sign language translation for deaf and hard of hearing individuals, and how effectively mobile ATP could be made available on platforms such as smartphones to increase access to expert opinions, anytime, anywhere. ATP could also reduce many of the concerns that arise with the traditional use of in person interpreters such as limited availability of translation services which can lead to miscommunications between doctor and patient and compromised quality of care.

This is an exciting area for further research and clinical development and is one which challenges the traditional paradigms of in-person psychiatric care by promoting the asynchronous consultation model of care in an online environment. It is our view that ATP is a disruptive healthcare process that has the potential to markedly change the way we deliver mental health care.

4.4.1 Mobile Therapy

We start off with an asynchronous telemedicine example with this simple mobile application which functions as a mood tracker. At random times throughout the day the app pops up a "mood map" on the screen. It allows the user to drag a small dot around the screen to describe their current mood state. The collected data can be later viewed on a graph to track mood swings for each day or time frame. The app can also track and chart energy levels, foods eaten, sleep patterns and activities to help manage mood change influencers [22].

4.4.2 Mobile Mood Diary

This application is similar to the paper daily diary but on a Smartphone platform. Psychotherapists who treat patients suffering from clinical depression use Cognitive Behavioral Therapy CBT, which relies mainly on writing down daily activities, charting their moods and energy levels. Patients are asked to bring their recorded paper daily diary to discuss with the therapist on their weekly therapy sessions. Many patients either forget or stop doing their CBT for whatever reason. Even though research proves that patients who do their CBT homework and practice them benefit the most and more quickly from the treatment than others, many may become lazy to do them.

Psychotherapists have found huge improvements of using the Smartphone application, especially for teenagers, over the pen and paper technique. The new generation is used to texting and typing on their smartphones, and implementing that in their therapy leads to great benefits. Many teenagers rarely miss their daily homework therapy and many are surprised that they could use their own smartphone to help themselves in the treatment. As for the psychotherapist, a complete printout of the patient's moods, energy level, sleep patterns and any comments they may have had throughout their day. These printouts help psychotherapists tremendously in diagnosing and treating their patients.

Even psychiatrists find mobile mood diary greatly beneficial since they can look into graphs illustrating the patient's mood swings throughout the day. This can be of great help since they can decide whether to prescribe a certain medication or change their dosage or whatever treatment they may acquire. The smartphone application allows the psychiatrist to monitor the mood swings precisely and with accurate measurements [22].

4.4.3 CBT MobilWork

This smartphone application is targeted at severely depressed adults. The idea of the app designed by researchers from University of Pittsburgh and Carnegie Mellon University is to overcome anxiety, phobias, eating disorders and other mental health issues. In one example, a patient who may be severely depressed can hardly get out of bed. This app functions as a homework assignment where a message pops up on the screen each day saying "make your bed". After the patient successfully accomplishes the task, another message pops up promoting the next step of tasks. Even though this kind of app would require some kind of responsibility from the patient to follow instructions and perform the tasks, it will allow the therapist to monitor the behavior of the patient and consistency in performing the assigned tasks [22].

4.4.4 T2 Mood Tracker

T2 Mood Tracker allows users to monitor their moods on six pre-loaded scales (anxiety, stress, depression, brain injury, post-traumatic stress, general well-being). Custom scales can also be built. Users rate their moods by swiping a small bar to the left or to the right. The ratings are displayed on graphs to help users track their moods over time. Notes can be recorded to document daily events, medication changes and treatments that may be associated with mood changes, providing accurate information to help health care providers make treatment decisions.

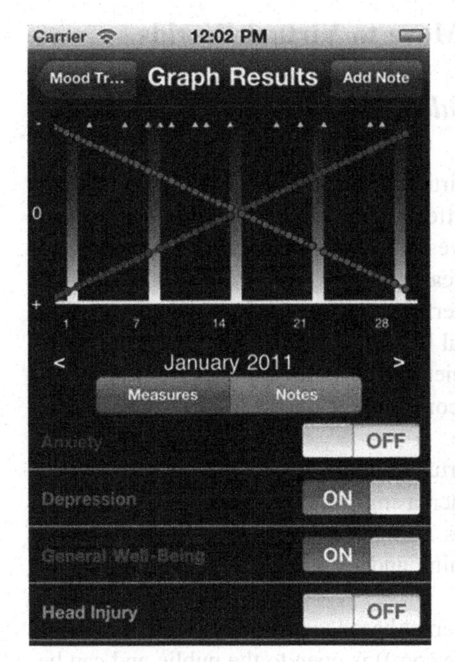

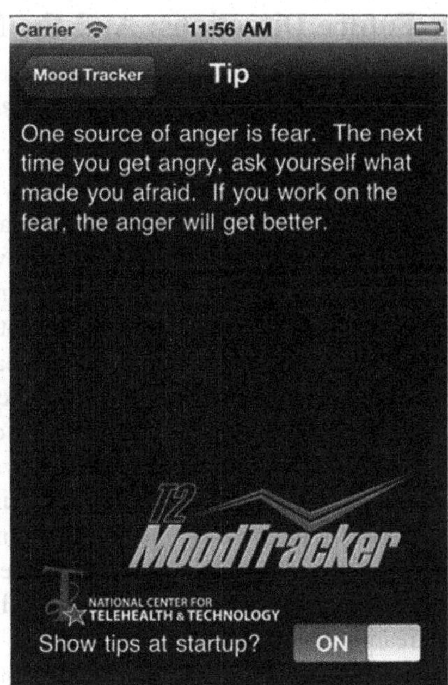

4.4.5 Mental Wellness Monitor

The Mental Wellness Monitor is a complete consumer-focused monitoring platform that aims to improve both the physical and mental health state of users by becoming integrated with their daily lives.

There are three separate parts to this monitor:

The Mods which is a biometric input/output device that is designed to be worn by the user collects and assesses biometric and environmental data and alerts the user when the data is getting off track from the user's goal.

The Trestle is the second part of the monitor which is the base station for Mods. It allows the monitor to be charged and transmit collected data through wireless connection. Some extended accessories can also be integrated with the system to monitor more variables of the body.

Finally, the cross platform software application, this can either be on the PC or a smartphone, that enables the users to study, manage and share their healthcare information according to their healthcare goals. All the information is personally customizable for best results.

4.5 Future Directions: And the Move to Virtual Worlds

4.5.1 Second Life and Virtual Reality

Virtual reality is the concept of being virtually but not physically at a specific place, and a number of virtual reality platforms have been developed in the past 20 years. Some of these platforms involve 3-dimensional imaging and surround audio that make the user feel like in the real world and allow the user to literally walk inside a room on which computer interfaces are screened on all surfaces. The user can go or do certain things that in real life might be difficult or impossible in these "caves" which have found many scientific and training uses from allowing biochemists to develop 3-D models of complicated molecules to helping train pilots in flight simulation environments.

Many companies have developed virtual reality platforms for games and entertainment on Tv's or the Internet. Increasingly though, it has been used in other professional fields with businesses using virtual reality applications to market their products, educators are teaching and for public awareness, and doctors treating their patients.

One of the leading and most popular internet based virtual reality applications is Second Life. Second Life (www.secondlife.com)) is open to the public and can be accessed free of charge. Fees are charged to purchase virtual "land" or server space, to use to build fantasy environments, and increasing numbers of players sell virtual objects and programs "inworld". Every user is assigned with an avatar that can be customized to reflect one self's physical appearance or character. Avatars can walk, run, or fly from one island to another. Some can go shopping, visit museums, or even go on a date. It all depends on the user's preference and liking. Some major businesses are investing in Second Life, since there are a lot of customers are checking out their online virtual reality stores.

Another type of a virtual reality platform is a fully immersive system. These fully immersive software systems give the user a full immersion in the virtual reality environment. This can take place in a virtual cave, which could be a three, four, five or six walled room with multiple projectors transmitting images on these walls. Some systems require a specific visual aid such as 3-dimensional glasses while others can be used with only the naked eye. A similar concept of fully immersive virtual reality environment is the use of specific glasses that has the 3-dimensional screen inside the device. These glasses are connected to a machine that transmits the virtual reality environment to the user with crispy images and sound. These immersive technologies are relatively costly which makes it less accessible to many providers and patients for treatment.

4.5.2 Treatment in Virtual Reality

One of the emerging uses of virtual reality in the medical field is used for psychiatry. Virtual reality can play a huge role in treating patients with many conditions including but not limited to: eating disorders, anxiety disorders, some autism spectrum disorders, stress management, pain management, strokes, brain injury, psychiatric disability, cognitive impairment, and dysfunctions of the central nervous system. Phobias and traumas can also be treated through virtual reality exposure therapy (VRE). VRE has proven to treat many patients by exposing them to visual and other sensory materials that represent the patient's feared object or traumatic event that was previously experienced. Many phobias including social phobias, fear of heights and flying, claustrophobia and fear of spiders have been proven to be treated through VRE. Many military organizations have also started utilizing VRE for post-traumatic stress disorders (PTSD) and other combat related disorders such as traumatic brain injury to treat soldiers and veterans suffering from these conditions.

An important aspect while treating in virtual reality is to look into the ethical implications of using such technology with patients. The rights and issues facing a patient in a virtual reality environment should not be any different than in real life. In a virtual reality environment, the user, whether the provider or the patient uses avatars to navigate through the virtual environment and will eventually face some obstacles and concerns similar to ones in real life. For example, the user might get in an argument with another person in the virtual environment but none of them probably ever met in their real lives but through their avatars they did. This means the user's emotions are involved, so any influence in the virtual environment is affecting the user directly. This also implies when the patient is going through a series of treatment techniques to overcome a type of phobia, claustrophobia for example. The patient's brain is having these symptoms and the brain is also controlling the avatar. This means that any changes to the avatar's status may affect the patient's treatment progress. When the avatar gets into a closed room, the patient will feel as if they were physically put into a closed room. The symptoms will be the same, but the consequences are less harmful as it is not so real.

Another ethical concern that is important to mention is medical practice boundaries. The rights for patients receiving the treatment in virtual environments should be as important as the ones in real life. Issues such as authentication, confidentiality, consent, and other clinical issues must be addressed to protect the patient and the provider. In case of a malpractice, licensing of providers should always be in the same state as the patient to assure protection in case of legal troubles. Similar to telemedicine consultations, the provider should be licensed in the same state where the patient is physically located, in this case wherever the patient is logged in from. An exception to this rule applies to providers working for the military, Veterans Affairs or the Indian Health Systems where clinicians are licensed to work in any of the facilities available nationwide. However, all policies and procedures used in the physical federal facility should be also used in the federal virtual reality facility [26].

4.5.3 Education in Virtual Reality

Second Life has become a strong emerging educational tool. Many universities, colleges, libraries and government bodies have adopted virtual reality software to educate and spread awareness. Many instructors and educators prefer Second Life over other distant learning methods because it is more personal and provides more opportunity for creativity. Research conducted in the U.K. in 2007 showed that over 80 % of United Kingdom's universities have developed teaching or learning tools in Second Life. It is also estimated that over 300 universities around the world teach courses or conduct researches in this platform [9, 12].

The benefits of using virtual reality platforms for educational purposes in the medical field are outstanding. Health educators can target many audiences and ethnic groups within virtual reality to promote health awareness. Diverse public audiences are wandering around these virtual reality platforms to find interesting and attention-grabbing activities. Games, billboards, and videos are simple approaches that can target big audiences. Healthcare providers can also use these virtual environments to educate their patients about certain diseases or conditions they may acquire. Instead of flipping through a brochure or going through web pages, virtual reality can offer important and beneficial sources of information with more appealing visual aid. This may lead to having the patient or family member spend more time learning about the specific topic while enjoying a fun virtual life.

References

1. Anthony, K., Nagel, D.M., Goss, S.: The Use of Technology in Mental Health: applications, ethics and practice. Charles C. Thomas, Springfield (2010)
2. Butler, T.N., Yellowlees, P.: Cost Analysis of Store-and-Forward Telepsychiatry as a Consultation Model for Primary Care. Telemed. J. E Health (2011). doi:10.1089/tmj.2011.0086
3. Cheung, K.M.: Patient-centered healthcare homes 'here to stay'. Fierce Healthcare. Retrieved 1 Dec 2011, from http://www.fiercehealthcare.com/story/patient-centered-healthcare-homes-here-stay/2011-09-27?utm_campaign=twitter-Share-NL (2011)
4. Deshpande, A., Khoja, S., Lorca, J., McKibbon, A., Rizo, C., Husereau, D., Jadad, A.R.: Asynchronous telehealth: a scoping review of analytic studies. Open Med. **3**(2), e69–e91 (2009)
5. Gruman, G.: The iPad's victory in defining the tablet: What it means. InfoWorld. Retrieved 16 Jan 2012, from http://www.infoworld.com/d/mobile-technology/the-ipads-victory-in-defining-the-tablet-what-it-means-431 (2011)
6. Heilman, K.J., Porges, S.W.: Accuracy of the LifeShirt (Vivometrics) in the detection of cardiac rhythms. Biol. Psychol. **75**(3), 300–305 (2007). doi:S0301-0511(07)00085-3. [pii]
7. Kouris, I., Mougiakakou, S., Scarnato, L., Iliopoulou, D., Diem, P., Vazeou, A., Koutsouris, D.: Mobile phone technologies and advanced data analysis towards the enhancement of diabetes self-management. Int. J. Electron. Healthc. **5**(4), 386–402 (2010). doi:Q2H73M6761826326. [pii]

8. Le, K.: Best iPad mental health applications—Relaxation, mind apps. Psychiatr. Disord. Retrieved from Suite101 website: http://kate-le-page.suite101.com/best-iphone-mental-health-applications—relaxation-mind-apps-a332094#ixzz1Yd511c6x
9. Livingstone, D., Kemp, J.: Second life education workshop 2007. Paper presented at the second life community convention, Chicago Hilton (2007)
10. Mahnke, C.B., Jordan, C.P., Bergvall, E., Person, D.A., Pinsker, J.E.: The Pacific Asynchronous TeleHealth (PATH) system: review of 1,000 pediatric teleconsultations. Telemed. J. E Health **17**(1), 35–39 (2011). doi:10.1089/tmj.2010.0089
11. Martin, J.C., Avant, R.F., Bowman, M.A., Bucholtz, J.R., Dickinson, J.R., Evans, K.L., Weber, C.W.: The future of family medicine: a collaborative project of the family medicine community (Research Support, Non-U.S. Gov't). Ann. Fam. Med. **2**(Suppl 1), S3–32
12. Michels, P.: Universities use second life to teach complex concepts. Retrieved from Government Technology website: http://www.govtech.com/education/Universities-Use-Second-Life-to-Teach.html (2008)
13. Muench, F.: Technology and Mental Health: Using Technology to Improve Our Lives. Psychology Today (2010)
14. National Center for Telehealth and Technology (n.d.-a): Introduction to Telemental Health. Telemental Health. Retrieved 1 Dec 2011, from http://t2health.org/sites/default/files/cth/introduction/intro_telemental_health_may2011.pdf
15. National Center for Telehealth and Technology (n.d.-b): Telemental Health Guidebook. Telemental Health. Retrieved 1 Dec 2011, from http://t2health.org/sites/default/files/cth/guidebook/tmh-guidebook_06-11.pdf
16. Oddsson, L.I., Radomski, M.V., White, M., Nilsson, D.: A robotic home telehealth platform system for treatment adherence, social assistance and companionship—an overview. Conf. Proc. IEEE Eng. Med. Biol. Soc. **2009**, 6437–6440 (2009). doi:10.1109/IEMBS.2009.5333744
17. Odor, A., Yellowlees, P.M., Hilty, D., Parish, M.B., Nafiz, N., Iosif, A.M.: PsychVACS: a system for asynchronous telepsychiatry. Telemed. J. E Health **17**(4), 299–303 (2011). doi:10.1089/tmj.2010.0159
18. Ogawa, H., Yonezawa, Y., Maki, H., Hahn, A.W., Caldwell, W.M.: An electronic location safety support system. Biomed. Sci. Instrum. **43**, 122–127 (2007)
19. Prociow, P.A., Crowe, J.A.: Development of mobile psychiatry for bipolar disorder patients. Conf. Proc. IEEE Eng. Med. Biol. Soc. **2010**, 5484–5487 (2010). doi:10.1109/IEMBS.2010.5626759
20. Prociow, P.A., Crowe, J.A.: Towards personalised ambient monitoring of mental health via mobile technologies. Technol. Health Care **18**(4–5), 275–284 (2010). doi:F7772070772P1W60. [pii]
21. Starfield, B., Shi, L.: The medical home, access to care, and insurance: a review of evidence (Research Support, U.S. Gov't, P.H.S. Review). Pediatrics, **113**(5 Suppl), 1493–1498 (2004)
22. Trudeau, M.: Mental health apps: Like a "Therapist In Your Pocket". Mental Health, (May 24, 2010). Retrieved from NPR website: http://www.npr.org/templates/story/story.php?storyId=127081326
23. U.S. Food and Drug Administration (n.d.): Is The Product A Medical Device? Medical Devices. Retrieved January 16, 2012, from http://www.fda.gov/MedicalDevices/DeviceRegulationandGuidance/Overview/ClassifyYourDevice/ucm051512.htm
24. University of California–San Diego: Wearable technology helps monitor mental illness. Sci. Daily. Retrieved 1 Dec 2011, from http://www.sciencedaily.com/releases/2007/05/070518160743.htm (2007)
25. Yellowlees, P.M., Hilty, D., Odor, A., Iosif, A.-M., Parish, M.B., Nafiz, N., Sanchez, R.: Transcutural Psychiatry Made Simple: Asynchronous telepsychiatry as a disruptive innovation. Telemed. J. E Health **19**(4), 259–264 (2011). Apr 2013
26. Yellowlees, P.M., Holloway, K.M., Parish, M.B.: Therapy in virtual environments: clinical and ethical issues. Telemed. e-Health J.

27. Yellowlees, P.M., Odor, A., Parish, M.B., Iosif, A.M., Haught, K., Hilty, D.: A feasibility study of the use of asynchronous telepsychiatry for psychiatric consultations. Psychiatr. Serv. **61**(8), 838–840 (2010). doi:61/8/838. [pii]
28. Yellowlees, P.M., Odor, A., Patrice, K., Parish, M.B., Nafiz, N., Iosif, A.M., Hilty, D.: Disruptive innovation: the future of healthcare? Telemed. J. E Health **17**(3), 231–234 (2011). doi:10.1089/tmj.2010.0130
29. Yellowlees, P.M., Odor, A., Parish, M.B.: Cross-lingual asynchronous telepsychiatry: disruptive innovation? Psychiatr. Serv. **63**(9), 945 (2012)

Chapter 5
Speech Analysis for Mental Health Assessment Using Support Vector Machines

Insu Song and Joachim Diederich

5.1 Introduction

Common measures of Speech and Language disorder (SLD) are observer-rated scales, such as TLC and CLANG, as they provide for a broad assessment of symptoms of mental health problems, such as schizophrenia [1, 2]. Common SLD rating items include phenomenological assessments (e.g., poverty-of-speech) and linguistic assessments (e.g., excess phonetic-association). These observer-rated scales are subjective in nature and require intensive human effort. In addition, inter-rater reliability of these scales is also a problem, as it is time consuming to establish and assess. Therefore, the use of observer-rated scales in clinical assessment of mental health conditions has been limited. Automated speech and language assessment methods (e.g., [3]) have shown a possibility of providing an accurate discrimination of groups.

In this chapter, we evaluate the use of N-gram concept features and Support Vector Machines (SVMs) for predicting the following SLD assessment items automatically from speech samples: the Thought, Language and Communication (TLC) rating items [1] and the Clinical Language Disorder Rating Scale (CLANG) rating items [2]. TLC has 18 items for evaluating schizophrenia speech, such as Poverty of Speech and Loss of Goal. CLANG has 17 items, such as Excess Phonetic Association and Abnormal Syntax. The sum of the prediction value of each of the items was then used to predict the underlying mental health condition. This is a two-level hierarchical classifier that predicts specific SLD items (e.g., poverty of speech) at the first level via a set of SVM classifiers and provides the

I. Song (✉)
School of Business and IT, James Cook University,
Singapore Campus, Singapore 574421, Singapore
e-mail: insu.song@jcu.edu.au

J. Diederich
School of Information Technology and Electrical Engineering,
The University of Queensland, Brisbane, QLD 4072, Australia

M. Lech et al. (eds.), *Mental Health Informatics*,
Studies in Computational Intelligence 491, DOI: 10.1007/978-3-642-38550-6_5,

final decision at the second level by combining the results of the first level. Importantly, the intermediate results (predictions based on the SLD items) at the first level serve as explanations of the final decision.

The TLC and CLANG items are evaluated on 5 or 4 point Likert scales, but for our purpose the scales were converted to 2 point scales: −1 for no point and +1 for any points in the original ratings. The transcribed speech samples of 46 participants (19 schizophrenia patients and 27 controls) were used to evaluate the N-gram concept features and SVM classifiers in predicting TLC and CLANG ratings. For each item, we applied C-SVC (Soft-Margin SVM classifiers) for prediction: +1 for any points to an item (i.e., rating > 0) and –1 for no points (i.e., rating $= 0$).

Although our sample size was small, the results suggest the possibility of using N-gram concept features and SVM for providing an accurate discrimination of groups: schizophrenia patients and controls.

5.2 Support Vector Machines

In this section, we describe a general purpose machine learning algorithm, Support Vector Machines (SVMs). SVMs offer a novel approach to machine learning. The subject was first suggested in 1979 by Cortes and Vapnik [4], but it has only recently been receiving increasing attention since its introduction by Vapnik in 1995 [5]. Burges provided a tutorial on Support Vector Machines and their applications to pattern recognition [6]. Joachims et al. [7] reported that SVMs outperformed all other major classifiers in text classification. Although SVMs are naturally binary-classifiers, Rennie and Rifkin applied SVM in multi-class text classification and compared them with naive Bayesian classifier [8]. In their experiment, SVM gave much lower error scores than Naive Bayes.

SVMs are based on the structural risk minimization (SRM) principle which overcomes the overfitting problems. SVMs find optimal hyperplanes by finding maximal margin hyperplanes separating two classes in data. This is done by limiting the minimum distance between a hyperplane and data points, which in turn limits the capability of the hypothesis space (hence, it is called structural risk minimization approach) while minimizing empirical errors. This leads to minimizing upper bound on expected risk (actual error rates $R[h]$). This is in contrast to other machines learning approaches, such as Neural Network, which minimize the empirical risk (error rates $R_{\mathrm{emp}}[h]$ on samples) [9].

In summary, given a linearly separable training data set comprised of two classes, there may be infinite number of hyperplanes that separate the two classes. SVM searches for the best hyperplane that minimizes expected risk by finding the hyperplane with the largest margin (largest distance between hyperplane and data points), i.e., maximum marginal hyperplane (MMH).

5.2.1 Maximal Margin Hyperplane

In the following, bold typefaces will be used to indicate vector or matrix quantities; normal typefaces will be used for scalars. A hyperplane can be defined by a weight vector **w** and a bias b:

$$\mathbf{w} \cdot \mathbf{x} + b = 0 \tag{5.1}$$

where **w** is a normal vector of the hyperplane. The equation says that the dot product of a feature vector **x** with a constant vector **w** is always the same constant $-b$. We use this hyperplane to separate our features into two classes: +1 and −1. However, we want this hyperplane to be the optimal one. The criteria for being optimal are now defined. A hyperplane is optimal if the hyperplane is a maximal margin hyperplane. A hyperplane is a maximal margin hyperplane if the following conditions are met:

1. All +1 class features satisfy this: $\mathbf{w} \cdot \mathbf{x} + b \geq m|\mathbf{w}|$, where m is the distance between the positive margin plane and the hyperplane.
2. All −1 class features satisfy this: $\mathbf{w} \cdot \mathbf{x} + \mathrm{b} \leq -m|\mathbf{w}|$, where m is the distance between the negative margin plane and the hyperplane.

If we choose $|\mathbf{w}|$ to be 1/m, then the conditions become:

1. All +1 class features satisfy this: $\mathbf{w} \cdot \mathbf{x} + b \geq +1$, where $1/|\mathbf{w}|$ is the distance between the positive margin plane and the hyperplane.
2. All +1 class features satisfy this: $\mathbf{w} \cdot \mathbf{x} + b \leq -1$, where $1/|\mathbf{w}|$ is the distance between the negative margin plane and the hyperplane.

The hyperplane is optimal if $2/||\mathbf{w}||^2$ is maximal such that the above two conditions are met. Now, this quadratic optimization problem is stated formally below:

1. Minimize $||\mathbf{w}||^2/2$
2. Subject to $c_i(\mathbf{w} \cdot \mathbf{x}_i + b) \geq 1$ for all feature vectors $\mathbf{x}_i$, where c_i is the class label: +1, −1.

The distance between any points in the feature space and the hyperplane can be obtained using the following equation:

$$d(\mathbf{w}, b; \mathbf{x}) = \frac{\mathbf{w} \cdot \mathbf{x} + b}{||\mathbf{w}||} \tag{5.2}$$

The offset b is determined using support vectors found because the equality equation holds for support vectors: $c_i(\mathbf{w} \cdot \mathbf{x}_i + b) = 1$, that is $b = c_i - \mathbf{w} \cdot \mathbf{x}_i$. To improve accuracy, we can obtain an average over all support vectors:

$$b = -\frac{1}{2}\mathbf{w} \cdot (\mathbf{x}_{s+} + \mathbf{x}_{s-})$$

$$b = c_i - \mathbf{w} \cdot \mathbf{x}_i \tag{5.3}$$

$$b = \frac{1}{N_{sv}}\sum_{i}^{Nsv}(c_i - \mathbf{w} \cdot \mathbf{x}_i)$$

The decision function is $\mathbf{w} \cdot \mathbf{x}_i + b$, formally

$$\text{Hard function: } f(\mathbf{x}) = sign(\mathbf{w} \cdot \mathbf{x} + b)$$

$$\text{Soft function: } h(\mathbf{x}) = h(\mathbf{w} \cdot \mathbf{x} + b) \begin{cases} +1 & z > 1 \\ z & -1 \leq z \leq 1 \\ -1 & z < -1 \end{cases} \tag{5.4}$$

In summary, our optimal hyperplane has the following properties:

The hyperplane : $\mathbf{w} \cdot \mathbf{x}_i + b = 0$ conditions: $\mathbf{w} \cdot \mathbf{x}_i + b \geq c_i$ or $c_i(\mathbf{w} \cdot \mathbf{x}_i + b) \geq 1$

$$b = \frac{1}{N_{sv}}\sum_{i}^{Nsv}(c_i - \mathbf{w} \cdot \mathbf{x}_i)$$

$$f(\mathbf{x}) = sign(\mathbf{w} \cdot \mathbf{x} + b) \tag{5.5}$$

5.2.2 C-Support Vector Classification (C-SVC): Soft Margin Classification

In general, not all data are linearly separable due to noises and outliers in data. To be able to find solutions in this case, we can allow some feature vectors to fall behind margin hyperplanes by introducing slack variables ξ_i. This changes the conditions as follows:

$$c_i(\mathbf{w} \cdot \phi(\mathbf{x}_i) + b) \geq 1 - \xi_i, \tag{5.6}$$

$$\xi_i \geq 0 \tag{5.7}$$

To favor fewer features falling behind the hyperplanes, we add a penalty function to the objective function:

$$Penalty(\xi) = C\sum_{i=1}^{l}\xi_i \tag{5.8}$$

The problem can then be defined as follows:

$$\min\left(\frac{1}{2}\mathbf{w}\cdot\mathbf{w}+C\sum_{i=1}^{l}\xi_i\right)$$
$$\text{subject to: } c_i(\mathbf{w}\cdot\phi(\mathbf{x}_i)+b)\geq 1-\xi_i,\ \xi_i\geq 0 \tag{5.9}$$

where $\phi(\mathbf{x}_i)$ is a mapping function that maps $\mathbf{x}_i$ into a higher dimension and C is a penalty cost value. The larger C is, the more severe the penalty is for the features falling behind the margin planes.

The structure error function then becomes:

$$\varphi(\mathbf{w},b,\xi,\alpha,\beta)=\frac{\mathbf{w}\cdot\mathbf{w}}{2}+C\sum_{i=1}^{l}\xi_i-\sum_{i}\alpha_i(c_i(\mathbf{w}\cdot\mathbf{x}_i+b)-1+\xi_i)-\sum_{i}\beta_i\xi_i \tag{5.10}$$

where the new Lagrange multipliers β_i are introduced for the new conditions $\xi_i\geq 0$. The solution (minimizing $\mathbf{w}\cdot\mathbf{w}$) is obtained by minimizing $\varphi(\mathbf{w}, b, \alpha, \beta)$ with respect to $\mathbf{w}$, b, and ξ, and maximizing with respect to α and β.

The hyperplane in the higher dimension is $\mathbf{w}\cdot\phi(\mathbf{x}_i)+b=0$. We have the same decision function: $\text{sign}(w\cdot\phi(\mathbf{x}_i)+b)$ and b:

$$b=\frac{1}{N_{sv}}\sum_{i}^{Nsv}(c_i-\mathbf{w}\cdot\phi(\mathbf{x}_i)). \tag{5.11}$$

5.3 Language Features

In this section, we review various language features that have been used for building classifiers for discriminating subtle language differences in individual–individual or individual-group.

5.3.1 Term-Frequency Based Features

Commonly used features for text document analysis are surface features of language, such as term-frequency (TF) and term-frequency weighted inverse document frequency (TF*IDF) [10]. In this approach, each document is represented as a vector of term frequencies (TFs) or one of its derived forms:

$$tf=tf\quad tfidf=tf\times\log\frac{N}{n} \tag{5.12}$$

$$ntf = \frac{tf}{|d|} \quad tf\max = \frac{tf}{t\max} \tag{5.13}$$

where *tf* is the term frequency of a vocabulary term of a collection of documents, |*d*| is the L2-norm of the document vector, *tmax* is the maximum frequency of the term, *N* is the number of documents in the collection, and *n* is the number of documents containing the term.

In this approach documents are compared using pairwise or tuple-wise co-occurrences and no use is made of any semantic relations or syntactic relations, such as word order. However, these simple features have shown good performance results in many applications, such as keyword extraction [11], information retrieval [10], and cosine-based document similarity measure [12].

5.3.2 Semantics Measures

5.3.2.1 Latent Semantic Analysis

Latent Semantic Analysis (LSA) is a semantic-based similarity measure. Simple TF measures (e.g., pairwise or tuple-wise co-occurrences) cannot provide similarity measures of word–word, word-passage and passage–passage that are well correlated with human cognitive phenomena such as association or semantic similarity. LSA goes beyond simple contiguity frequencies, co-occurrence counts, or correlations used to simulate human meaning-based judgments [13].

LSA does not make use of word order and thus may result in incorrect judgments when, for example, syntactic relations must be considered for word meaning disambiguation [13].

LSA can be described as decomposition of a corpora of text documents into a few prototypical text passages. Thus, any text document could be represented as a linear combination of the prototypical text passages. To achieve this, given a set of text documents, LSA uses singular value decomposition (SVD) to find eigen-text-passages. Each text is then mapped to a few selected eigen-text-passages. Each word or text-passages then can be represented as a vector of eigenvalues.

5.3.2.2 AnalogySpace

As with LSA, AnalogySpace [14] is a generalized similarity measure that finds other relevant concepts that are similar. AnalogySpace was shown to perform better than other semantic-based similarity measures including LSA. As in LAS, it uses semantic relations between terms to measure similarity between terms, sentences, and/or documents.

However, instead of using a vector of TFs as a representation of a word or documents, AnalogySpace uses data from the Open Mind Common Sense (OMCS) project [15], which represents each word or passage *t* (e.g., "cake") as a feature vector $c = \text{concept}(t)$ where each feature is a commonsense property of the concept (e.g., "IsA dessert"). This is done by finding the usage of the conceptual term in the ConceptNet [16].

5.3.3 Syntactic and N-Gram Features of Communication

Traditionally syntactic and semantic processing approaches have been used for dialogue classification (e.g., dialog act classification), but they are error prone [17]. Such approaches require intensive human effort in defining linguistic structures and developing grammar.

Recently, a simple template-based syntactic relation analysis has shown promising results in keyword extraction [18]. For example, given two words A and B, a rule can be defined so that "A of B" and "B of A" could be treated as the same phrases. However, such methods would also require significant human effort in defining such linguistic structures.

Various modern advanced automated natural language parsing tools, such as MontyLingua [19], are now available making use of n-gram likelihoods as well as an extensive database of common sense knowledge to parse English sentences. It is now reasonably straightforward to extract basic sentences, called predicates (e.g., subject-verb-object pairs) from complex sentences. However, these tools still require text to have clear sentence boundaries and structure. Unstructured text documents without clear sentence boundaries (e.g., free conversation or conversations of non-native speakers) cannot be easily analyzed using such automated natural language parsing tools.

In comparison, almost all probabilistic classifiers make a "term independence assumption", which states that each word in a document is independent of all other words in the document. This assumption is fundamental in removing the intractability of determining which word pairs are relevant and which word pairs are not.

Fukada et al. (20) reported that performance enhancement from term order information (Unigram vs. Bigram) was not significant in dialog act classification. That is, most of the information was in terms, but not in the order of the terms for dialog analysis.

An advantage of the probabilistic approaches over the traditional syntactic and semantic processing approaches is that no expensive and error-prone deep processing is involved.

5.4 Automated Speech and Language Analysis Using SVM

5.4.1 Participants

We used speech samples collected by psychology students at the James Cook University, Singapore campus. The students transcribed the English speech samples recorded from interviews of 46 participants ($N = 46$, 19 schizophrenic patients and 27 controls) into an electronic format. Schizophrenic subjects were recruited from two centers of the Singapore Association of Mental Health (SAMH). Non-psychotic participants were recruited from a batch of first year psychology students of James Cook University, Singapore campus.

All of the participants were non-native English speakers, such as Singaporeans, Malays, and students from other countries. The participants were asked to freely talk about some subjects and, thus, the transcriptions were not well structured. They contained many non-English words and chunks of text with no clear sentence boundaries.

For more detailed description of this data set, see Chap. 11 where the complete set of the data was analyzed and compared with speech and language disorder measures.

5.4.2 *Comparison of SVM with Linear Discriminant Analysis*

In the first experiment, we compared LDA with SVM in classification performance. In this experiment, the input features were normalized frequencies of words. Recordings of interviews were transcribed into text documents, and each document was segmented into a list of words. Words in the whole corpora were ranked and infrequent words were discarded. The normalized frequency (normalized to the length of the documents) of each word in the ranked list of words were then used as input features of each document. That is, an input feature $\mathbf{x} = (v_1,\ldots,v_d) \in \Re^d$ is a d-dimensional vector and each feature value vi is a normalized frequency of a word:

$$v_i = (\text{Frequency of the } i\text{th Word}) / (\text{The Length of Document}) \qquad (5.14)$$

where the length of document is the L2-Norm of word frequencies in a document. Two sample input feature vectors comprising of only 7 most frequent words are shown in Table 5.1.

The task was then to find a function $f: \mathbf{x} \rightarrow \mathrm{C}$ that maps the input feature vector $\mathrm{x}\in\Re^d$ to a class label $C \in \{+1, -1\}$. When the dimensionality of the input features is small, a simple Linear Discriminant Analysis (LDA) can be applied to find a linear classifier. For example, if we use only two most frequent words as features, the function can be described using a few coefficients:

Table 5.1 Example feature vectors for control and schizophrenia samples

Class label	"just"	"know"	"think"	"time"	"see"	"person"	"get"
Control	0.166	0.152	0.069	0.180	0.180	0.290	0.166
Schizo	0.330	0.088	0.000	0.132	0.088	0.110	0.110

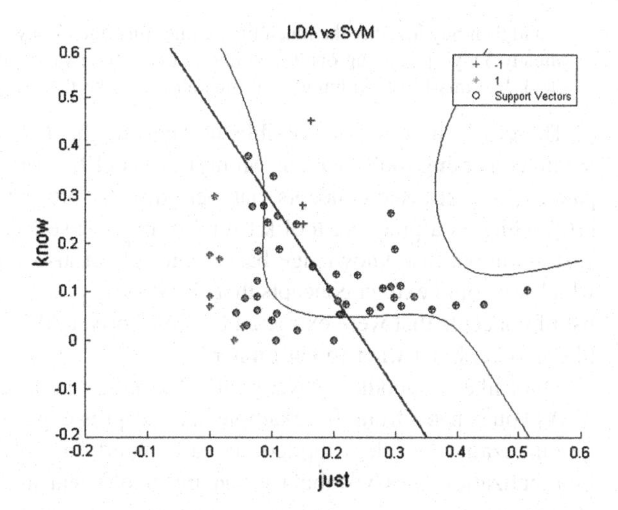

Fig. 5.1 Decision boundary for two features. The *straight line* is a decision function learned using LDA and the *curved lines* represent the decision function learned using SVM

$$f(\mathbf{x}) = a \times v_{\text{just}} + b \times v_{\text{know}} \tag{5.15}$$

Fisher's linear discriminant using two features achieved an accuracy of 68.5 % and AUC of 0.79 whereas SVM achieved the accuracy of 77.7 % and AUC of 0.76. Figure 5.1 illustrates the decision boundaries obtained using LDA and SVMs.

When the dimensionality of data is too large or the normal probability distribution cannot be assumed for input features, Discriminant Analysis methods, such as Fisher's linear discriminant, are not applicable. In contrast, SVMs do not assume a particular probability distribution and find a classification function that minimizes the true error rate rather than minimizing the empirical error rate. SVMs can also easily handle large number of features. In this sense, SVM can be considered as a nonparametric counterpart of LDA. In addition, SVMs can find more generalized classifiers by minimizing the true error rate and are able to handle data with much larger dimensionality.

5.4.3 N-Gram Concepts

In this section, three types of features for analyzing speech and language are discussed. These features were used to develop SVM classifiers for binary classifications (schizophrenic vs. control) using the transcribed speech samples.

The transcripts were comprised of large chunks of ill-formed (e.g., misspellings, missing verbs, missing punctuation) English text. There were no clear sentence boundaries nor clear sentence structures. An excerpt from text samples is shown below:

…and then buy together the lunch time dinner time then I buy noodle then run downstairs already Ya ya just go up one time only no every time ya ya Hmm I think have eleven o clock like this I rest Ya hmm what time ah three like that I I rest then I go…

Therefore, it was not possible to analyze the text using automated natural language parsing tools, such as MontyLingua [19]. Instead of relying on syntactic parsing, we extracted concepts that were directly present in text using ConceptNet [16], which is a practical tool kit for Commonsense Reasoning. In addition to its vast commonsense knowledge base, ConceptNet also provides Python APIs with which we could extract concepts that are directly present in text. The following is a list of concepts that were extracted by ConceptNet API from the sentence "I don't like noodle, but I want to eat dinner":

["not like", "noodle", "want eat", "want", "eat dinner", "eat", "dinner"]

As you can see from this example, a concept is expressed in one or more words. Lemmatization is also applied to each word to remove inflectional endings. Lemmatization uses vocabulary and morphological analysis of words to reduce inflectional forms of a word to the base form of a word, called the lemma.

We extract concepts from the transcribed speech samples to build a concept vocabulary. In the vocabulary, the concepts are ranked according to corpora frequency (the total number of times that each concept was encountered). Concepts occurring less than two times were removed. Using this approach, we generated three datasets:

1. Concept1: Concepts comprising a maximum of 1 word.
2. Concept3: Concepts comprising a maximum of 3 words (i.e., N-gram).
3. Concept3n: the 46 samples were divided into smaller samples (approximately 100 word length text documents) and each concept comprised a maximum of 3 words.

Concept1 vocabulary V comprised a total of 2,064 concepts that were collected from the 46 transcribed speech samples in this manner: $|V| = 2{,}064$.

5.4.3.1 Feature Extraction

For each transcribed speech sample d_i, the number of occurrences of each concept was counted. This is called the (concept) term frequency (TF) of a concept. We also measured the length of document as the sum of the TF of each concept in the document. The TFs of each concept were then normalized to the document length. These normalized TFs were then used as document features. That is, a document is a vector $\mathbf{x} = \{f_1, f_2, \ldots, f_{|V|}\}$ of normalized TFs: $\mathbf{x} \in \Re^{|V|}$.

5.4.3.2 Experiment Result

Leave-One-Out (LOO) cross validation method is used to evaluate the performance of SVM. In this method, one sample is held out for testing and the rest of the samples were used for training. That is, a total of 46 tests were performed. In each test, 45 samples were used to generate a SVM classification model, and one sample was used to test the model. The number of correct and incorrect classification results was then counted for the 46 tests to generate the following performance measures: accuracy, recall, specificity, precision, and balanced accuracy. Recall is also called true positive rate or sensitivity. Specificity is also called true negative rate (1 −false_negative_rate). These are defined below:

Recall = True Positive / (True Positive + False Negative)
Specificity = True Negative / (True Negative + False Positive)
Precision = True Positive / (True Positive + False Positive)where True Positive is the number of positive samples that are classified as positive, False Negative is the number of positive samples that are classified as negative, True Negative is the number of negative samples that are classified as negative, False Positive is the number of negative samples that are classified as positive. C-SVC (Support Vector Classification) of LibSVM [21] was used for the evaluation with the regularization parameter $C = 300$.

The LOO evaluation results for the three SVM classifiers ($SVM_{Concept1}$, $SVM_{Concept3}$, $SVM_{Concept3N}$) are shown in Table 5.2.

Figures 5.2, 5.3, and 5.4 show the Receiver Operating Curve (ROC) of the AUC values. The ROC shows the tradeoff between specificity and False Negative rate (i.e., 1-Sensitivity). In our experiments, we used the approach of adjusting the bias term b after the n-fold cross validation results. We used receiver-operating-curve (ROC) and balanced accuracy (BAC) as the heuristics for finding the optimal adjustment amount of the bias term.

5.4.4 Predicting Phenomenological Features of TLC

The Thought, Language and Communication (TLC) scale [1] is a phenomenological approach [22] to assessing SLD of patients. It consists of 18 items. We used the transcribed speech samples to generate SVM classifiers for the following 10 TLC items: poverty of speech, poverty of content, pressure of speech, distractibility, tangentiality, derailment, incoherence, illogicality, circumstantiality, and loss of goal, and preservation. Because of the lack of sufficient examples, the following TLC items were excluded in this experiment: neologisms, word-approximations, stilted-speech, clanging, echolalia, blocking, and self-reference. There were too few positive cases for these symptoms.

The Concept3 dataset was used to build the classifiers. The task was to predict the ratings given by the psychology students who interviewed the patients and

Table 5.2 C-SVC performance result on transcribed speech samples

Data Set	+1	−1	ACC	PREC	REC	SPEC	BAC	AUC
Concept1	19	27	0.96	0.95	0.95	0.96	0.95	0.99
Concept3	19	27	0.93	0.86	0.99	0.89	0.94	0.99
Concept3n	127	406	0.90	0.74	0.89	0.90	0.90	0.96

Three datasets were generated (Concept 1, Concept 3, Concept 3n) from the transcribed speech samples of schizophrenics (+1) and controls (−1) to generate three SVM classifiers: $SVM_{Concept1}$, $SVM_{Concept3}$, and $SVM_{Concept3N}$. C-SVC with C = 300 were evaluated. The table shows LOO performance results: accuracy (*ACC*), precision (*PREC*), recall (*REC*), specificity (*SPEC*), balanced accuracy (*BAC*), and area under curve (*AUC*)

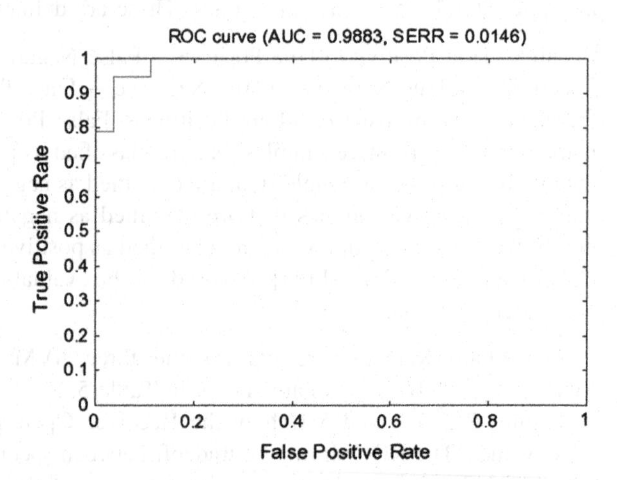

Fig. 5.2 Receiver operating curves (*ROCs*) of the C-SVC performance results for dataset Concept1

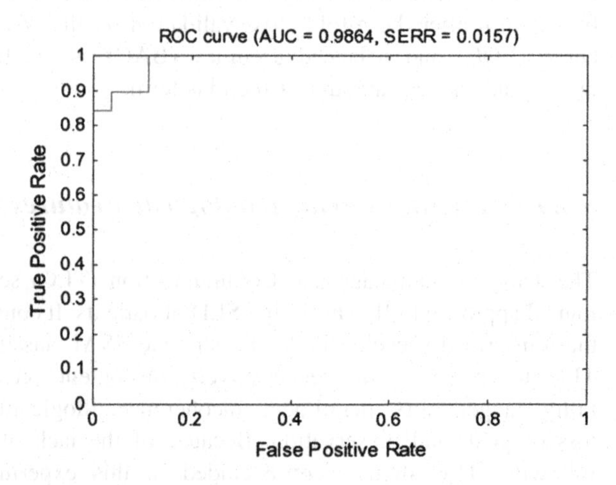

Fig. 5.3 Receiver operating curves (*ROCs*) of the C-SVC performance results for dataset Concept3

controls. Table 5.3 shows the results in predicting the 10 TLC items using the learned SVM classifiers. It includes classifiers for predicting the global rating provided by the psychology students, the observer predictions (predictions made

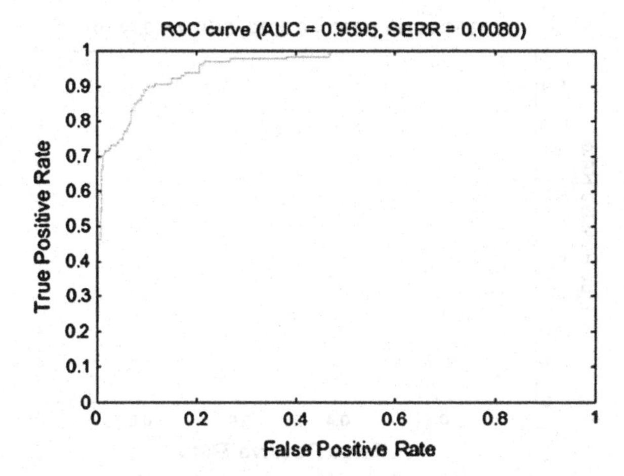

Fig. 5.4 Receiver operating curves (*ROCs*) of the C-SVC performance results for dataset Concept3n

Table 5.3 TLC component prediction using SVM

TLC Lables	+1	−1	ACC	PREC	REC	SPEC	BAC	AUC
Poverty of speech	15	31	0.89	0.81	0.87	0.90	0.88	0.90
Poverty of content of speech	15	31	0.76	0.60	0.80	0.74	0.77	0.78
Pressure of speech	3	43	0.43	0.10	0.99	0.40	0.70	0.54
Tangentiality	9	37	0.87	0.64	0.78	0.89	0.83	0.88
Derailment	12	34	0.89	0.77	0.83	0.91	0.87	0.87
Incoherence	4	42	0.83	0.33	0.99	0.81	0.90	0.87
Illogicality	4	42	0.78	0.29	0.99	0.76	0.88	0.86
Circumstantiality	6	40	0.87	0.50	0.16	0.97	0.57	0.65
Loss of goal	5	41	0.83	0.39	0.99	0.80	0.90	0.89
Perserveration	6	40	0.78	0.37	0.99	0.75	0.87	0.87
Global rating	17	29	0.93	0.84	0.99	0.90	0.94	0.98
Observer prediction (+1, −1)	17	29	0.93	0.85	0.99	0.90	0.95	0.98
Actual class (+1, –1)	19	27	0.93	0.86	0.99	0.88	0.94	0.99

by the psychology students as to whether the participant was schizophrenic patient or not), and the actual class labels using. Figures 5.5, 5.6, 5.7, 5.8, 5.9, 5.10, 5.11, 5.12, 5.13, 5.14, 5.15, and 5.16 show ROC curves of the 13 SVM classifiers. Except for the items "Pressure of speech" and "Circumstantiality", the SVM classifiers achieved more than 80 % balanced accuracy.

The sum, S_{TLC}, of the SVM prediction values of each of the 8 TLC items (circumstantiality and pressure of speech were excluded because of their poor performance) were used to predict the observer prediction and the actual class labels. Using S_{TLC}, the participants were classified as schizophrenic if S_{TLC} was greater than a threshold value T_{TLC}.

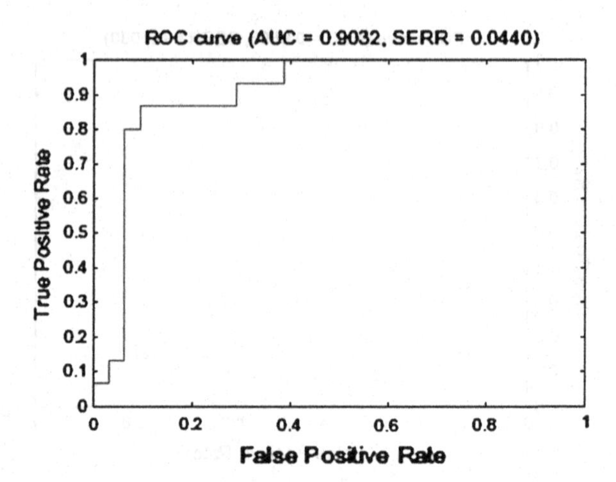

Fig. 5.5 ROC *curve* for TLC poverty of speech

$$f(\mathbf{x})_{TLC} = \begin{cases} +1 & S_{TLC} > T_{TLC} \\ -1 & S_{TLC} \leq T_{TLC} \end{cases} \quad (5.16)$$

S_{TLC} achieved AUC values of 0.92 and 0.94 for predicting the observer predictions and the actual class labels, respectively. Figures 5.17, 5.18 show the ROC curves of S_{TLC}. The 95 % confidence interval (0.860, 1.00) of the AUC value 0.94 of S_{TLC} captures the AUC value 0.99 of the $SVM_{Concetp3}$, meaning their differences were not significant.

5.4.5 Predicting Linguistic Features of CLANG

The Clinical Language Disorders Rating Scale (CLANG) utilizes 17 SLD items described in linguistic terms. We used the transcribed speech samples to generate SVM classifiers for the following 12 CLANG items: abnormal syntax-structure, lack of semantic association, discourse failure, excess details, lack of details, a prosodic speech, abnormal prosody, pragmatics disorder, dysfluency, dysarthria, poverty of speech, and pressure of speech.

The following items could not be modeled due to too few positive cases in the sample: excess phonetic-association, excessive syntactic-constraints, referential failures, neologisms, and paraphasic error.

Concept3 dataset were used to build the classifiers. The task was to predict the ratings given by the psychology students who interviewed the patients and controls. Table 5.4 shows the SVM performance results in predicting the 12 CLANG items plus the following three additional items: global ratings given by the students, observer predictions given by the students, and the actual classes. Figures 5.19, 5.20, 5.21, 5.22, 5.23, 5.24, 5.25, 5.26, 5.27, 5.28, 5.29, 5.30 shows the ROC curves of the SVM classifiers for the 12 CLANG items. For CLANG,

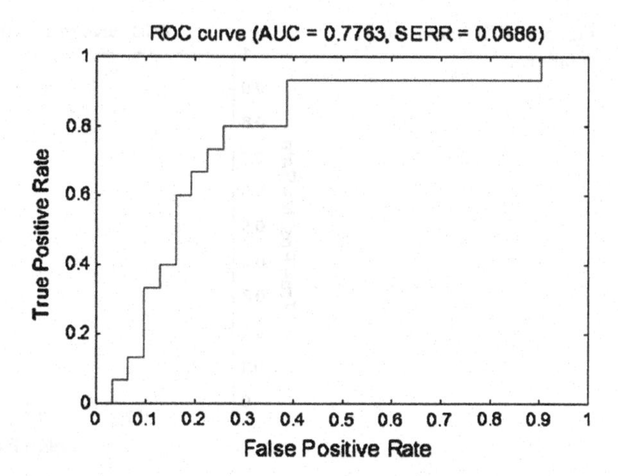

Fig. 5.6 ROC *curve* for TLC poverty of content of speech

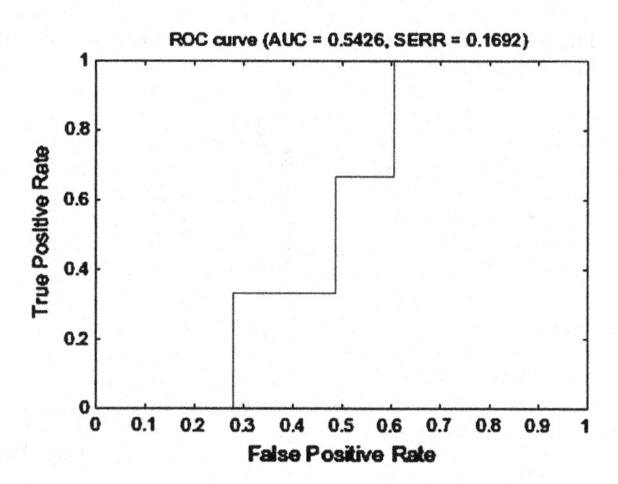

Fig. 5.7 ROC *curve* for TLC pressure of speech

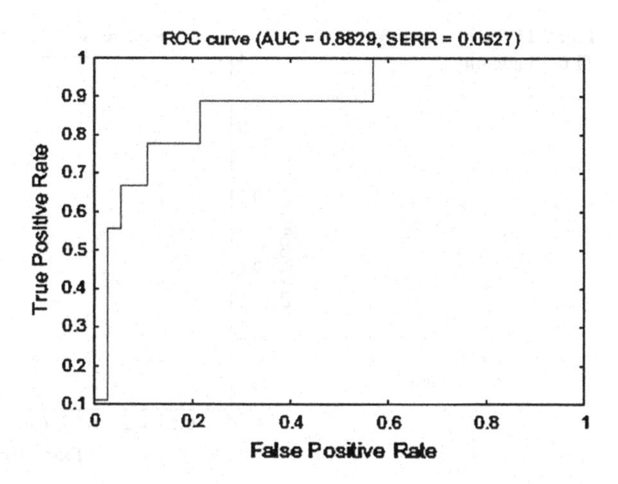

Fig. 5.8 ROC *curve* for TLC tangentiality

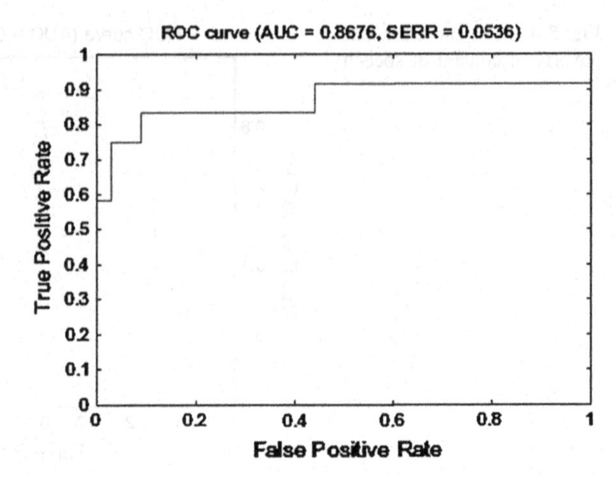

Fig. 5.9 ROC *curve* for TLC derailment

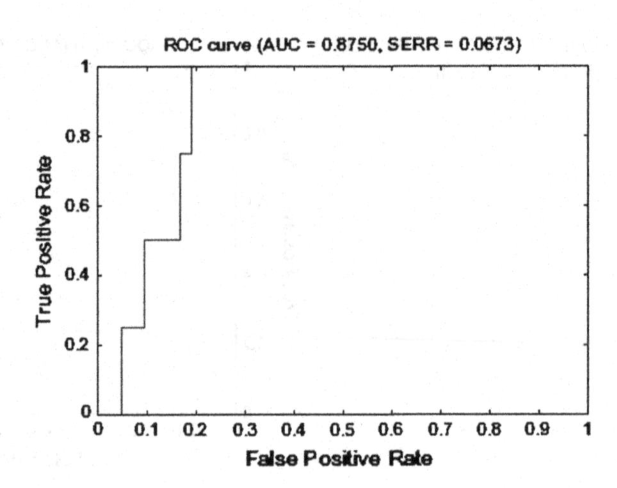

Fig. 5.10 ROC *curve* for TLC incoherence

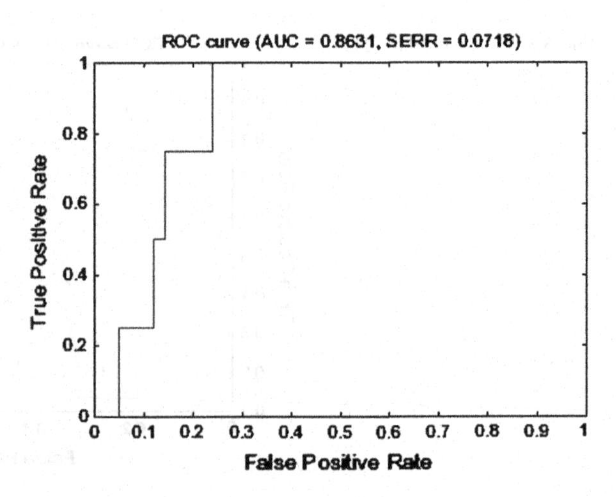

Fig. 5.11 ROC *curve* for TLC illogicality

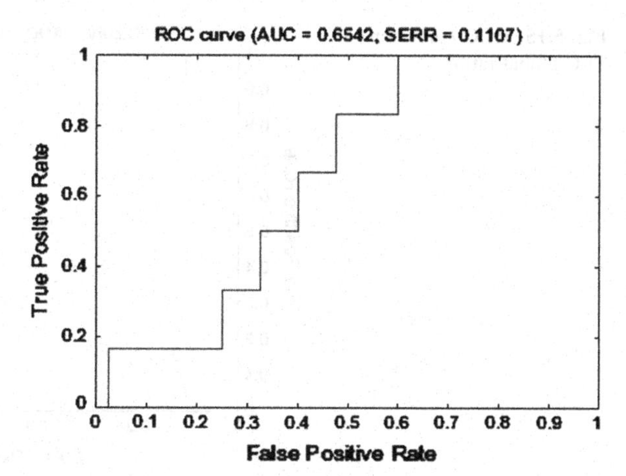

Fig. 5.12 ROC *curve* for TLC circumstantiality

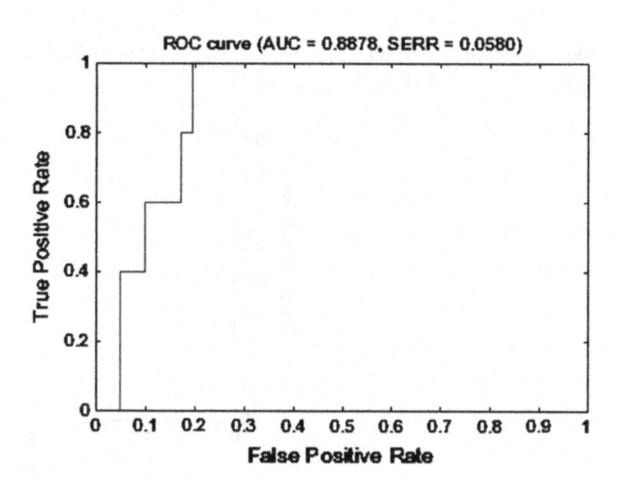

Fig. 5.13 ROC *curve* for TLC loss of goal

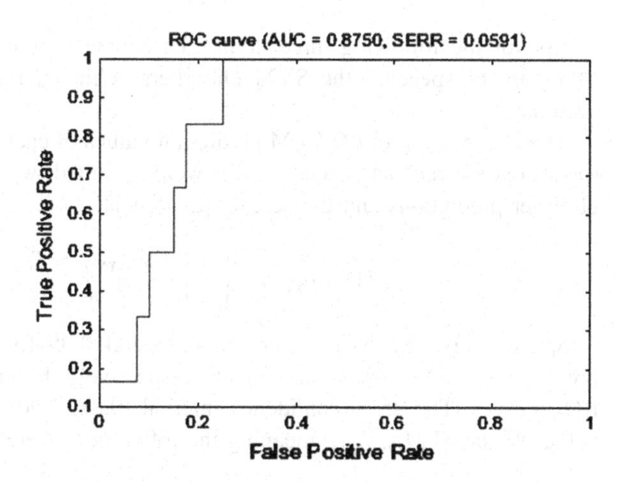

Fig. 5.14 ROC *curve* for TLC perserveration

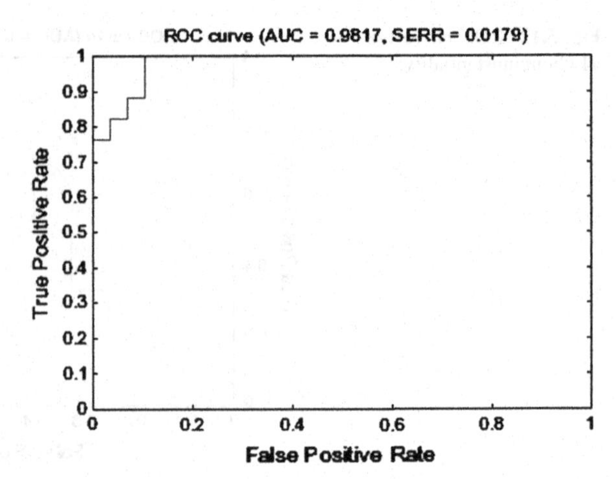

Fig. 5.15 ROC *curve* for TLC global rating

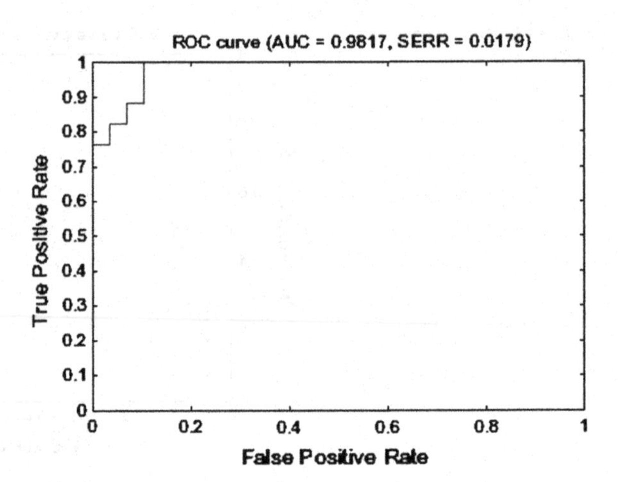

Fig. 5.16 ROC *curve* for TLC observer prediction

except for the following three items "Discourse failure," "Excess details," and "Pressure of speech," the SVM classifiers achieved more than 80 % balanced accuracy.

The sum S_{CLANG} of the SVM prediction values of each of the 10 CLANG items (pressure of speech and excess details were excluded) were also used to predict the observer predictions and the actual class labels.

$$f(\mathbf{x})_{CLANG} = \begin{cases} +1 & S_{CLANG} > T_{CLANG} \\ -1 & S_{CLANG} \leq T_{CLANG} \end{cases} \tag{5.17}$$

S_{CLANG} achieved AUC values of 0.96 and 0.95 for predicting the observer predictions and the actual class labels, respectively. Figures 5.31, 5.32 show their ROC curves. The 95 % confidence interval (0.88, 1.00) again captures the AUC values of the $SVM_{Concept3}$, meaning the differences were not significant.

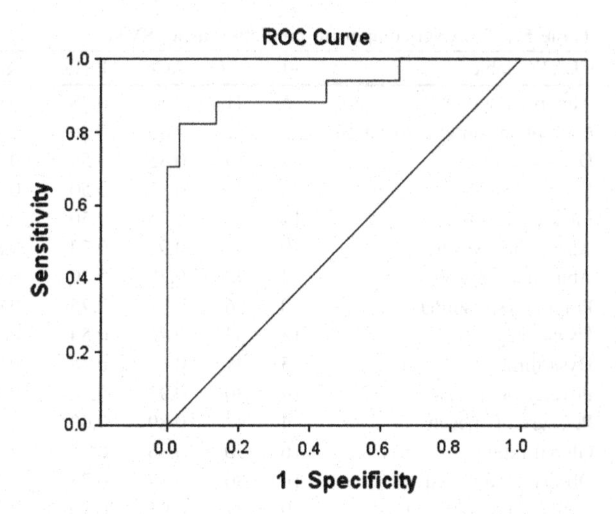

Fig. 5.17 ROC *curve* for the SVM classifier that predicts the observer rated classes using S_{TLC} (the sum of SVM prediction values of the 8 TLC items: poverty of speech, poverty of content, distractibility, tangentiality, derailment, incoherence, illogicality, loss of goal, and preservation). AUC = 0.92, Std Err = 0.046, 95 % confidence interval (0.83, 1.00)

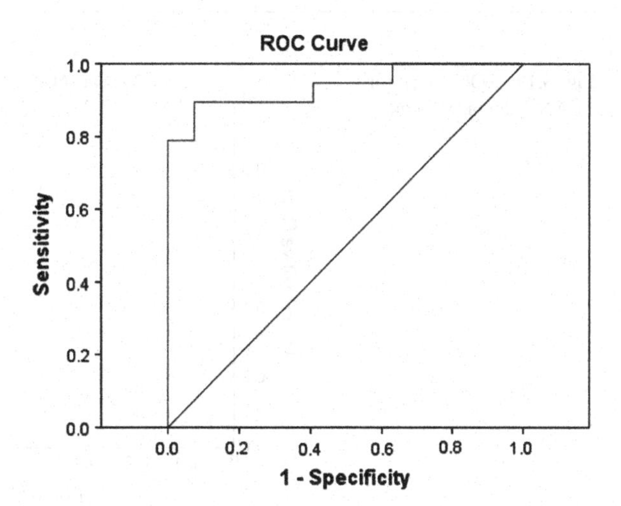

Fig. 5.18 ROC *curve* for the SVM classifier that predicts the actual classes using S_{TLC} (the sum of SVM prediction values of the 8 TLC items: poverty of speech, poverty of content, distractibility, tangentiality, derailment, incoherence, illogicality, loss of goal, and preservation). AUC = 0.92, Std Err = 0.046, 95 % confidence interval (0.83, 1.00)

5.4.6 *Predicting Schizophrenia Using TLC and CLANG Features*

The total of 17 SLD items (8 TLC and 10 CLANG less one common item: poverty of speech) were combined into SSLD: the sum of 17 SVM prediction values of the SLD items.

$$f(\mathbf{x})_{SLD} = \begin{cases} +1 & S_{TLC} + S_{CLANG} > T_{SLD} \\ -1 & S_{TCL} + S_{CLANG} \leq T_{SLD} \end{cases} \tag{5.18}$$

The combined SLD items also showed good performance in predicting schizophrenia. The combined predictor achieved AUC of 0.94 with the 95 %

Table 5.4 CLANG component prediction using SVM

CLANG lables	+1	−1	ACC	PREC	REC	SPEC	BAC	AUC
Abnormal syntax	5	41	0.82	0.38	0.99	0.80	0.90	0.86
Lack of semantic association	5	41	0.83	0.38	0.99	0.80	0.90	0.91
Discourse failure	7	39	0.85	0.50	0.71	0.87	0.79	0.78
Excess details	6	40	0.87	0.50	0.17	0.98	0.57	0.66
Lack of details	11	35	0.76	0.50	0.91	0.71	0.81	0.78
Aprosodic speech	9	37	0.91	0.73	0.89	0.92	0.90	0.92
Abnormal prosody	4	42	0.78	0.29	0.99	0.77	0.88	0.80
Pragmatics disorder	10	36	0.91	0.75	0.90	0.92	0.90	0.91
Dysfluency	13	33	0.76	0.54	0.99	0.66	0.83	0.80
Dysarthria	5	41	0.82	0.38	0.99	0.80	0.90	0.86
Poverty of speech	16	30	0.93	0.88	0.94	0.93	0.94	0.93
Pressure of speech	4	42	0.89	0.00	0.00	0.98	0.49	0.51
Global rating	16	30	0.86	0.73	0.99	0.80	0.90	0.96
Observer predicted	16	30	0.87	0.73	0.99	0.80	0.90	0.96
Actual Class (+1, −1)	19	27	0.93	0.86	0.99	0.89	0.94	0.99

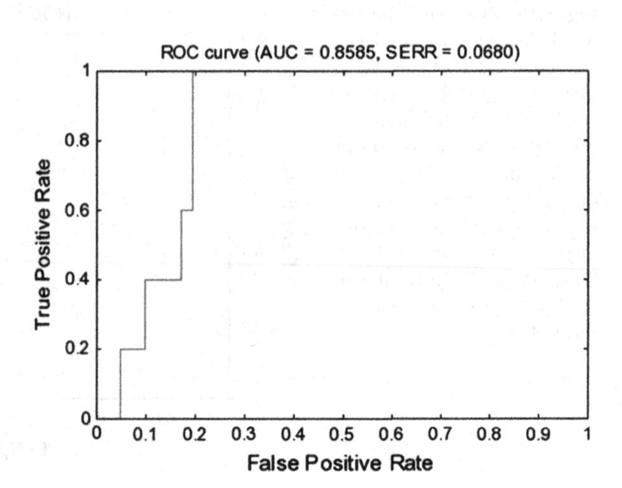

Fig. 5.19 ROC *curve* for CLANG abnormal syntax

confidence interval of (0.87, 1.00). Figure 5.33 shows the ROC curve of the TCL and CLANG combined prediction result.

5.5 Discussion

The simple bag-of-words representation (Concept1) of the speech samples achieved the best performance (AUC = 0.99) in predicting schizophrenia. However, the differences were not significant ($\alpha = 0.05$). Although the size of our dataset was small, the results indicate that automated method of predicting mental

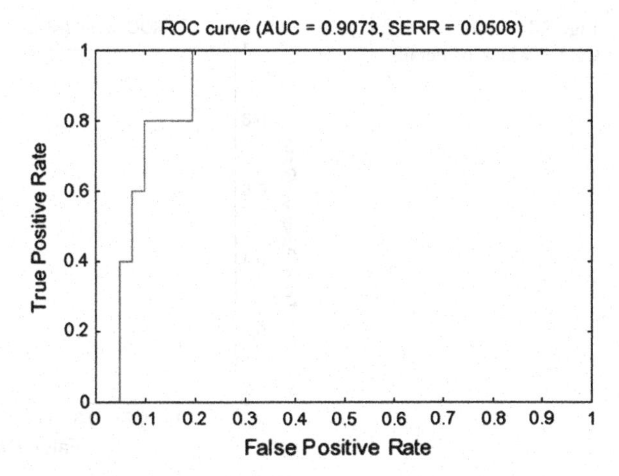

Fig. 5.20 ROC *curve* for CLANG lack of semantic association

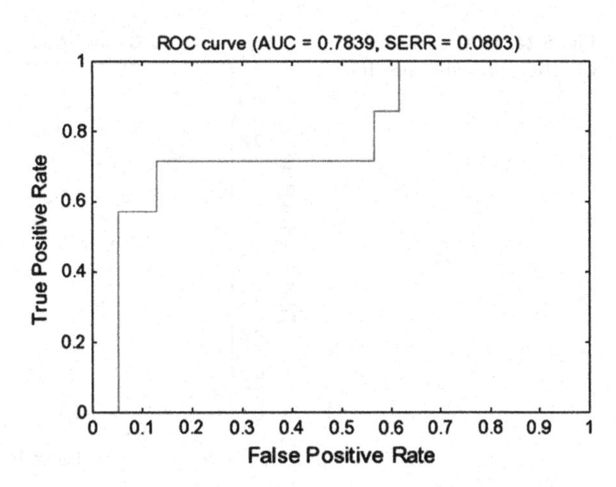

Fig. 5.21 ROC *curve* for CLANG discourse failure

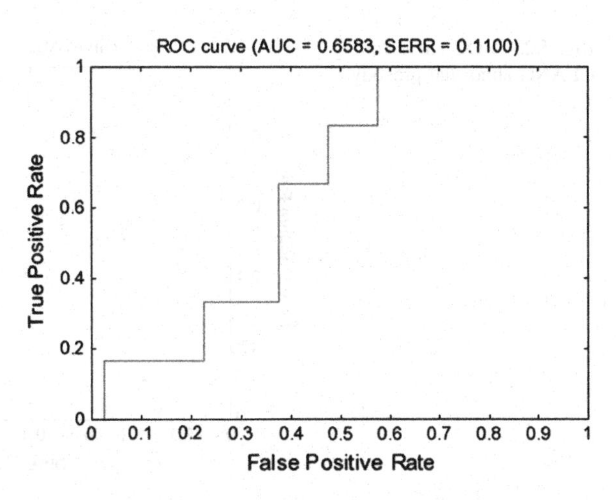

Fig. 5.22 ROC *curve* for CLANG excess details

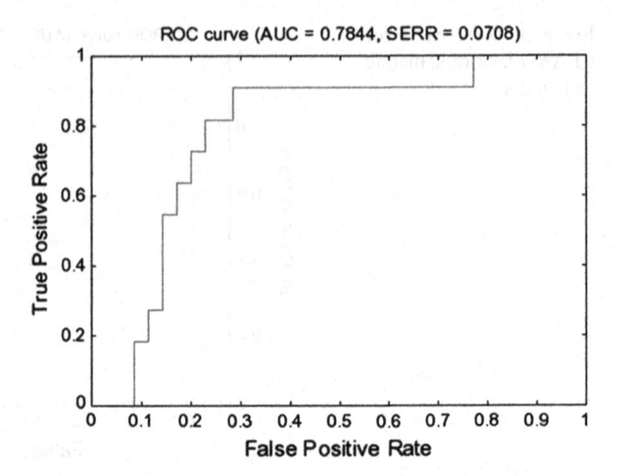

Fig. 5.23 ROC *curve* for CLANG lack of details

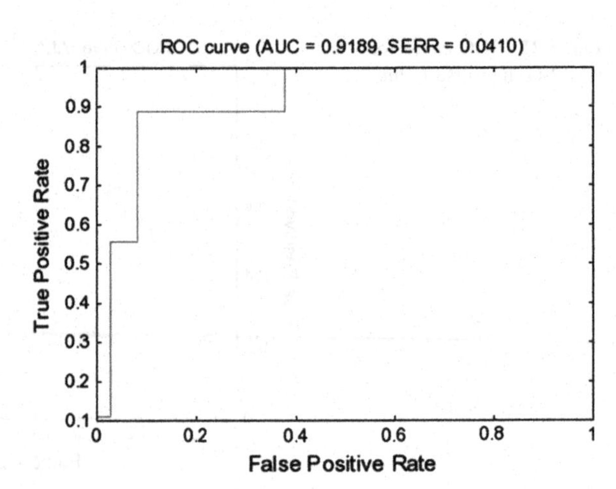

Fig. 5.24 ROC *curve* for CLANG aprosodic speech

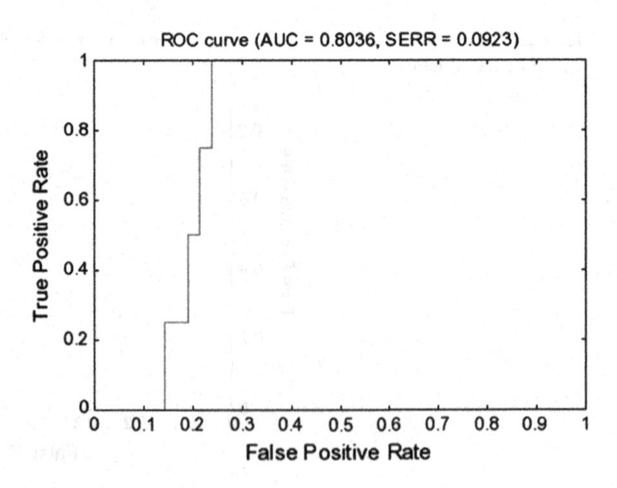

Fig. 5.25 ROC *curve* for CLANG abnormal prosody

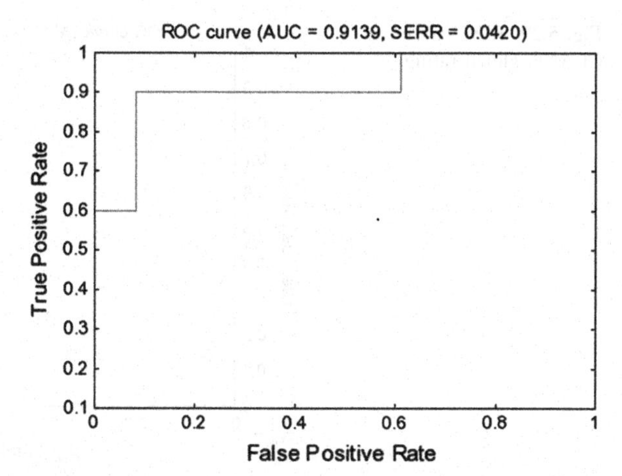

Fig. 5.26 ROC *curve* for CLANG pragmatics disorder

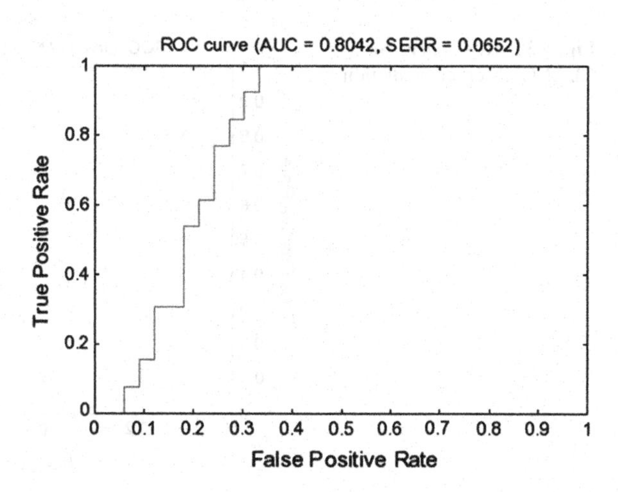

Fig. 5.27 ROC *curve* for CLANG dysfluency

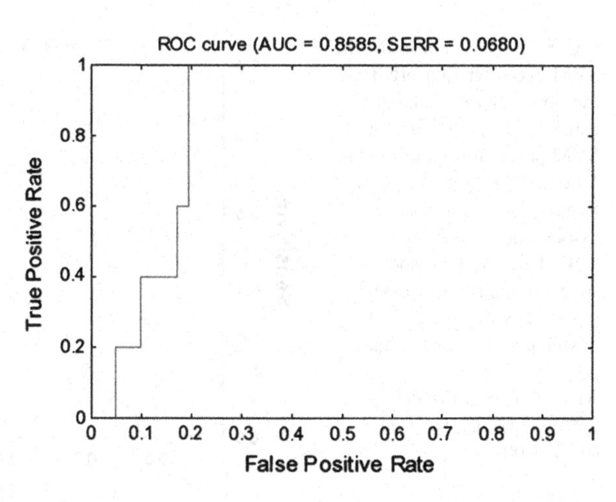

Fig. 5.28 ROC *curve* for CLANG dysarthria

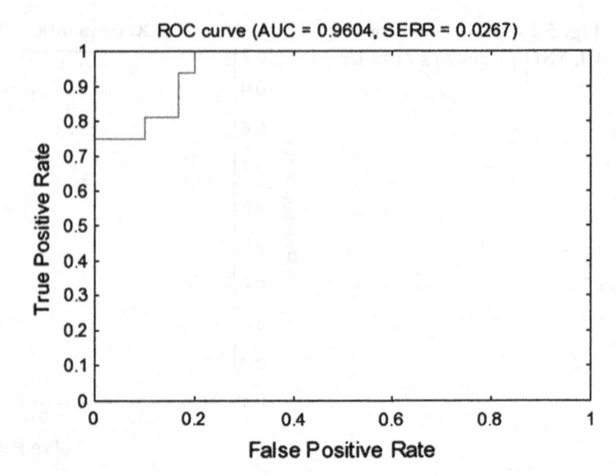

Fig. 5.29 ROC *curve* for CLANG global rating

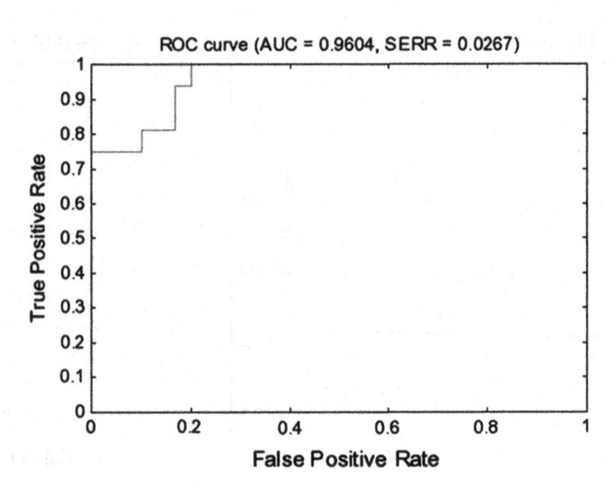

Fig. 5.30 ROC *curve* for CLANG observer prediction

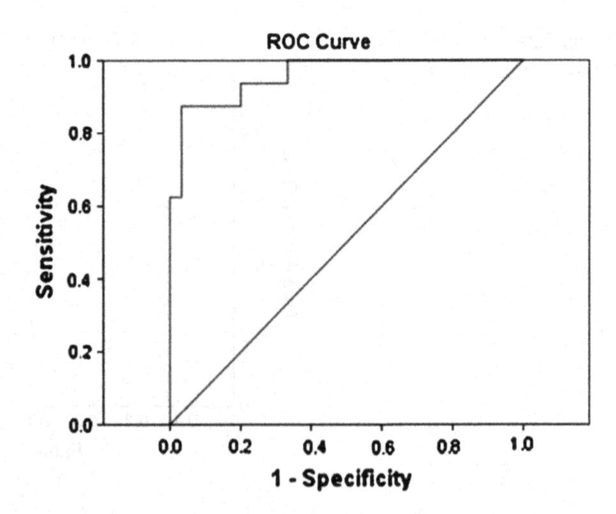

Fig. 5.31 ROC *curve* for the SVM classifier that predicts the observer rated classes using S_{CLANG} (the sum of SVM prediction values of the 10 CLANG items: abnormal Syntax, lack of semantic association, discourse failure, lack of details, aprosodic speech, abnormal prosody, pragmatics disorder, dysfluency, dysarthria, and poverty of speech). AUC=0.96 Std.Err=0.03, 95% confidence interval (0.90, 1.00)

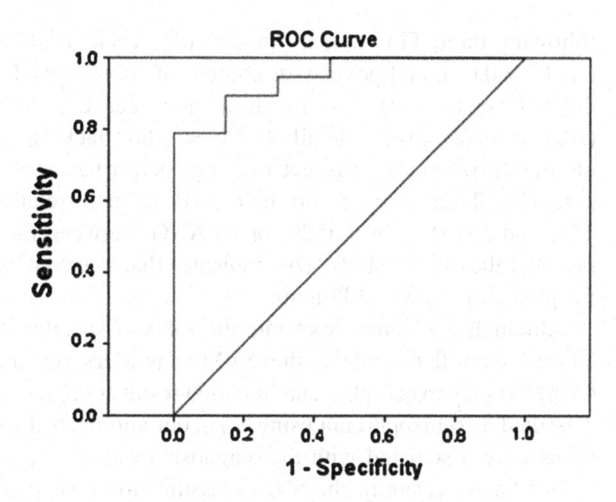

Fig. 5.32 ROC *curve* for the SVM classifier that predicts the actual classes using S_{CLANG} (the sum of SVM prediction values of the 10 CLANG items: abnormal Syntax, lack of semantic association, discourse failure, lack of details, aprosodic speech, abnormal prosody, pragmatics disorder, dysfluency, dysarthria, and poverty of speech). AUC=0.95 STD=0.03, 95% confidence interval (0.88, 1.00)

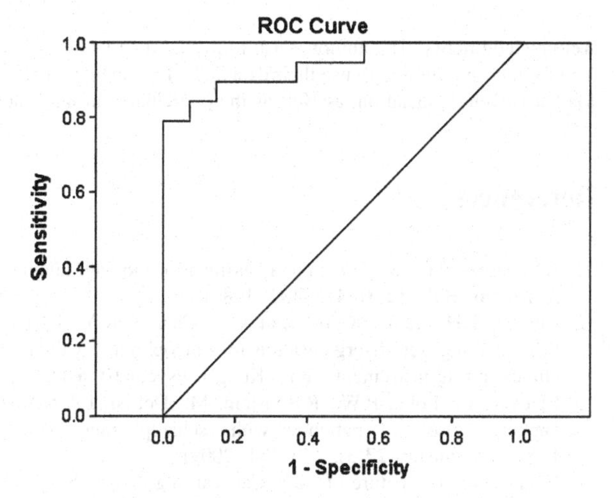

Fig. 5.33 ROC of the sum S_{SLD} of SVM prediction values of both TCL and CLANG in predicting the actual classes. AUC = 0.94, STD = 0.04, 95 % confidence interval (0.87, 1.00)

health conditions and SLD items (both phenomenological and linguistic) from speech can provide an accurate discrimination of the groups.

Concept3 features were based on n-gram concept terms (e.g., "don't know" and "looks like") that preserve word order for meaning disambiguation. This feature combines the following three types of language features: surface feature (e.g., counts of words and phrases), statistical language features (e.g., n-gram likelihood), and semantic features (e.g., checking the concepts against the commonsense database). In addition, the features can be used to test vocabulary knowledge of participants. SVM will use combinations of the features to model each of the tasks of predicting the 17 SLD items and the actual class labels.

SVM performed equally in predicting TLC items (average AUC = 0.81) and CLANG items (average AUC = 0.81). SVM did not perform well for the following three TLC items: pressure of speech (AUC = 0.54), circumstantiality (AUC = 0.65), and poverty of content of speech (AUC = 0.78). Additionally, it did not perform well for the following four CLANG items: discourse failure (AUC = 0.78), excess details (AUC = 0.66), lack of details (0.78), and pressure of speech (0.51). We suspect the poor performance was due to lack of positive cases, but there were no correlations (Pearson correlation $r = 0.32$, $p = 0.37$ for TLC and $r = 0.40$, $p = 0.20$ for CLANG) between the number of positive samples and the AUC values. This indicates that Concept3 features were not suitable for predicting those SLD items.

Although we cannot associate the roles of specific language features with the learned classifier models, the SVM classifiers for the SLD items (TLC and CLANG) may explain the classification results of S_{SLD}. That is, if a participant was classified as schizophrenia using S_{SLD}, our approach could tell which specific SLD items were associated with the diagnosis result.

In Chapter [Debra], the SVM classification results are compared with manual TLC and CLANG rating results.

Acknowledgments The authors wish to thank Anne Debra Tilaka, Lynette Tham, and Sabrina Yeo for their permission to use their data and all the mental health professionals at the Singapore Mental Health Association, as well as the participants in this study.

References

1. Andreasen, N.C.: Scale for the assessment of thought, language, and communication (TLC). Schizophr. Bull. **12**(3), 473–482 (1986)
2. Chen, E.Y.H., Lam, L.C.W., Kan, C.S., Chan, C.K.Y., Kwok, C.L., Nguyen, D.G.H., Chen, R.Y.L.: Language disorganisation in schizophrenia: validation and assessment with a new clinical rating instrument. Hong Kong J. Psychiatry **6**(1), 4–13 (1996)
3. Elvevag, B., Foltz, P.W., Rosenstein, M., DeLisi, L.E.: An automated method to analyze language use in patients with schizophrenia and their first-degree relatives. J. Neurolinguistics **23**(3), 270–284 (2009)
4. Vapnik, V.: The nature of statistical learning theory. Springer (1999)
5. Cortes, Corinna, Vapnik, V.: Support-vector networks. Mach. Learn. **20**(3), 273–297 (1995)
6. Burges, C.J.C.: A tutorial on support vector machines for pattern recognition. Data Min. Knowl. Disc. **2**(2), 121–167 (1998)
7. Joachims, T., Nédellec, C., Rouveirol, C.: Text categorization with support vector machines: learning with many relevant features In: Machine Learning: ECML-98, Lecture Notes in Computer Science, vol. 1398, pp 137–142. Springer, Berlin/Heidelberg (1998)
8. Rennie, J.D.M., Rifkin, R.: Improving Multiclass Text Classification with the Support Vector Machine (2001)
9. Gunn, S.R.: Support Vector Machines for Classification and Regression (1998)
10. Manning, C., Raghavan, P., Schtze, H.: Introduction to Information Retrieval. Cambridge University Press (2008). doi:citeulike-article-id:4469058
11. Matsuo, Y., Ishizuka, M.: Keyword extraction from a single document using word co-occurrence statistical information. Int. J. Artif. Intell. Tools **13**(1), 157–169 (2004). doi:citeulike-article-id:573187
12. Baeza-Yates, R., Ribeiro-Neto, B.: Modern Information Retrieval. Addison-Wesleym, Harlow, England (1999). doi:citeulike-article-id:6580677

13. Landauer, T., Foltz, P., Laham, D.: An introduction to latent semantic analysis. Discourse Processes **25**, 259–284 (1998). doi:citeulike-article-id:2243850
14. Speer, R., Havasi, C., Lieberman, H.: AnalogySpace: reducing the dimensionality of common sense knowledge. In: AAAI'08: Proceedings of the 23rd National Conference on Artificial Intelligence, Chicago, Illinois, 2008, pp 548–553. AAAI Press (2008). doi:citeulike-article-id:6873905
15. Singh, P., Lin, T., Mueller, E., Lim, G., Perkins, T., Zhu, W.: Open mind common sense: knowledge acquisition from the general public (2002). doi:citeulike-article-id:311042
16. Liu, H., Push, S.: Conceptnet: a practical commonsense reasoning toolkit. BT Technol. J. **22**, 211–226 (2004)
17. Reithinger, N., Engel, R., Kipp, M., Klesen, M.: Predicting Dialogue Acts for a Speech-To-Speech Translation System, vol 2. ICSLP-96, Philadelphia, PA (1996)
18. Kim, S.N., Medelyan, O., Kan, M.-Y., Baldwin ,T.: SemEval-2010 task 5: automatic key phrase extraction from scientific articles. Paper Presented at the Proceedings of the 5th International Workshop on Semantic Evaluation, Los Angeles, California 2010
19. Liu, H.: MontyLingua: an end-to-end natural language processor with common sense. Available at: http://web.media.mit.edu/~hugo/montylingua (2004)
20. Fukada, T., Koll, D., Waibel, A., Tanigaki, K.: Probabilistic dialogue act extraction for concept based multilingual translation systems. Proceedings of the ICSLP, ISCA (1998)
21. Chang, C.-C., Lin, C.-J.: LIBSVM: a library for support vector machines. ACM Trans. Intell. Syst. Technol. **2**(3), 1–27 (2011). doi:10.1145/1961189.1961199
22. McKenna, P., Oh, T.M.: Schizophrenic Speech: Making Sense of Bathroots and Ponds that Fall in Doorways. Cambridge University Press, Cambridge (2005)

Chapter 6
Social Networks and Automated Mental Health Screening

Insu Song and John Vong

6.1 Introduction

According to a survey done in 2008, most Americans (up to 80 %) rely on the Internet to find health information they use to make their health care decisions [1]. Indeed, in 2008, the Internet rivaled physicians as a source of health information [2]. Indeed, this heightened reliance on the Internet manifests itself in patients increasingly turning to the Internet for emotional support and to acquire clinical knowledge for self-care. The massive production of social media enabled by Web 2.0 offers patients a wealth of clinical knowledge, thereby providing an efficient platform for patients to support each other. The platform, also known as Health Social Network or Health 2.0, has fuelled great interest and shown massive potential to empower patients' self-care. Some prominent examples include PatientsLikeMe[1] and the IBM Patient Empowerment System.[2] These newly emerged patient-driven health care services are outreach efforts to harmonize the plethora of existing frameworks and new ideas. They aim to serve as a reliable communication channel for information exchange and better collaboration among patients and doctors. The services provided by health social networks include: (a) emotional support and information sharing, (b) physician Q & As, and (c) self-tracking of conditions, their symptoms, treatment options, and other biological information [3].

---

1 http://www.patientslikeme.com/all/patients
2 http://www-03.ibm.com/press/us/en/pressrelease/33944.wss

I. Song (✉) · J. Vong
School of Business and IT, James Cook University Australia, Singapore Campus, Singapore 574421, Singapore
e-mail: insu.song@jcu.edu.au

J. Vong
e-mail: john.vong@jcu.edu.au

M. Lech et al. (eds.), *Mental Health Informatics*,
Studies in Computational Intelligence 491, DOI: 10.1007/978-3-642-38550-6_6,

Advances in Internet technology and the proliferation of social media, such as blogs and social networking sites, are overwhelming to the point that it is difficult to keep abreast of current affairs and growing information. With the vast amount of information on the internet, conventional methods of searching via keywords or descriptors have become laborious and mundane. For new patients, medical assessments or discussions are often overloaded with jargon, making them difficult to explore and find relevant communities. In particular, mental health descriptions and medical assessment reports contain sensitive information, and, therefore, most existing document similarity measures, such as the popular cosine-based similarity measure [4] and latent semantic analysis (LSA) [5] are not suitable, since those methods either require the entire source medical report or a large number of features that are confidential and can possibly give away patients' sensitive information.

We have developed a method of generating a small number of relevant keywords or codes that can distinguish patients based on their health conditions and that can be used as a similarity measure of patients' underlying health conditions to reduce the risk of revealing sensitive personal information.

6.1.1 Background

This work is based on social networking, text mining, and, in particular, text classification. The following section provides a brief overview of the core techniques, focusing on social networking and similarity measures.

6.1.1.1 Health Social Networks

A health social network is an online information service which facilitates information sharing between closely related members of a community. Also known as social media on the Internet, or Health 2.0, a health social network empowers patients and health service providers by promoting collaboration between patients, their caregivers, and clinicians [6]. At its basic level, a health social network provides emotional support by allowing patients to find others in similar health situations. They can also share information about conditions, symptoms, and treatments [3]. Other services include physician Q & A, and self-tracking of conditions, symptoms, treatments, and other biological information [3]. The self-supporting community is particularly important to sustainability in the case of lifelong conditions, such as autism.

6.1.1.2 Recommendation Systems

The main means of finding patients with similar health conditions involves labor-intensive methods, such as searching through the Internet, keywords in community titles, and descriptions of other members in communities [7]. Over the years, many recommender systems and similarity measurement methods have been developed [8]. These approaches can be broadly classified into two categories: content matching based on available semantic information and a collaborative filtering approach based on overlapping membership of pairs of communities [7]. In this paper, we focus on content matching based on semantic similarity of words, since our source of information relies on descriptions of health conditions, such as online messages on Internet health forums.

6.1.1.3 Cosine-Based Similarity Measure

One of the popular similarity measures for text documents is the cosine similarity measure [4]. The cosine similarity measure between two feature vectors $\mathbf{a}, \mathbf{b} \in \Re^d$ can be defined as a normalized dot product between the two vectors:

$$\cos im(\mathbf{a}, \mathbf{b}) = \frac{\mathbf{a} \cdot \mathbf{b}}{|a||b|} \tag{6.1}$$

where $|\mathbf{a}|$ and $|\mathbf{b}|$ are L2-norms of the feature vectors. Commonly used features for text document similarity measures are TF (term-frequency) and TFIDF (term-frequency weighted inverse document frequency) [4]. We define four types of features based on TF and TFIDF:

$$tf = tf \tag{6.2}$$

$$tfidf = tf \times \log\frac{N}{n} \tag{6.3}$$

$$ntf = \frac{tf}{|d|} \tag{6.4}$$

$$tft\max = \frac{tf}{t\max} \tag{6.5}$$

where tf is the term frequency of a vocabulary term of a collection of documents, $|d|$ is the L2-norm of the document vector, t max is the maximum frequency of the term, N is the number of documents in the collection, and n is the number of documents containing the term.

6.1.1.4 AnalogySpace-Based Similarity Measure

AnalogySpace is a generalized similarity measure that finds other relevant concepts that are similar [9]. This has been shown to be superior to other semantic-based similarity measures, such as latent semantic analysis (LSA) [5]. It uses semantic relations between terms to measure similarity between terms, sentences, and/or documents.

AnalogySpace, using data from the Open Mind Common Sense (OMCS) project [10], represents each term c (e.g., "cake") as a feature vector $\mathbf{c} = concept(t)$, where each feature is a commonsense property of the concept (e.g., IsA dessert). This is done by finding the usage of the conceptual term in the ConceptNet. Using the feature vectors of concepts, AnalogySpace represents knowledge as a matrix of concepts [9]. For instance, each column may represent a concept and each row represents a property. This is a sparse matrix of very high dimension. The question is then how do we measure similarity between two new concepts using the AnalogySpace. Similarly to the eigenface decomposition of a human face [11], we can decompose a concept feature vector $\mathbf{c}$ into eigenconcepts and project the new concepts onto the eigenconcepts to obtain a low dimension vector $\mathbf{a}_c = analogy(\mathbf{c})$ of coefficients. The similarity measure between two concepts c_1 and c_2 is then defined as a dot product of the normalized coefficient vectors:

$$u(c_1, c_2) = \overline{\mathbf{a}_{c_1}} \cdot \overline{\mathbf{a}_{c_2}} \tag{6.6}$$

where $\overline{\mathbf{a}_{c_1}}$ is the normalized vector of the coefficient vector $\mathbf{a}_{c1}$.

6.1.1.5 Mental Health Informatics

In recent years, machine learning techniques, such as support vector machines (SVMs), have shown significant potential for supporting the practice of medicine and psychiatric classification [12, 13]. The application of machine learning techniques in mental health diagnosis has significant merits because of the potential to provide early diagnosis and more standardized objective diagnosis. In mental health assessment, conventionally, expert psychiatrists consciously and unconsciously analyze the body language of their patients to make clinical diagnoses using diagnostic classification schemas, such as the DSM IV [14] and ICD 10 [15]. Although the DSM-IV and ICD-10 guidelines are helpful to clinicians in their diagnostic process, the effectiveness of their utilization depends on the level of experience of the clinicians [16].

Mental health conditions, such as autism, are usually lifelong conditions such that long-term treatment planning and support from family and communities are crucial. Social networking for health care may empower parents and other family members of children with mental health conditions to conveniently share information with their counterparts and collaborate more easily with doctors.

6.1.1.6 Support Vector Machines

Cortes and Vapnik [17] introduced support vector machines which were a novel approach to machine learning. SVMs are based on the structural risk minimization principle in order to overcome the overfitting problems. Support vector machines find the hypotheses out of the hypothesis space H of a learning system which approximately minimizes the bound on the actual error by controlling the empirical error using training samples and the complexity of the model using the VC-dimension of H. SVMs are universal learning systems [Joachims: 99]. In their basic form, SVMs learn maximal margin hyperplanes (linear threshold functions). A hyperplane can be defined by a weight vector $\mathbf{w}$ and a bias b:

$$\mathbf{w} \cdot \mathbf{x} + b = 0 \tag{6.7}$$

The corresponding threshold function for an input vector x is then given by:

$$f(\mathbf{x}) = sign(\mathbf{w} \cdot \mathbf{x} + b) \tag{6.8}$$

However, it is possible to learn polynomial classifiers, radial basis function (RBF) networks, and three or more layered neural networks by mapping input data $\mathbf{x}$ to some other (possibly infinite dimensional) feature space $\phi(\mathbf{x})$ and using kernel functions $K(\mathbf{x}_i, \mathbf{x}_j)$ to obtain dot products, $\phi(\mathbf{x}_i) \cdot \phi(\mathbf{x}_j)$, of feature data.

6.1.2 Overview

In the next section, we propose a social networking framework for parents of autistic children that utilizes mobile phone-based ubiquitous computing. The remainder of the paper summarizes experiments and their results: text classification, discriminant keyword generation for mental health descriptions, statistical analysis on the model parameters that are generated for mental health descriptions (autism and ADHD descriptions), and social linking using keywords.

6.2 Parent Network Framework

We propose a parent social network framework, where health service providers can actively engage in facilitating information sharing and social links between parents. Figure 6.1 shows how hospitals can facilitate communities of parents. Parents can obtain preliminary assessment tools from hospitals via their mobile phones. They can then fill in standard assessment questionnaires to obtain preliminary diagnoses and information on how to get help. Upon the first consultation with a clinician, the parents' mobile agent can provide the clinicians' agent the completed questionnaires and other preliminary diagnosis results, thereby improving the clinicians' effectiveness and efficiency. Clinicians then can provide treatment plan and tasks that parents can follow on the parent agent. The assessment report is then stored in the data mining server to generate keywords and parent link information. Subsequent visits to the hospital then will provide more refined treatment plans and information to communities who can share their experiences and facilitate learning in order to meet the communities' needs, such as for emotional support and clinical knowledge.

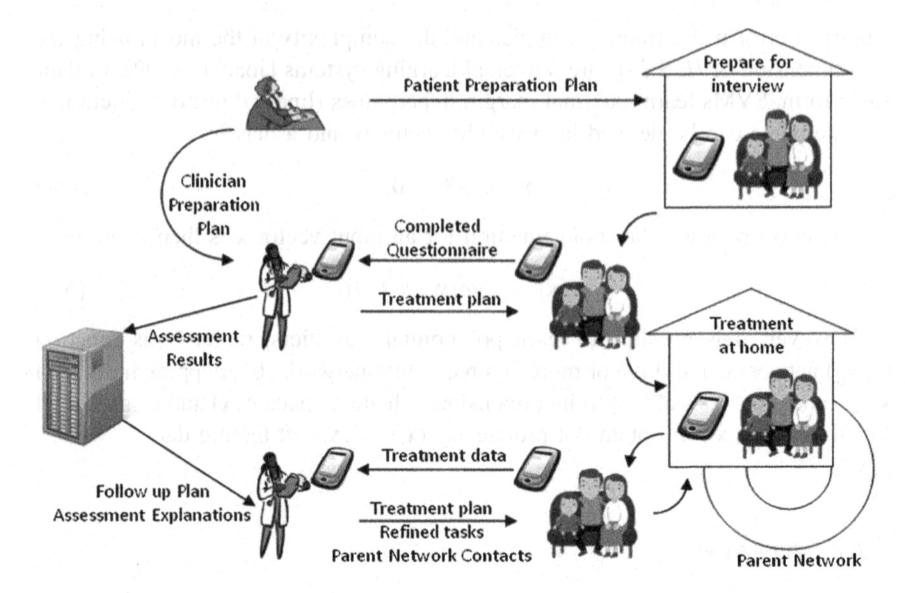

Fig. 6.1 Parents of autistic children collaborate with hospitals and the community to share experiences and learning in order to address their needs. The hospital engages with the community by providing links between parents whose children share similar health descriptions. Families are matched based on similarity of their health descriptions

6.3 Mental Health Database and Feature Extraction

To evaluate our similarity measure, we utilized two sets of text documents used in [12, 13]. The two sets of non-overlapping text documents were collected from various Internet health forums where parents of children with mental health conditions, such as Autism and ADHD (attention deficit hyperactivity disorder), exchange their stories. The first data set (Dataset A) was obtained from Internet forums where parents exchange their experiences and stories using letter-like communications. Therefore, the contents were well written and structured. This data set consisted of a total of 50 text documents: 25 autism descriptions and 25 ADHD descriptions. The second data set (Dataset B) was obtained from different Internet forums where parents exchange their stories informally. Thus, the contents were less well-written, often containing spelling errors and incomplete sentences. This data set consisted of a total of 200 text documents: 100 autism descriptions and 100 ADHD descriptions.

The text documents were segmented into words, each word was lemmatized, and functional words (such as "to" and "the") were removed. The words were then mapped into conceptual words using ConceptNet [18]. For example, the sentence "My son still struggles with self control" was converted to a set {'son', 'still', 'struggles', 'self', 'control'}. The conceptual words were ranked according to corpora frequency (frequency of words in the collection of documents), and words with less than two corpora frequency were removed. The selected words were then used as attributes. Thus, each text document was represented as a vector of the frequencies of conceptual words. Four sets of feature files were generated: term frequency (TF), term frequency weighted with inverse document frequency(TF-IDF), normalized TF (NTF), and TFMAX (tf/t max) as defined in Sect. 6.1.1.3. The NTF feature was used for generating SVM models.

In the SVM feature file (i.e., the NTF feature), the input features were normalized to the length of the documents. That is, an input feature vector is a *d*-dimensional vector and each feature value is a normalized frequency of a conceptual word. The classification task was to find a function f: $\mathbf{x} \rightarrow C$ by using SVM learning that maps the input feature vector x to a class label C = {Autism, ADHD}.

To generate keywords for health conditions, the text documents of the mental health conditions were preprocessed using the same procedure as above. The extracted feature vectors of the text documents were classified into a class label using the SVM model. Then, a small number of top N most contributing conceptual words were selected as the keywords of the patients. The set of keywords were then compared with other patients' keywords for similarity in the AnalogySpace using Eq. (6.6).

6.4 Methodology

6.4.1 Classification Model

Figure 6.2 illustrates the overall procedure for generating a small number of keywords for mental health descriptions. The training and testing were done using the Leave-one-out (LOO) cross validation method. For Dataset A (health forum with well-structured contents), a total of 50 SVM models were generated using the linear kernel. Thus, each model was used to classify one document. The performance results of classification are presented in Table 6.1. The ROC curve of the classification of Dataset B is shown in Fig. 6.3.

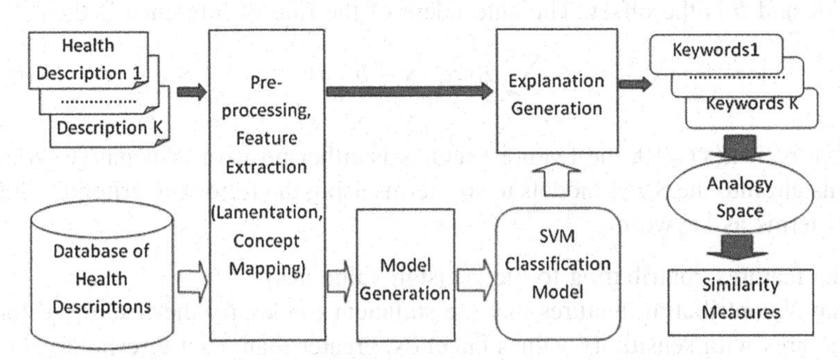

Fig. 6.2 Block diagram of generating keywords for similarity measure and recommender system

Table 6.1 Linear SVM classification performance

Dataset	Accuracy (%)	Recall	Precision	AUC
Dataset A	84	0.80	0.87	0.88
Dataset B	88	0.87	0.89	0.94

Autism versus ADHD classification performance using linear SVM classifier and normalized term frequency (*NTF*) feature. AUC values are the area under the Receiver Operating Curve (*ROC*)

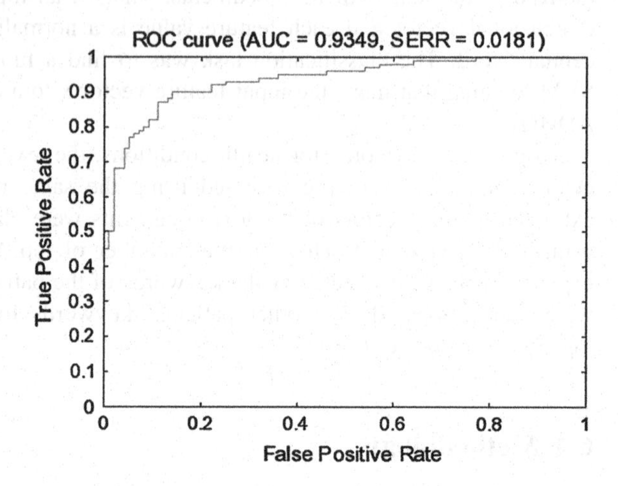

Fig. 6.3 ROC *curve* of classification of data B (informal health-forum): true positive rate versus false positive rate

6.4.2 Keyword Generation

An SVM model is defined by support vectors $\mathbf{x}_i$ and associated parameters. The decision value of a text sample (represented as a feature vector $\mathbf{x}$) is then obtained as follows:

$$d(\mathbf{x}) = \sum_{i \in SV} \alpha_i y_i K(\mathbf{x}_i, \mathbf{x}) + b \tag{6.9}$$

where $\mathbf{x}_i$ are support vectors and $\mathbf{x}$ is the feature vector, α_i are Lagrangian multipliers, and b is the offset. The antecedent of the rule of inference is then:

$$\sum_{i \in SV} \alpha_i y_i \mathbf{x}_i \cdot \mathbf{x} + b \geq 0 \tag{6.10}$$

That is, if $d(\mathbf{x}) \geq 0$, the feature vector $\mathbf{x}$ is either positive or negative. We use this insight into the SVM models to sort terms using the following criteria to select top-N terms as keywords:

1. The features contributing to the decision value $d(\mathbf{x})$.
2. Top-N contributing features that are sufficient to classify the feature vector.
3. Features with sensitivity values $\partial d(\mathbf{x})/\partial \mathbf{x}_j$ greater than a set threshold value.

Technical details on generating each set of keyword type are described in Sect. 6.4.4.

6.4.3 Sim: Similarity Measure

A small selection of the top-N terms was used as conceptual terms (keywords) for each patient. The keywords were used to measure similarities between health conditions based on AnalogySpace and ConceptNet[3] (a common sense database). The similarity measure was then used to connect the communities and patients. The method involves scoring each keyword in one health description with each keyword in another health description. In this approach, the similarity between two descriptions is given by determining contributions made by keywords and semantic relationships between terms. The similarity between two sets of keywords, A and B, is defined as follows:

$$Concept\ 1_{i,j} = \frac{1}{|A||B|} \sum_{i \in A} \sum_{j \in B-\{i\}} u(i, j) \tag{6.11}$$

$$Concept\ 2_{i,j} = \frac{1}{|A||B|} \sum_{i \in A} \sum_{j \in B-\{i\}} u(i, j) |d(\mathbf{A})_i d(\mathbf{B})_j s(\mathbf{A})_i s(\mathbf{B})_j| \tag{6.12}$$

$$Concept\ 3_{i,j} = \frac{1}{|A||B|} \sum_{i \in A} \sum_{j \in B} u(i, j) \tag{6.13}$$

where $u(i,j)$ is the semantic similarity function defined in Eq. (6.6), which measures how close the term i in the set **A** of keywords is to the term j in the set **B** of keywords where $i \neq j$ for Concept 1 and Concept 2, $d(A)_i$ and $d(B)_j$ are the amount of contributions of the features i and j, respectively, and $s(\mathbf{A})_i$ and $s(\mathbf{B})_j$ are the sensitivity of the features i and j, respectively. For Concept 2 measure, the dot products of two concept vectors are weighted with contributions of terms. To test whether different terms in the keywords can provide similarity information using semantic information, we exclude cases where two terms are identical: $i \neq j$.

Using this similarity measure, we can recommend a patient p to a community among a set C of communities by selecting the community with the maximum average-similarity between the parent p and all parents p' in a community c:

$$R(p, C) = \arg\max_{c \in C} \frac{1}{|c|} \sum_{p' \in c} Concept\ 2_{p,p'} \tag{6.14}$$

[3] Used ConceptNet v2.1 from the Common Sense Computing Initiative at the MIT Media Lab (http://csc.media.mit.edu).

6.4.4 Generating Keywords from SVM Models

In order to calculate the contribution values of each feature of a feature vector **x**, we use the centroid **C** of the population, which is estimated using the centroid $\mathbf{C}_{sv}$ of the support vectors of the SVM classification model:

$$\mathbf{C}_{sv} = \frac{1}{Nsv} \sum_{i \in SV} \phi(\mathbf{x}_i) \tag{6.15}$$

where N_{sv} is the number of support vectors. We can then calculate the deviation of a feature vector **x** from the estimated population centroid:

$$\mathbf{D}(\mathbf{x}) = \phi(\mathbf{x}) - \mathbf{C}_{sv} \tag{6.16}$$

Suppose C_{sv} is on the hyperplane: $\mathbf{w} \cdot \mathbf{C}_{sv} \approx -b$. Then, we can obtain the decision value $d(\mathbf{x})$ using the deviation $\mathbf{D}(\mathbf{x})$:

$$d(\mathbf{x}) \approx (\mathbf{w} \cdot (\phi(\mathbf{x}) - \mathbf{C}_{sv})) = \sum_{i \in SV} \alpha_i y_i [K(\mathbf{x}_i, \mathbf{x}) - K(\mathbf{x}_i, \mathbf{C}_{sv})] \tag{6.17}$$

If K is the linear kernel, we can estimate the contribution of each jth feature $\mathbf{x}_j$ as follows:

$$C_{sv,j} = \frac{1}{Nsv} \sum_{i \in SV} x_{i,j} \tag{6.18}$$

$$d(\mathbf{x})_j = \sum_{i \in SV} \alpha_i y_i x_{i,j} (x_j - C_{sv,j}) \tag{6.19}$$

Now, for a feature vector **x**, we can explain why a sample is positive (negative) by listing the feature elements that contribute to the decision value. That is, we can rank the features of a feature vector according to the contribution made by the features.

This method can be extended to non-linear SVM models with convex decision boundaries. Applying the K-NN algorithm, N number of support vectors can be selected as a reference point forming a centroid and a hyperplane in the input space. This new hyperplane is now a linear SVM model that can be used to generate keywords with regard to the selected support vectors.

6.4.5 Experimental Results

Figure 6.4 compares three Sim similarity measures and four cosine-based similarity measures. It shows that all Sim similarity measures performed better with a small number of selected keywords. For Dataset A, when top-N = 1 (i.e., only one term was used for similarity measure), the average similarity within group was

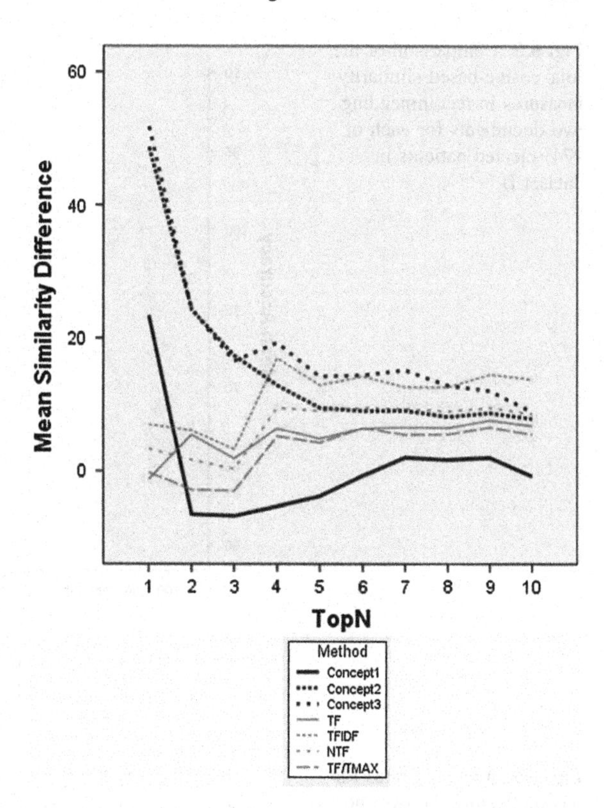

Fig. 6.4 Comparison of the seven similarity measures in recommending two documents for each of 40 selected patients in dataset A: 20 Autism and 20 ADHD

significantly larger than average similarity between groups for both Concept 1 ($p < 0.395$) and Concept 2 ($p < 0.001$). The differences were significant for all top-N values for Concept 2 and Concept 3.

Cosine-based similarity measures performed well when a large number of features were used as shown in Fig. 6.5, but degraded quickly as the number of features used was reduced. Since our objective was to use a small number of keywords that were possibly disjoint among patients, this clearly indicates that cosine-based approaches are not suitable for our purpose.

In comparison, Sim similarity measures performed well with a small number of keywords. Figure 6.6 shows accuracy rates for recommending the two most similar patients for each of 38 patients in Dataset A. Sim similarity measures significantly outperformed the cosine-based similarity measure when a small number of chosen explanatory terms were used. We should note that unlike cosine-based similarity measures, Sim generated a set of keywords for each patient that was possibly disjoint. Instead of comparing for frequency of exact same terms, Sim measures similarity between all possible keyword pairs between two patients using semantic similarity.

Figure 6.7 shows accuracy rates for recommending the two most similar patients for each of 178 selected patients in Dataset B. Two Sim similarity

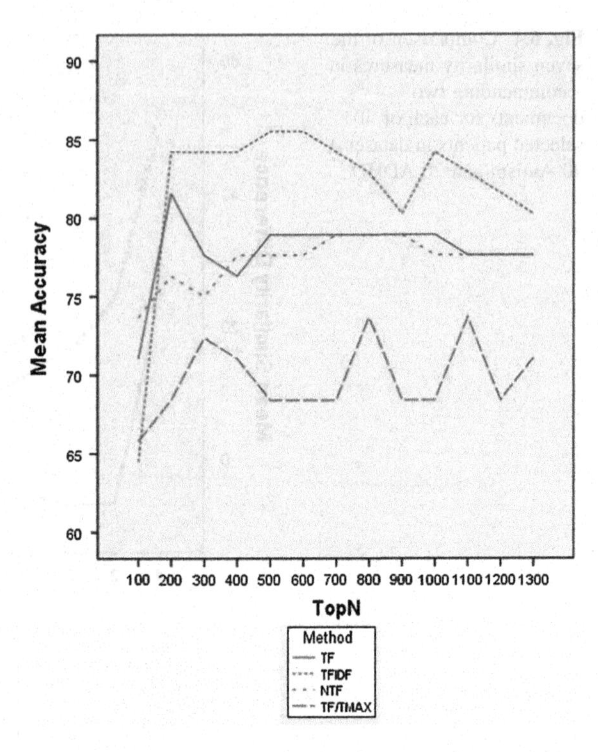

Fig. 6.5 Comparison of the four cosine-based similarity measures in recommending two documents for each of 174 selected patients in dataset B

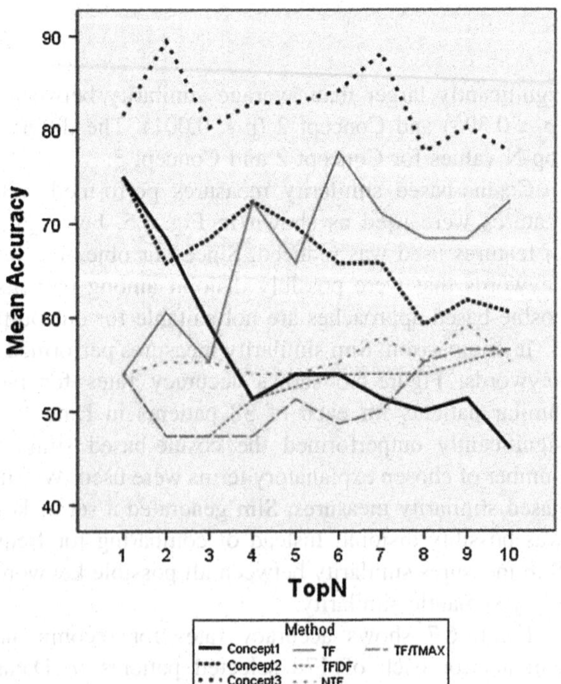

Fig. 6.6 Accuracy rates for recommending the two most similar patients for each of 38 patients in dataset A

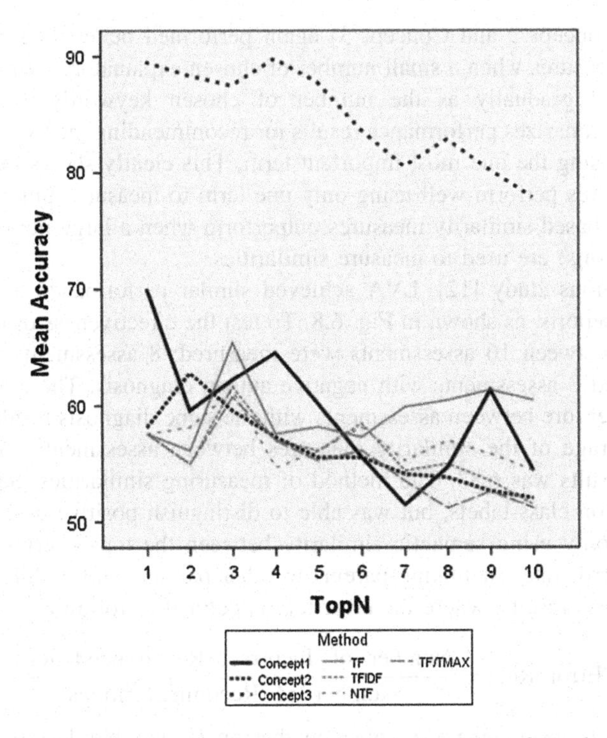

Fig. 6.7 Accuracy rates for recommending the two most similar patients for each of 178 selected patients in dataset B

Table 6.2 Performance results for recommending the two most similar documents using the one most important term

Data	Method	Acc	Prec	Spec
A	Concept 1	0.75	0.77	0.78
A	Concept 2	0.75	0.75	0.77
A	Concept 3	0.81	0.86	0.86
A	TF	0.53 (0.81)	0.44 (0.91)	0.55 (0.90)
A	TFIDF	0.54 (0.85)	0.44 (0.91)	0.55 (0.91)
A	NTF	0.54 (0.79)	0.42 (0.94)	0.55 (0.93)
A	TFMAX	0.54 (0.72)	0.44 (0.89)	0.55 (0.85)
B	Concept 1	0.70	0.60	0.67
B	Concept 2	0.58	0.87	0.70
B	Concept 3	0.90	0.89	0.90
B	TF	0.57 (0.75)	0.41 (0.86)	0.56 (0.83)
B	TFIDF	0.57 (0.81)	0.42 (0.82)	0.56 (0.82)
B	NTF	0.58 (0.74)	0.42 (0.88)	0.56 (0.85)
B	TFMAX	0.58 (0.77)	0.42 (0.84)	0.56 (0.82)

Numbers in the brackets are maximum performance results among all possible top-N > 100 values. Precision = total number of correct autism patients recommended/total number of recommendations for autism patients. Specificity = total number of correct ADHD patients recommended/total number of recommendations for ADHD patients measures (Concept 2 and Concept 3) again performed better than cosine-based similarity measures when a small number of chosen explanatory terms were used, but degraded gradually as the number of chosen keywords was increased. Table 6.2 summarizes performance results for recommending the two most similar documents using the one most important term. This clearly shows that Sim similarity measures perform well using only one term to measure similarities. However, cosine-based similarity measures outperform when a large number of terms (over 100 terms) are used to measure similarities.

In a previous study [12], LVA achieved similar performance on the autism assessment reports, as shown in Fig. 6.8. To test the effectiveness of this method, similarities between 16 assessments were measured: 8 assessments with autism diagnosis and 8 assessments with negative autism diagnosis. The average of the similarity measure between assessments with the same diagnosis results was 8.66, and the average of the similarity measures between assessments with different diagnosis results was 6.83. The method of measuring similarities did not utilize information on class labels, but was able to distinguish positive cases from negative cases only using semantic similarity between the top-N terms. Figure 6.8 shows the error rates of linking parents to other parents whose children had the same diagnosis results, where the error rate is defined as follows:

$$\text{Error Rate} = \frac{\text{Number of Incorrect Recommendations}}{\text{Number of Recommendations}} \tag{6.20}$$

The parents were linked by selecting the top-K most similar assessments. It shows that when one parent was linked to 32 % or less proportions of the total community, the error rate was less than 35 %, and errors consistently decreased as

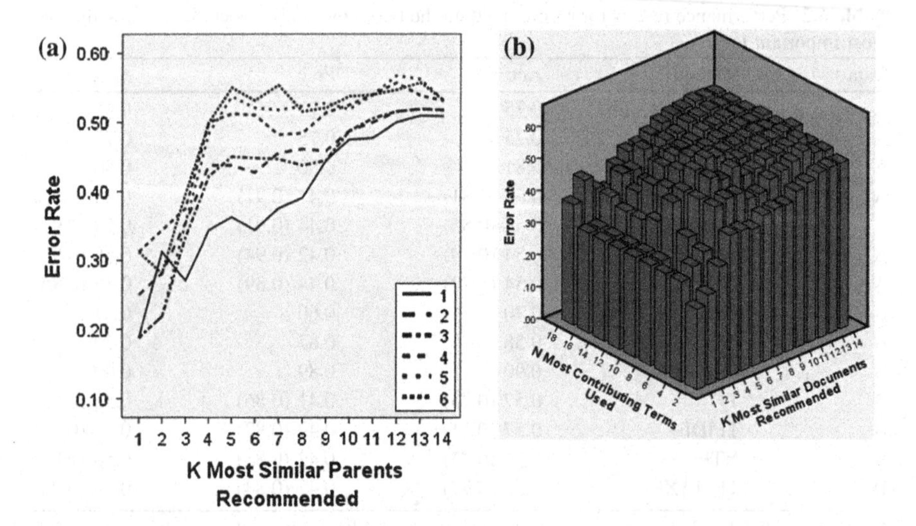

Fig. 6.8 Error rates of linking 18 autism assessment reports to the top-K most similar assessment reports using top-N most contributing terms. **a** Average error rates over top-N terms. **b** Average error rate matrix

K decreased. The average error rate matrix in Fig. 6.8b clearly indicates that a small number of selected terms can provide good link information and that the relevance information of the terms is useful.

6.5 Discussion and Conclusions

The performance results of the two Sim similarity measures, Concept 1 and Concept 2, showed that the selected keywords were semantically related to each other. This is because Concept 1 and Concept 2 do not compare conceptual terms that are identical. That is, the keyword generation method chose terms that were semantically related to each other in the AnalogySpace. It is not exactly clear why there exists a link between AnalogySpace and the keywords generated using SVM models. This may be due to their co-occurrences in the same document or in the same context. However, since a large number of words were shared between the two groups of documents (Autism and ADHD), random selections of words would not show significant differences in similarity measures within groups and between groups. To test this, error rates and differences in relative similarities were obtained using randomly selected keywords. The random keyword selection method performed worse on both Dataset A and Dataset B as compared to the cosine-based similarity measures. Figure 6.9 shows that the error rates of using randomly selected keywords is no better than chance. Therefore, the keyword

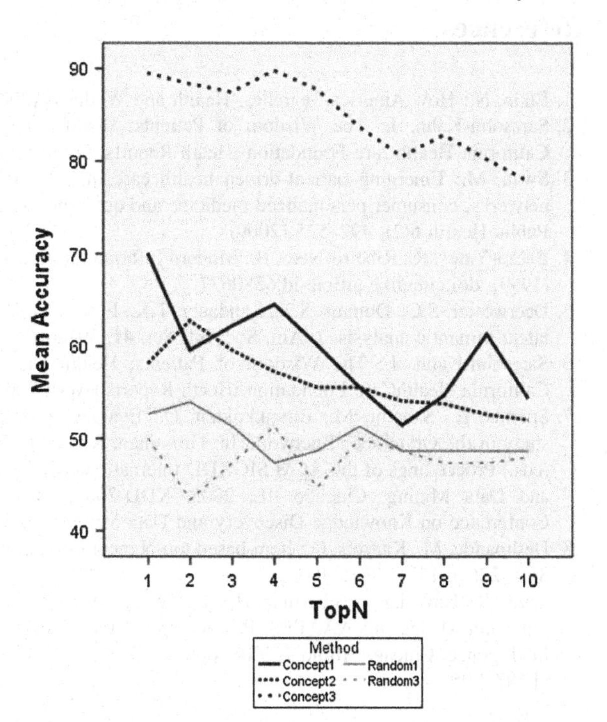

Fig. 6.9 The error rates and differences in relative similarities obtained using randomly selected terms. The random keyword selection method performed worse on both dataset A and B as compared to the cosine-based similarity measures

generation method preferred to select semantically related words (even if they were different words) for patients with common mental health conditions. We believe this is an interesting finding which requires further study.

The semantic similarity measure between keywords of mental health descriptions has great potential for discovering close social communities of parents who can support each other for lifelong conditions such as autism. Such long term disabilities pose a heavy burden to families. Thus, it is essential that health care services actively participate in communities to support patients' families. Sim is an ideal method for health care organizations to use to facilitate such social linking because of its anonymous indexing feature. The community suggestion method facilitates social linking between parents whose children share similar mental health descriptions to allow relevant and useful information to be acquired through social networking. It can also be used to discover potential hidden communities of patients and parents on the Internet. In general, there is massive potential for incorporating these sophisticated information extraction technologies in social networking.

Acknowledgments We would like to thank Yi Pin Song for collecting text documents from various Internet health forums. This work was supported by JCU Research Grant JCUS/003/2011/IS, a grant from the Bill & Melinda Gates Foundation through the Grand Challenges Explorations Initiative (Grant Number: OPP1032125), and T-BOP PTE LTD (http://www.t-bop.com).

References

1. Elkin, N.: How America Searches: Health and Wellness (2008)
2. Sarasohn-Kahn, J.: The Wisdom of Patients: Health Care Meets Online Social Media. California HealthCare Foundation iHeath Reports (2008)
3. Swan, M.: Emerging patient-driven health care models: an examination of health social networks, consumer personalized medicine and quantified self-tracking. Int. J. Environ. Res. Public Health **6**(2), 492–525 (2009)
4. Baeza-Yates, R., Ribeiro-Neto, B.: Modern Information Retrieval. Addison-Wesley, England (1999). doi:citeulike-article-id:6580677
5. Deerwester, S.C., Dumais, S.T., Landauer, T.K., Furnas, G.W., Harshman, R.A.: Indexing by latent semantic analysis. J. Am. Soc. Inf. Sci. **41**, 391–407 (1990)
6. Sarasohn-Kahn, J.: The Wisdom of Patients: Health Care Meets Online Social Media. California HealthCare Foundation iHeath Reports (April 2008)
7. Spertus, E., Sahami, M., Buyukkokten, O.: Evaluating similarity measures: a large-scale study in the Orkut social network. In: Grossman, R.L., Bayardo, R., Bennett, K., Vaidya, J. (eds.) Proceedings of the ACM SIGKDD International Conference on Knowledge Discovery and Data Mining, Chicago, IL, 2005. KDD-2005: 11th ACM SIGKDD International Conference on Knowledge Discovery and Data Mining, pp. 678–684 (2005)
8. Deshpande, M., Karypis, G.: Item-based top-N recommendation algorithms. ACM Trans. Inf. Syst. **22**(1), 143–177 (2004)
9. Speer, R., Havasi, C., Lieberman, H.: AnalogySpace: reducing the dimensionality of common sense knowledge. In: AAAI'08: Proceedings of the 23rd National Conference on Artificial Intelligence, Chicago, Illinois, 2008, pp. 548–553. AAAI Press (2008). doi:citeulike-article-id:6873905

10. Singh, P., Lin, T., Mueller, E., Lim, G., Perkins, T., Zhu, W.: Open mind common sense: Knowledge acquisition from the general public (2002). doi:citeulike-article-id:311042
11. Turk, M., Pentland, A.: Eigenfaces for recognition. Cogn. Neurosci. **3**, 71–86 (1991)
12. Song, I., Dillon, D., Goh, T.J., Sung, M.: A health social network recommender system. In: Agents in Principle, Agents in Practice—14th International Conference, PRIMA 2011. Lecture Notes in Computer Science, pp 361-372. Springer (2011)
13. Song, I., Marsh, N.V.: Anonymous indexing of health conditions for a similarity measure. IEEE Trans. Inf. Technol. Biomed. **16**(4), 737–744 (2012)
14. DSM-IV: Diagnostic and Statistical Manual of Mental Disorders. American Psychiatric Association, Washington (1994)
15. ICD10: International Statistical Classification of Disease and Related Health. World Health Organization, Geneva (1992)
16. Klin, A., Lang, J., Cicchetti, D.V., Volkmar, F.R.: Brief report: Interrater reliability of clinical diagnosis and DSM-IV criteria for autistic disorder: results of the DSM-IV autism field trial. J. Autism Dev. Disord. **30**(2), 163–167 (2000)
17. Cortes, C., Vladimir, V.: Support-vector networks. Mach. Learn. **20**(3), 273–297 (1995)
18. Liu, H., Push, S.: Conceptnet: A practical commonsense reasoning toolkit. BT Technol. J. **22**, 211–226 (2004)

Chapter 7
Generating Explanations from Support Vector Machines for Psychological Classifications

Insu Song and Joachim Diederich

7.1 Introduction

In recent years, machine learning techniques, such as support vector machines (SVMs), have shown significant potential as aids to the practice of medicine and to psychiatric classification [1]. The application of machine learning techniques in psychiatric diagnosis has significant merit, because of the lack of standardized biological diagnostic tests. Conventionally, expert psychiatrists, consciously and unconsciously analyze the language of their patients for assessment purposes using diagnostic classification systems, such as DSM IV [9] and ICD-10 [12]. To provide a more objective clinical diagnosis, SVMs have been applied to conversations of patients and clinicians [1].

However, an explanation capability is crucial in security-sensitive domains, such as medical applications. Although support vector machines (SVMs) have shown superior performance in a range of classification and regression tasks, SVMs, like artificial neural networks (ANNs), lack an explanatory capability. There is a significant literature on obtaining human-comprehensible rules from SVMs and ANNs in order to explain how a decision was made or why a certain result was achieved [8].This chapter proposes a novel approach for SVM classifiers.

The experiments reported below describe a first attempt at generating textual and visual summaries for classification results. Learned model parameters are analyzed to select informative features, and filtering is applied to generate explanation terms by selecting subsets of more relevant and reliable features for

I. Song (✉)
School of Business and IT, James Cook University Australia, Singapore Campus,
Singapore 574421, Singapore
e-mail: insu.song@jcu.edu.au

J. Diederich
School of Information Technology and Electrical Engineering,
The University of Queensland, Brisbane, QLD 4072, Australia
e-mail: j.diederich@uq.edu.au

M. Lech et al. (eds.), *Mental Health Informatics*,
Studies in Computational Intelligence 491, DOI: 10.1007/978-3-642-38550-6_7,

each case. We show that this approach is applicable to both linear and non-linear SVM classifiers.

To generate textual explanations (a set of sentences), a natural language parser is used to convert each text sample into a set of basic concept-constructs called basic-sentences (verb-subject-object tuples) that make up the sentences. For example, a sentence "I have a dog that is 9 years old" can be decomposed into two basic-sentences: "I have a dog" and "The dog is 9 years old" In some literatures, such basic-sentences are also referred to as grounded predicates. Generated explanation terms are used to rank relevant basic-sentences using a similarity measure function, which is based on a common sense database called ConceptNet. The ranked basic-sentences are used to generate textual explanations of SVM classifications. Unlike previous text summarization approaches, the generated text summaries explain why the particular sample is classified as positive or negative.

The generated explanations (informative features) are consistent in the sense that an explanation term does not appear in two separate explanations which are used to explain inconsistent samples. We define the accuracy of the explanation terms and show that the accuracy of an SVM model is bounded by the accuracy of explanation terms. That is, the accuracy of an explanation term is always greater or equal to the accuracy of an SVM model.

7.2 Background

The following section provides a brief overview of the core techniques, focusing on support vector machines (SVMs), the significance of generating human-comprehensible explanations from SVMs, and what it means to explain the decision-making process of a machine learning system to a human user who may not be a domain expert or familiar with methods in information technology.

7.2.1 Support Vector Machines

Cortes and Vapnik [7] introduce Support Vector Machines (SVMs) which are a novel approach to machine learning. SVMs are based on the structural risk minimization principle in order to overcome the overfitting problems. SVMs generate the hypotheses out of the hypothesis space H of a learning system which approximately minimizes the bound on the actual error by controlling the empirical error using training samples and the complexity of the model using the VC-dimension of H. SVMs are universal learning systems [13]. In their basic form, SVMs learn maximal margin hyperplanes (linear threshold functions). A hyperplane can be defined by a weight vector w and a bias b:

$$\mathbf{w} \cdot \mathbf{x} + b = 0 \quad (7.1)$$

The corresponding threshold function for an input vector x is then given by:

$$f(\mathbf{x}) = sign(\mathbf{w} \cdot \mathbf{x} + b) \tag{7.2}$$

However, it is possible to learn polynomial classifiers, radial basis function (RBF) networks, and three or more layered neural networks by mapping input data $\mathbf{x}$ to some other (possibly infinite dimensional) feature space $\phi(\mathbf{x})$ and using kernel functions $K(\mathbf{x}_i, \mathbf{x}_j)$ to obtain dot products, $\phi(\mathbf{x}_i) \cdot \phi(\mathbf{x}_j)$, of feature vectors.

7.2.2 Explanations: The Foundation

To illustrate why it is important to add an explanation capability to SVMs, let us consider the case where medical doctors tell patients a diagnosis by use of test results or descriptions of symptoms. It is essential that doctors also use comprehensible explanations. The explanations may be via deductive arguments which include a list of patients' observed symptoms, a list of possible causes, and modus ponens (the rule of inference) for deriving the conclusion.

Thagard and Litt [19] illustrate several major approaches to generating explanations. The classical view is that explanations are deductive arguments that include background knowledge and inference rules, such as modus ponens. The inference rules allow the sequential application of if–then-else statements in order to justify explanatory targets. Whenever no precise knowledge is available, explanatory schemas or probabilistic rules can be used.

Cawsey [6] used a very simple definition of explanation: In general, explanations make knowledge clear to the hearers. Explanations is complete when the hearers are satisfied with the reply and understand the piece of knowledge. Hence, explanation is based on an information need.

7.2.3 Generating Explanations from SVMs

Much of the work that aims at providing an explanation capability to SVMs has focused on rule extraction techniques [8], following in the footsteps of efforts to obtain human-comprehensible rules from artificial neural networks (ANNs). One approach to classifying rule extraction methods is the translucency dimension which includes decompositional and pedagogical (or learning based) techniques as extremes [3].

The decompositional approach relies on the degree to which the internal representation of the ANN is accessible to the rule extraction technique. The basic strategy of decompositional techniques is to extract rules at the level of each individual hidden and output unit within the trained ANN. In general, decompositional rule extraction techniques incorporate some form of analysis of the weight vector and associated bias (threshold) of each unit in the trained ANN. Then, by treating each unit in the ANN as an isolated entity, decompositional techniques initially generate rules in which the antecedents and consequents are expressed in terms which are local to the unit from which they are derived.

In contrast to the decompositional approaches, the strategy of the pedagogical approaches is to view the trained ANN at the minimum possible level of granularity, i.e., as a single entity or alternatively as a black box. The focus is on finding rules that map the ANN inputs (i.e., the attribute-value pairs from the problem domain) directly to outputs [22]. In addition to these two main categories, Andrews et al. [3] also proposed a third category which they labeled as eclectic to accommodate those rule extraction techniques which incorporate elements of both the decompositional and pedagogical approaches.

7.2.4 Translucency and Explanation Quality Applied to Explanation Extraction from SVMs

It is very easy to illustrate the limitations of current studies on rule extraction from SVMs by use of an example: text classification. SVMs can achieve good performance with very simple text representation formats such as the "bag-of words" (BOW) technique. BOW methods use a document-term matrix such that rows are indexed by the documents and columns by the terms (e.g. words). SVMs allow the classification of texts of differing lengths; hence, document vectors may differ greatly in the number of elements.

A disadvantage of the BOW representation is that after successful classification, it may not be obvious what has been learned. For instance, an author or speaker may have a preference for certain topics and, as a result, an SVM trained on an authorship identification problem may, in reality, perform topic detection. In the case of author or speaker verification, this problem has led to various techniques to eliminate content from the BOW input, for instance, by replacing content words with lexical tags (categories).

Given the fact that it is not at all obvious what contributes to classification in the case of a BOW input representation, rule extraction from support vector machines is presented with a special opportunity. However, the number of features in input or support vectors can be very large given, the number of words that exist in a given natural language. While a combination of words constitutes meaning in a natural language, a BOW representation is based on words in isolation. This is a significant problem for rule quality: The antecedents in a rule include individual words completely out of context. As the set of antecedents includes completely unrelated words, human or semantic comprehensibility is low.

7.2.5 Evaluation of the Quality of Extracted Explanations

Rule extraction from neural networks adopted criteria for the quality of the extracted rules. The set of criteria for evaluating rule quality includes [3]:

1. accuracy
2. fidelity
3. consistency, and
4. comprehensibility of the extracted rules.

A rule set is considered to be accurate if it can correctly classify a set of previously unseen examples from the problem domain [22]. Similarly, a rule set is considered to display a high level of fidelity if it can mimic the behavior of the neural network from which it was extracted by capturing all of the information represented in the ANN. An extracted rule set is deemed to be consistent if, under differing training sessions, the neural network generates rule sets which produce the same classification of unseen examples. Finally, the comprehensibility of a rule set is determined by measuring the size of the rule set (in terms of the number of rules) and the number of antecedents per rule [22].

7.2.6 Overview

The reminder of this chapter summarizes experiments and their results: classification of text and image data, explanation generation for classification results, and technical details of methods with statistical analysis on the model parameters that are generated for depression poems. Then, in Sect. 7.5, we show how explanation terms can be used to generate textual summaries of the classification results.

7.3 Experimental Evaluation

Figure 7.1b shows how our method can be used to provide explanation assisted Fig. 7.1a illustrates an overview of our approach of generating explanations for psychological assessments using Support Vector Machines (SVMs). Explanation terms are extracted from assessment documents using both SVM models and classification results. Figassessment of autism and other mental health issues. For example, the explanations can highlight the main issues that were used to differentiate autism cases from normal cases.

7.3.1 Methodology: Explanation Term Generation

A preliminary study was undertaken on generating explanations of classification results of depression poems, online text messages, autism descriptions, facial expressions, and facial palsy. Poems were obtained from the Internet (Poetry-America.com) and comprise a total of 76 poems: 56 depression poems and 20

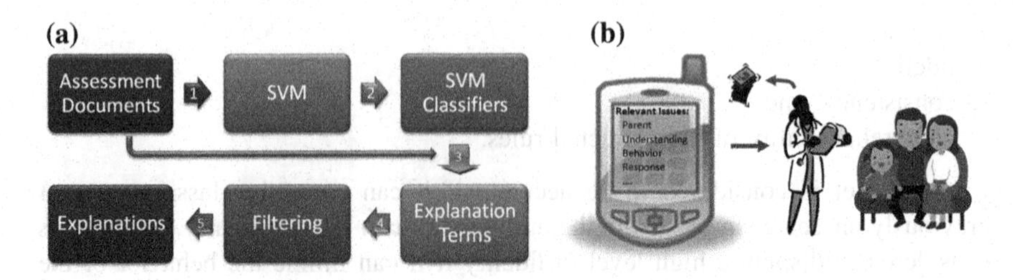

Fig. 7.1 **a** Illustrates the overall process of generating textual explanations to classification results. **b** Shows an example use of the explanation method, where a clinician make use of textual explanations to previous or current mental assessments, such as Autism. Mobile devices, such as smart phones, can be used to record interview questions and provide on the spot classification and explanations, resulting in more objective mental health assessments

funny poems. The online text messages were obtained from Usenet news groups and comprise a total of 350 sentences: 297 open questions and 53 closed questions. The autism descriptions were obtained from autism forums (http://www.autism-pdd.net) and ADHD (Attention Deficit Hyperactivity Disorder) forums (http://www.addforums.com) where parents discuss problems of their children. The autism data comprise a total of 200 descriptions: 100 autism descriptions and 100 ADHD descriptions.

For the text data sets, the resulting text documents are represented as attribute-value vectors (bag of words representation) where each distinct word corresponds to a feature whose value is the frequency of the word in the text sample: a text document is represented as a feature vector $\mathbf{x} = (x_{1,}., x_{j,} \ldots, x_L)$ where x_j is the jth feature. Values were transformed with regard to the length of the sample. For the poem and autism data sets, functional words were removed, and each word was converted into its lemma form (its base form without inflections). In addition, words that were not present in ConceptNet [16][1] were removed. For the question data set, all words were used. In summary, input vectors for machine learning consist of attributes (the words used in the sample) and values (the transformed frequency of the words). Outputs are depression versus funny, open question versus closed question, and autism versus ADHD, that is, binary decision tasks were learned. Clearly, the expressive power of the resulting explanations is limited by this bag-of-words representation.

For LOO (leave-one-out) cross validation, 76, 350, and 200 SVM models were generated using the linear kernel for the poem, online message, and autism text data sets, respectively. Thus, each model was used to classify one document. An SVM model is defined by support vectors x_i and associated parameters. The decision value of a text sample (represented as a feature vector x) is then obtained as follows:

[1] Used ConceptNet v2.1 from the Common Sense Computing Initiative at the MIT Media Lab (http://csc.media.mit.edu).

$$d(x) = w \cdot \phi(x) + b = \sum_{i \in SV} \alpha_i y_i K(x_i, x) + b \tag{7.3}$$

where $\mathbf{x}_i$ are support vectors and $\mathbf{x}$ is the feature vector, α_i are Lagrangian multipliers, y_i are the labels (+1, −1) of the support vectors, and b is the offset. The support vectors and the Lagrangian multipliers can be found by solving a quadratic programming problem. A popular setup of an SVM quadratic programming problem that allows some classification errors in the solution [7] is shown below:

$$\begin{gathered} \min\left(\frac{1}{2}w^T w + C\sum_{i=1}^{l}\xi_i\right) \\ \text{subject to: } y_i(w^T\phi(x_i) + b) \geq 1 - \xi_i, \quad \xi_i \geq 0 \end{gathered} \tag{7.4}$$

where C is the penalty for errors and ξ_i are slack variables for allowing errors. This particular formula isn't important here. The important thing is that the antecedent of the rule of inference is $d(x) \geq 0$. That is, if $d(x) \geq 0$, then the feature vector x is positive or else negative. Unlike previous rule extraction approaches, for each sample x, we formulate textual summaries to explain why $d(x) \geq 0$ or $d(x) < 0$. We start with generating an explanation (a set of explanation terms) for each classification result. An explanation term is a selected feature that is considered to be informative in explaining why $d(x) \geq 0$ or $d(x) < 0$. For text documents, an explanation term can be a word. For image data, an explanation term can be a region in the image. In Sect. 7.5, we extend this method to generate textual summaries. Features are filtered according to their sensitivity and contributions to the decision value $d(x)$ with respect to a reference point $\mathbf{C} = (c_1, c_2, \ldots, c_\mathrm{L})$ in the input space. We define three types of explanations for a classification result of a feature vector $\mathbf{x}$, where each explanations comprise a subset of features x_j of the feature vector $\mathbf{x} = (x_1, x_2, \ldots, x_\mathrm{L})$:

1. Explanation A comprising all the features x_j contributing to the decision value $d(\mathbf{x})$ with its feature value x_j greater than a reference point c_j:

   - For $d(\mathbf{x}) > 0$, this includes all the features x_j with positive contribution values $d(\mathbf{x})_j > 0$ and a feature value x_j greater than a reference point c_j.
   - For $d(\mathbf{x}) > 0$, this includes all the features x_j with negative contribution values $d(\mathbf{x})_j > 0$ and afeature value x_j greater than a reference point c_j.

2. Explanation B comprising top-N contributing features that are sufficient to classify the feature vector:

   - For $d(\mathbf{x}) > 0$, the sum of contributions of the features included in B is greater than the absolute value of the sum of all the negative contributions from the other features of the feature vector $\mathbf{x}$:

$$\sum_{x_i \in B} d(\mathbf{x})_i + \sum_{d(x)_j < 0} d(\mathbf{x})_j > 0 \tag{7.5}$$

where $d(\mathbf{x})_i > 0$ are the positive contributions of the ith features that are included in B and $d(\mathbf{x})_j < 0$ are the negative contributions.

3. Explanation C comprising top-N contributing features that also have their sensitivity values, $|\partial d(x)/\partial x_j|$, greater than a threshold value c.

Technical details on generating each explanation types are described in Sect. 7.4. This approach is clearly decompositional in nature: analysis of the model parameters to select informative features and selecting subsets of more relevant features. Figure 7.2 summaries the significance of each type of explanation. It plots sensitivity, contribution, and word rank of all features of the depression poem and autism-ADHD text data sets. It shows that sample features having higher ranking order (more frequent words in the text corpus) and higher sensitivity values tend to have larger absolute contribution values. This suggests that features having higher sensitivity values and higher ranking orders provide greater information in decision making than other features. It also shows that most of large contributions are made by more frequent words (high rank words).

In Sect. 7.4, we show that the accuracy of explanation terms is positively correlated with the accuracy of the SVM model: the accuracy of explanation terms increases as the accuracy of the SVM model increases.

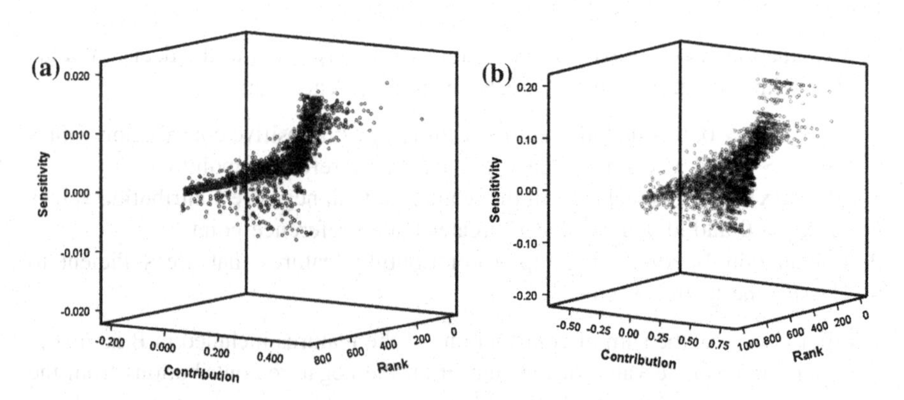

Fig. 7.2 Relationship between sensitivity, contribution (*deviation*), and word ranks. Each point is a feature that contributes to the decision of a feature vector. If a feature vector is a positive (*negative*) case, only the features having positive (*negative*) contributions are plotted. Rank 1 represents the most frequent feature (*vocabulary term*)

7.3.2 Results of Explanation Generation

7.3.2.1 Explanations of Text Classifications

Support vector machines trained on the poem and online text message data sets achieved accuracies of 94 and 98 %, respectively. The sensitivity values were adjusted manually to obtain reasonable numbers of explanation terms for Explanation type C. Sample explanations of a depressive poem are provided below:

1. Explanation A: dont (56 53), call (23 44), tear (21 50), know (17 18), fall (16 37), leave (16 35), cut (16 27), dark (14 24), sad (10 17), cold (10 16), face (10 20), smile (8 13), belong (5 7), letter (4 7), star (4 7), say (4 9), grave (2 3), shell (2 3), mold (1 2), useless (1 1).
2. Explanation B: dont (56 53), call (23 44), tear (21 50), **know** (17 18), fall (16 37), leave (16 35), cut (16 27), **dark** (14 24), **sad** (10 17), **cold** (10 16), **face** (10 20).
3. Explanation C: dont (56 53), call (23 44), tear (21 50), fall (16 37), leave (16 35), cut (16 27).

The numbers (*d*, *q*) in the brackets indicate relative contribution values *d* to the decision value *d*(x) and sensitivity values *q*, respectively. For positive cases, if the sensitivity value of a feature is positive, an increase in the frequency of the feature contributes to the decision value. Sensitivity filtering (Explanation C) eliminates some of less sensitive terms (bold-faced terms) from Explanation B. Sample explanations of a funny poem are provided below:

1. Explanation A: always (−45 −25), food (−34 −38), guy (−34 −38), come (−23 −32), name (−22 −24), good (−18 −21), im (−18 −25), same (−11 −14), best (−10 −11), go (−9 −13), mouth (−7 −8), true (−5 −5), happy (−2 −2), bad (−2 −2)
2. Explanation B: always (−45 −25), food (−34 −38), guy (−34 −38), come (−23 −32), name (−22 −24)
3. Explanation C: always (−45 −25), food (−34 −38), guy (−34 −38), come (−23 −32)

Explanation terms for negative cases have negative contribution values to derive $d(\mathbf{x})$ below zero. For negative cases, the sensitivity values of features must be negative. That is, the increase in the frequency of a feature contributes to deriving a decision value $d(\mathbf{x})$ below zero.

The explanations of the question data sets are much shorter (please note that this is a binary decision problem, that is, the task is to decide whether this is an open or closed question). Explanations for open questions (e.g., What is the dolphin species seen in most of Oceania?) are provided below:

1. Explanation A: what (539 166), species (34 8), most (15 3), in (7 2).
2. Explanation B: what (539 166)
3. Explanation C: what (539 166)

The corresponding explanations of a closed question (Do dolphins live shorter lives in captivity?) are provided here:

1. Explanation A: dolphins (−156 −35), live (−73 −15)
2. Explanation B: dolphins (−156 −35)
3. Explanation C: {empty}

As expected, questions are explained by the presence or absence of question words, such as what, why, or how.

Support vector machines trained on the autism description data set achieved an accuracy of 93 %. Sample explanations of the autism data are shown below with the sample sentences from the descriptions:

1. Explanation A for Autism description: speech (97 23), boy (91 45), begin (90 42), month (64 33), old (61 45), therapy (51 24), issue (50 23), train (48 22), school (39 25), year (38 26), soon (23 11), good (23 11), cream (10 4), improve (8 4), receive (4 1)
   - "…receives **speech therapy** in…. In recent **months**, his **speech** has **improved** greatly…. we will begin the… process very soon."
2. Explanation A for ADHD description: entire (−74 −24), sit (−60 −20), still (−52 −19), wall (−33 −11), pen (−26 −8), crayon (−21 −6), use (−11 −4), hour (−8 −2)
   - "…**uses** all the handwash to wash his hands, has drawn over his **entire wall** with **pen** and **crayon**…… and can **sit still** for **hours**."

The explanation terms are highlighted on the descriptions to provide contexts. This can assist clinicians to better understand their assessments more quickly during consultations as illustrated in Fig. 7.1b.

7.3.2.2 MPEG-7 Annotations for Explaining Facial Expressions and Facial Palsy

Figure 7.3 shows preliminary results of generating MPEG-7 annotations for explaining why a face image in a video frame is smiling or classified as facial palsy. The experiments shown here are to highlight that our method can be used to understand and verify learned classifier models. For example, in one attempt, we observed from the visual explanations that our classifier achieved good accuracy simply by learning different lightning conditions in the forehead facial regions. After equalizing image histograms, the SVM classifier learned more relevant features as shown in Fig. 7.3a, b, where it now highlights facial expression regions. For the expression classification task, we utilized facial expressions of one of the authors. The facial palsy images were obtained from Mater Misericordiae Health Services in Brisbane, which was previously used in [1]. Support vector

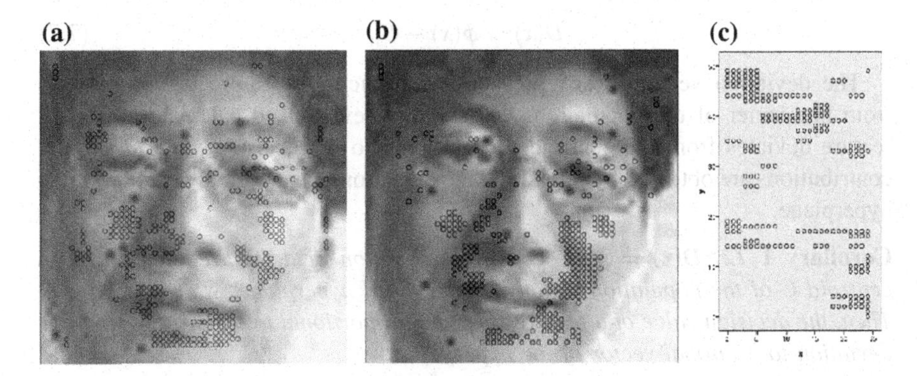

Fig. 7.3 Explaining image classification: (**a**) is a normal expression and (**b**) is a smiling expression. The dots represent explanation points. The last picture (c) shows explanation points of a facial palsy patient, highlighting the parts of face with deformities (the patient's face image removed for privacy reasons)

machines trained on the facial palsy images achieved an accuracy of 78 % and AUC of 0.84. For the facial expression classification task, the images were down sampled to 30 by 30 gray scale image features. For the facial palsy classification task, we used hamming distances between the right and left halves of each face image. Similarly to the method of generating textual explanations, learned SVM model parameters were analyzed to select informative features (pixels for facial expressions and hamming distances for facial palsy) and filtering was applied to select subsets of more relevant and reliable features. Further, the selected features were clustered to form explanation regions, which were then used to explain the classification of a region of interest in a video frame as shown in Fig. 7.3.

7.4 Generating Explanations from SVM Models

In order to calculate the contribution values of each feature of a feature vector **x**, we use the centroid **C** of the population as the reference point, which is estimated using the centroid $\mathbf{C}_{sv}$ of the support vectors:

$$C_{sv} = \frac{1}{Nsv} \sum_{i \in SV} \phi(x_i) \tag{7.6}$$

where N_{sv} is the number of support vectors. We use the estimated centroid as the neutral point where no clear decisions can be made. When the classifier is a non-linear classifier, we can identify K nearest support vectors in the input space and use them to form a centroid and a linear SVM model as shown in Fig. 7.9. Using the centroid, we can calculate the deviation of a feature vector x from the estimated population-centroid:

$$D(x) = \phi(x) - C_{sv} \tag{7.7}$$

The deviation vector **D(x)** represents how much the feature vector deviates from the center of the population. We use this deviation to calculate how each feature deviates from the centroid to contribute to the decision value $d(\mathbf{x})$. The contributions are obtained by projecting the deviation to the normal vector **w** of the hyperplane.

Corollary 1 *Let* $\mathbf{D(x)} = \phi(\mathbf{x}) - \mathbf{C}$ *be the deviation of a feature vector from a centroid C of the population which is on an SVM hyperplane*: $\mathbf{w} \cdot \phi(\mathrm{x}) + b = 0$. *Then, the decision value of a feature vector is proportional to the projection of the deviation to a normal vector of the hyperplane*:

$$d(x) = w \cdot D(x) = a \frac{w}{||w||} \cdot D(x) \tag{7.8}$$

where a is a positive constant.

Proof Since **C** is on the hyperplane, we have $\mathbf{w} \cdot \mathbf{C} = -b$. Then, we can obtain the decision value $d(\mathbf{x})$ using the deviation **D(x)** as follows:

$$\begin{aligned} d(x) &= w \cdot (D(x) + C) + b = w \cdot D(x) \\ &= a \frac{w}{||w||} \cdot D(x) \end{aligned}$$

where a = || **w** ||.

For linear SVMs, we can obtain the contributions of the j th feature as shown below:

Corollary 2 *Let* $\mathbf{D(x)} = \mathbf{x} - \mathbf{C}$ be *the deviation of a feature vector from a centroid* **C** *of the population which is on a linear SVM hyperplane:* $\mathbf{w} \cdot \mathbf{x} + b = 0$. Then, the deviation $\mathbf{D(x)}_j$ of the jth feature x_j of the feature vector **x** is proportional to the contribution $d(\mathbf{x})_j$ of the jth feature to the decision value $d(\mathbf{x}) = \mathbf{w} \cdot \mathbf{x} + b$:

$$d(x)_j = w_j D(x)_j \tag{7.9}$$

where w_j is the jth component of the weight vector **w**.

Proof According to Corollary 1, the decision value of the feature vector is proportional to the projection of the deviation to a normal vector of the hyperplane:

$$d(x) = w \cdot D(x)$$

If K is the linear kernel, we can estimate the contribution of each jth feature x_j as follows:

$$\begin{aligned} d(x)_j &= \sum_{i \in SV} \alpha_i y_i x_{i,j} (x_j - C_j) \\ &= (x_j - C_j) \sum_{i \in SV} \alpha_i y_i x_{i,j} \\ &= w_j D(x)_j \end{aligned} \tag{7.10}$$

where $w_j = \sum_{i \in SV} \alpha_i y_i x_{i,j}$ is the jth component of the weight vector $\mathbf{w}$.

For linear SVMs, we can directly use Corollary 2 to generate explanations. For non-linear classifiers with a convex hull, such as the elliptical decision boundary shown in Fig. 7.9, we can identify a subset of support vectors as reference points, which form both a centroid $\mathbf{C}'$ and a linear hyperplane with weight vector $\mathbf{w}'$ in the input space. The weight vector $\mathbf{w}'$ of the reference hyperplane can then be used with Corollary 2 to generate explanations for non-linear classifiers. The explanations will then be with respect to the reference point $\mathbf{C}'$. Figure 7.9 illustrates this procedure.

7.4.1 Consistency of Explanations

By the definition of Explanation A, if a sample is classified as positive (negative), a feature x_j is included in Explanation A as an explanation term only if $d(x)_j > 0$ ($d(x)_j < 0$), respectively. If a feature x_j is included in an explanation with $D(x)_j > 0$ for a sample, it means that the feature is included as an explanation term because the feature appears more frequently in the sample than the centroid C_j of the corresponding feature. Naturally then, for our explanations to be consistent, the same feature should not be included in an explanation to explain an opposite class. We now show that Explanations A, B, and C are consistent. Consistency is one of the criteria for evaluating rule quality [3].

Theorem 1 *Explanations A, B, and C are consistent: Given a feature vector x and its classification, let* A(**x**) *be its Explanation* A. *For Explanations* A, B, and C, *the following holds*:

1. If a feature vector $\mathbf{x}$ is classified as positive and $x_j \in A(\mathbf{x})$, then $x_j \notin A(\mathbf{x}')$ for all feature vectors $\mathbf{x}'$ that are classified as negative.
2. If a feature vector $\mathbf{x}$ is classified as negative and $x_j \in A(\mathbf{x})$, then $x_j \notin A(\mathbf{x}')$ for all feature vectors $\mathbf{x}'$ that are classified as positive.

Proof We first show that condition (1) holds. Suppose a sample x is classified as positive and x_j is included in Explanation A. By the definition of Explanation A, $d(\mathbf{x})_j = w_j \mathbf{D}(\mathbf{x})_j > 0$ and $\mathbf{D}(\mathbf{x})_j > 0$. Thus, $w_j > 0$. Now, we also suppose that the same feature x_j is included in Explanation A for a negative sample $\mathbf{x}'$, then by the definition of Explanation A $d(\mathbf{x}')_j = w_j \mathbf{D}(\mathbf{x}')_j < 0$ and $\mathbf{D}(\mathbf{x}')_j > 0$. This means that $w_j < 0$. Contradiction! Therefore, condition (1) must hold. Condition (2) can be proved similarly. B and C are subsets of A, and thus B and C are consistent as well.

The above theorem is applicable to certain non-linear SVM models by defining a reference point and a new linear hyperplane in the input space as shown in Fig. 7.9.

7.4.2 Accuracy of Explanation Terms

Another important criterion for evaluating rule quality is accuracy [3]. Conventionally, the accuracy of a binary classifier is defined as follows:

$$A_M = \frac{TP + TN}{N} \tag{7.11}$$

where N is the total number of samples, TP is the number of true-positive classification results, and TN is the number of true-negative classification results. Unfortunately, it is not that straightforward to define accuracy of explanation terms. However, we find that the following definition is the most natural way of defining the concept of accuracy of explanation terms. We start by defining the error rate of an explanation term.

Definition 1 The error rate of an explanation term x_j is the number of times that the term x_j is used incorrectly in an explanation divided by the number of explanations generated.

For Explanations A, B, and C, the number of times that x_j is used incorrectly in an explanation is the sum of the number of times that x_j is used for explaining negative samples with $d(x)_j > 0$ and the number of times that x_j is used for explaining positive samples with $d(x)_j > 0$.

Definition 2 Let M be a linear SVM model. Then, the empirical error rate $E_{j,M}$ of an explanation term x_j for Explanation A of the SVM model is

$$E_{j,M} = \frac{FP_{d(x)_j > 0} + FN_{d(x)_j < 0}}{N} \tag{7.12}$$

where N is the total number of samples, $FP_{d(x)j>0}$ is the number of explanations containing x_j for false-positive classification results, and $FN_{d(x)j<0}$ is the number of explanations containing x_j for false-negative classification results. The accuracy of an explanation term x_j is $A_{j,M} = 1 - E_{j,M}$.

With these definitions, we can now show that the accuracy of an SVM model is bounded by the accuracy of the explanation terms.

Theorem 2 *Let M be a linear SVM model. Then, the accuracy A_M of the SVM model M is bounded by the accuracy $A_{j,M}$ of explanation terms x_j:*

$$A_M \leq A_{j,M} \tag{7.13}$$

Proof The accuracy of an explanation term x_j is defined as follows:

$$\begin{aligned} A_{j,M} &= 1 - E_{j,M} \\ &= 1 - \frac{FP_{d(x)_j > 0} + FN_{d(x)_j < 0}}{N} \end{aligned}$$

By definition, the accuracy of the SVM model M is:

$$\begin{aligned} A_M &= \frac{TP + TN}{N} \\ &= 1 - \frac{FP + FN}{N} \end{aligned}$$

where FP is the number of false-positive classification results and FN is the number of false-negative results. By definition, the set of elements included in $FP_{d(x)j>0}$ ($FN_{d(x)j<0}$) is a subset of the set of elements included in FP (FN), respectively. Thus, $FP_{d(x)j>0} \leq FP$ and $FN_{d(x)j<0} \leq FN$. Furthermore, the following holds for any explanation term x_j:

$$\frac{FP_{d(x)_j > 0} + FN_{d(x)_j < 0}}{N} \leq \frac{FP + FN}{N}$$

Therefore, $A_M \leq A_{j,M}$ for any explanation term x_j.

7.4.2.1 Experimental Results of Accuracy of Explanation Terms

Figure 7.4 shows the distribution of the explanation term accuracy with the poem text data. As shown in Theorem 2, the minimum accuracy value is 0.94, which is the accuracy of the SVM model for the poem text data.

7.4.3 Fidelity of Explanations

In order to test the explanation capability of the explanation terms, we used all entries in Explanation A to generate a new feature set for the poem text data. By using explanation terms only for generating the new feature set, the vocabulary size was reduced from 1410 to 554. The ROC (Receiver Operating Curve) of the classification is shown in Fig. 7.5. Support vector machines trained on the new feature set achieved accuracy of 87 % and AUC (Area Under the Curve) of 0.89. The corresponding ROC (Receiver Operating Curve) is shown in Fig. 7.5.

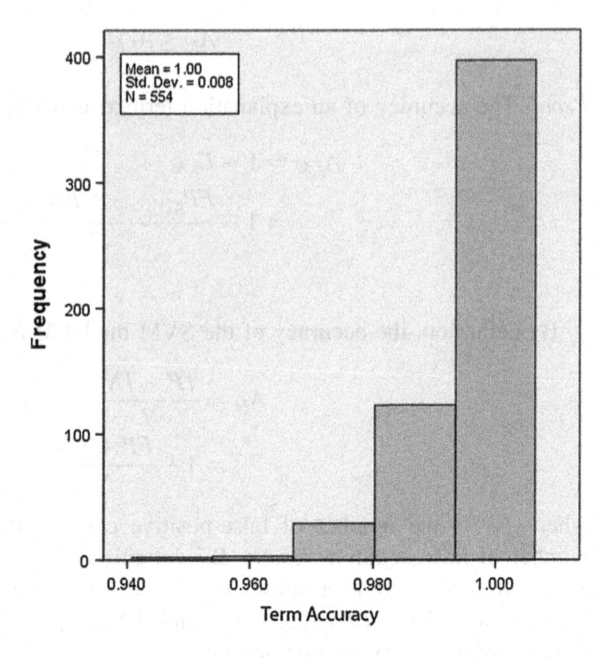

Fig. 7.4 Accuracy distribution of the explanation terms of the poem text data. The minimum accuracy value of the explanation terms is 0.94, which is the accuracy of the corresponding SVM model

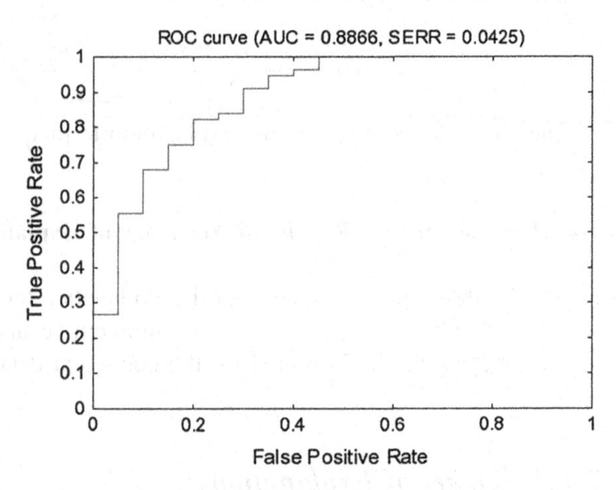

Fig. 7.5 True-positive rate versus false-positive rate of a linear support vector machine using an explanation-term vocabulary

The ROC curve for the SVM model using the full vocabulary is shown in Fig. 7.6. This clearly shows that the explanation terms are representative. That is, the explanations display a high level of fidelity because the explanation term set can mimic the behavior of the SVM model from which the explanation terms are extracted. According to Theorem 2, the explanation terms are also consistent. That is, if an explanation term is used to explain a positive case, then the same explanation term is not used to explain a negative case.

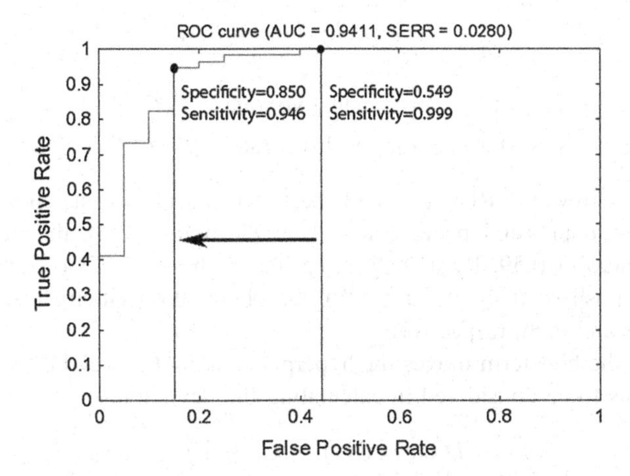

Fig. 7.6 ROC curve of the SVM model of the depression poem data. This illustrates that performance indicators can be adjusted by moving the threshold of the decision value. Specificity (recall) rate is increased from 0.549 to 0.85 by moving the decision threshold from 0 to 0.162. This effectively moves the estimated centroid of the population to produce more accurate explanations for imbalanced data

7.4.4 Optimization for Imbalanced Data

SVMs have been successfully applied to many text classification tasks, for example, to determine mental health problems using transcribed speech samples [1]. However, very few data sets are balanced: often the numbers of positive and negative samples are very different. This is particularly true for medical data, where few positive samples may be available, because positive cases are rare or there are a few negative examples only. For example, Autism assessment records contain very few negative cases, because most of the patients have been referred to Autism specialists by medical practitioners who have provided a first assessment. This imbalance can have a significant impact on the performance of machine learning algorithms. Furthermore, this imbalance in data can affect the accuracy of the estimated population-centroid. Thus explanations can become unreliable.

Various adjustments to SVMs have been proposed to improve the performance of SVMs with imbalanced data [14, 24]. Most of these approaches are based on the idea that the locations of the SVM hyperplanes can be adjusted to account for imbalanced data. One approach is to use separate cost factor measures C_+ and C_- for positive and negative samples, respectively [14]. Another approach is to adjust the bias term b [24] after n-fold cross validation to find optimal performance indicators.

In our experiments, we used the approach of adjusting the bias term b after n-fold cross validation. We used receiver-operating-curve (ROC) and balanced accuracy (BAC) as the heuristics for finding the optimal adjustment amount of the bias term.

$$BAC = \frac{specificity + sensitivity}{2}$$
$$specificity = \text{true\_negative\_rate} = P(O_-|L_-)$$
$$sensitivity = \text{true\_positive\_rate} = P(O_+|L_+)$$

Figure 7.6 shows the ROC curve of the LOO (leave-one-out) cross validation results for the depression poem data. Using the default bias, the model had a specificity value of 0.59. By adjusting the bias to b −0.17628 (i.e., a sample is classified as positive if $d(\mathbf{x}) > 0.17628$), we obtained specificity and sensitivity values of 0.8 and 0.96, respectively.

Adjusting the bias term moves the hyperplane along the weight vector **w**. This movement has to be considered in calculating the deviation.

$$D'(x) = \phi(x) - (C_{sv} + \Gamma) \tag{7.14}$$

where $\mathbf{\Gamma}$ is the adjustment to the centroid. If the adjustment value to the bias term is δ (i.e., a sample is classified as positive if $d(\mathbf{x}) > \delta$), $\mathbf{\Gamma}$ is defined as follows:

$$\Gamma = \delta \frac{w}{||w||^2} = \delta_n w \tag{7.15}$$

where $\delta_n = \delta/||\mathbf{w}||^2$ is the normalized adjustment of the hyperplane. For a hyperplane in the input space $\mathbf{w} \cdot \mathbf{x} + b = \delta$, we can estimate the contribution of each jth feature x_j as follows:

$$d'(x)_j = \sum_{i \in SV} \alpha_i y_i x_{i,j} (x_j - C_{sv,j} - \delta_n x_{i,j}) \tag{7.16}$$

7.4.5 Filtering Explanations with Sensitivity

Training a support vector machine for a data set of interest generates a hyperplane, which can be used to obtain the distance of a feature vector to the hyperplane. The distance is normal to the hyperplane. Thus, the importance of a feature can be measured as the rate of change of the distance with respect to the feature. This can be easily obtained for linear classifiers as follows:

$$\frac{\partial d(x)}{\partial x_j} = \sum_{i \in SV} \alpha_i y_i x_{i,j} = w_j \tag{7.17}$$

where $d(\mathbf{x})$ is the distance of a feature vector $\mathbf{x}$ to the hyperplane, x_j is the jth feature, x_i is the jth feature value of a support vector $\mathbf{x}_i$, and w_j is the jth component of the weight vector **w**.

Figure 7.7 shows a histogram of sensitivity and contribution values of features for the poem text data set. Greater population is centered at sensitivity value 0 and

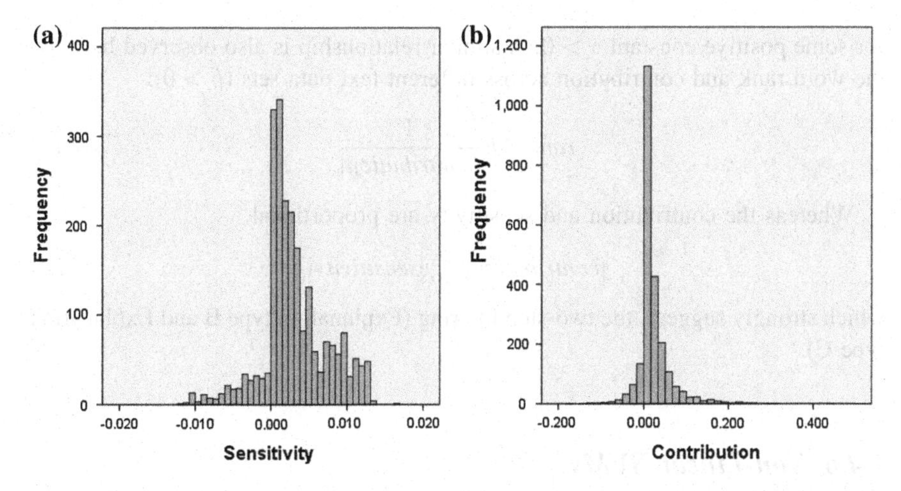

Fig. 7.7 Distribution of sensitivity and contribution values of the poem text data set

contribution value 0. This suggests that features having higher sensitivity and contribution values will provide more information on the decisions. It is also suggested in Fig. 7.2 that most of the contributions are made by terms with higher sensitivity values.

Figure 7.8 shows the relationship between word ranks and sensitivity values of sample features. Those with higher sensitivity values tend to have higher ranking order. The relationship between the word rank and sensitivity for the poem text data set can be summarized as follows:

$$rank \leq \alpha \frac{1}{|sensitivity|} \tag{7.18}$$

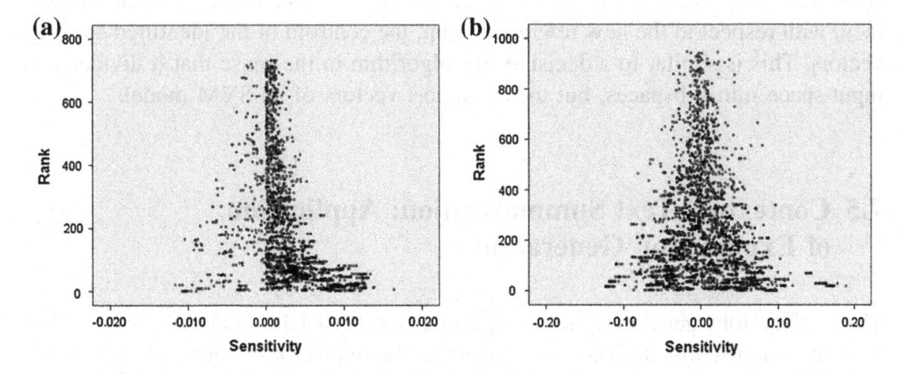

Fig. 7.8 Feature components with higher sensitivity values tend to have higher ranking orders (rank 1 is the highest rank and the most frequent term in the text corpus)

for some positive constant $\alpha > 0$. A similar relationship is also observed between the word rank and contribution across different text data sets ($\beta > 0$):

$$rank \leq \beta \frac{1}{|contribution|} \tag{7.19}$$

Whereas the contribution and sensitivity are proportional

$$|contribution| \leq \gamma |sensitivity| \tag{7.20}$$

which strongly suggests the two-step filtering (Explanation type B and Explanation type C).

7.4.6 Non-Linear SVMs

For non-linear cases, we have to obtain partial derivatives of kernels to obtain contribution and sensitivity values. As an example, let us consider the polynomial kernel: $K(\mathrm{x}_i \cdot \mathrm{x})_{\gamma,\mathrm{d}} = (\gamma \mathrm{x}_\mathrm{i} \cdot \mathrm{x} + r)^d$. The sensitivity of a feature x_j can be obtained as follows:

$$\begin{aligned} \frac{\partial d(x)}{\partial x_j} &= \sum_{i \in SV} \alpha_i y_i d\gamma x_{i,j} (\gamma x_i \cdot x + r)^{d-1} \\ &= d\gamma \sum_{i \in SV} \alpha_i y_i x_{i,j} K(x_i \cdot x)_{\gamma, d-1} \end{aligned} \tag{7.21}$$

This shows that the importance of the jth input feature for the hyperplane is a combination of other input features weighted by support vector elements. To avoid this, we can form a new hyperplane in the input space by identifying a subset of support vectors as shown in Fig. 7.9. The straight line in the figure is a newly formed hyperplane in the input space that separates the positive cases on the upper right side from the negative cases at the centre. The generated explanations are then, with respect to the new reference point, the centroid of the identified support vectors. This is similar to a decision tree algorithm in the sense that it divides the input space into subspaces, but using support vectors of an SVM model.

7.5 Contextual Text Summarization: Application of Explanation Generation

The explanations generated provide the relevance of each feature for a particular case. We can use this information to measure the relevance of each part of the text data to generate a textual summary with regard to a classification result. Unlike previous text summarization approaches, the textual summaries generated by the

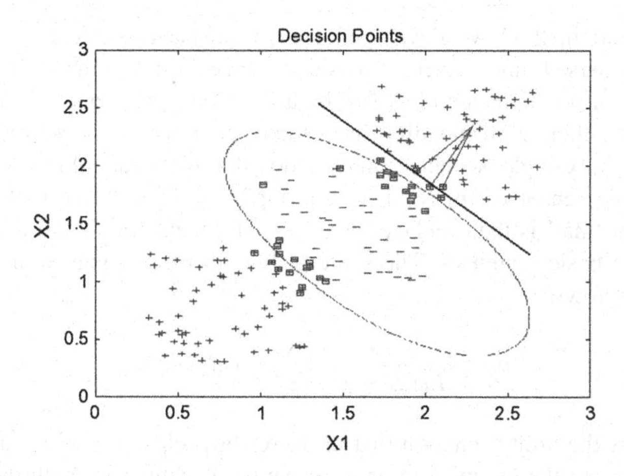

Fig. 7.9 K-NN (*nearest neighbour*) method of identifying a subset of support vectors (*square points*) to generate explanations for a convex non-linear decision boundary. In the figure, a positive data point at the upper right hand side is associated with the three nearest support vectors, and its distance to the centroid of the support vectors is used as an explanation. The support vectors form both a centroid and a new hyperplane in the input space

approach explained in this chapter aims at explaining why the particular sample is classified as positive or negative.

We start with a simple approach to generating a textual summary. The first method is scoring each sentence in a sample, using the explanation terms generated for the sample. In this approach, each sentence is given a score by determining contributions made by parts of the sentences. The score for the *k*th sentence in a sample text is defined as follows:

$$s_k = \frac{1}{|S_k||E|}\sum_{j\in X}\sum_{t\in S_k\cap E} u_j(t)d(x)_j q(x)_j \quad (7.22)$$

where *j* is a term included in explanation *X*, S_k is a set of terms in the *k*th sentence, *E* is the set of all explanation terms for the model, $u_j(t)$ is the utility function that measures how close the term *t* in $S_k \cap E$ is to term *j*, *d*(x) is the amount of contribution of the feature *j*, and $q(x)_j$ is the sensitivity of the feature *j*. The text summary is then generated by selecting a subset of sentences from the text using the scores as relevance measures. The ConceptNet analogy space [16] is used as the utility function. The following example shows similarity values for $j =$ 'frustration':

- u_j (end) = 0.269967456035
- u_j (miss) = 0.75678954875
- u_j (cry) = 0.599278222108
- u_j (tear) = 0.168901775853

The second method we developed uses more basic elements of text. Each sentence is parsed into a set of basic-sentences (verb-subject-object tuples). Antecedents of pronouns are identified by using ConceptNet and the pronouns are replaced with their corresponding antecedents to improve readability of basic-sentences. For example, sentence I have a dog that is 9 years old" is decomposed into two basic sentences: p_1 = "I have a dog" and p_2 = "That is 9 years old". The pronoun 'that' is then replaced with its antecedent 'dog'. We then calculate scores of the basic-sentences. The score of the *k*th basic-sentence in a sample is defined as follows:

$$p_k = \frac{1}{|P_k||E|}\sum_{j \in X}\sum_{t \in P_k \cap E} u_j(t)d(x)_j q(x)_j \tag{7.23}$$

where $u_j(t)$ is the utility function that measures how close the term t in the basic-sentence ρ_k is to the feature j in an explanation X. Similarly, with the sentence-based summarization, the text summary is generate0d by selecting a subset of the basic-sentences using the scores as relevance measures.

7.5.1 Result of Text Summarization

The following is an example sentence-based text summary that is generated for a depression poem by selecting the top-5 most relevant sentences out of a total of 28 sentences:

Time is the only one who can really tell us.
Then soon enough it will be the end I cry almost every minute.
So much pain so much hurt.
You may ask and look concerned wanting to know why I cry.

The following is a sample basic-sentence-based text summary generated for the same depression poem by selecting the top-5 most relevant basic-sentences:

It seem death. Death be me. You see. Who tell us

To evaluate the effectiveness of our approach, we measure similarities between each explanations and sentences of the poem text files. An explanation selects the top- K sentences that are most similar to the explanation. The error rate of this evaluation method is defined as follows:

$$error = \frac{\#\_of\_Incorrect\_Sentences\_selected\_in\_K}{K} \tag{7.24}$$

For an explanation of a depression (funny) poem, a sentence is incorrectly selected if the sentence is from a funny (depression) poem, respectively. This measures the degree to which an explanation of a depressing (funny) poem prefers sentences of depressing (funny) poems, respectively. This is an extrinsic method of measuring text summaries based on relevance prediction [5], which is shown to be less sensitive than and positively correlated with ROUGE scores [15]. This is also a multi-document summarization task, but significantly different from existing approaches, such as clustering based approaches [2]. Our approach automatically extracts key words that are relevant to a given classification task and uses the set of key words to measure similarities.

Figure 7.10 shows the average error rates of 18 explanations when the top-K most similar sentences were selected out of 90 sentences (45 sentences from depression poems and 45 sentences from funny poems). The left figure (the unit of K is 5) shows that the average error rate was below 35 % when fewer than the top 15 most similar sentences were selected using top 3 most contributing explanation terms. Figure 7.11 shows that within-class similarities (the average similarity between explanations and sentences of the same classes) are consistently better than between-class similarities (the average similarity between explanations and sentences of the different classes).

Similar performance is achieved by selecting the top-K documents that are most similar to an explanation: a below 35 % error rate when selecting fewer than 35 % of the total documents. This method can be used to recommend patients with similar assessments to specific doctors or social networking communities.

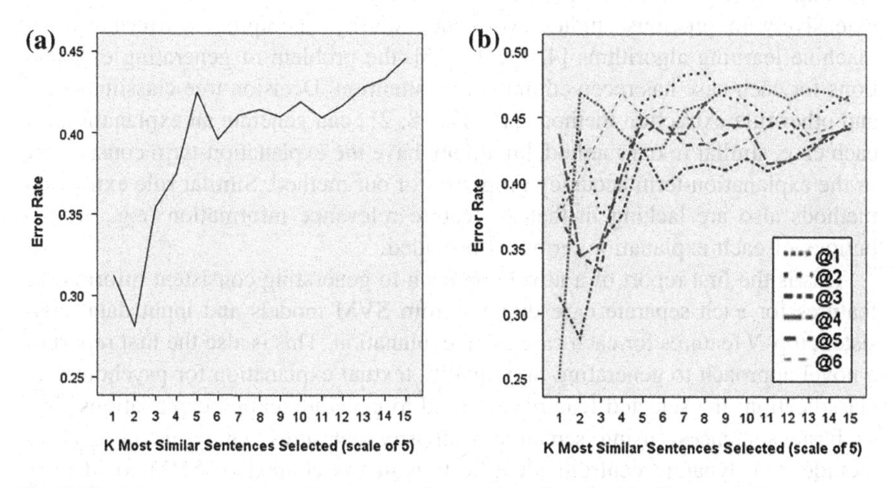

Fig. 7.10 Average error rates of text summaries are plotted against the K most similar sentences that were selected for each explanation. The figure on the left shows the average error rate when the top-3 most contributing terms are used to measure similarities. The figure on the right shows the average error rates for each of the top-N most contributing terms used ranging from 1 to 6 terms

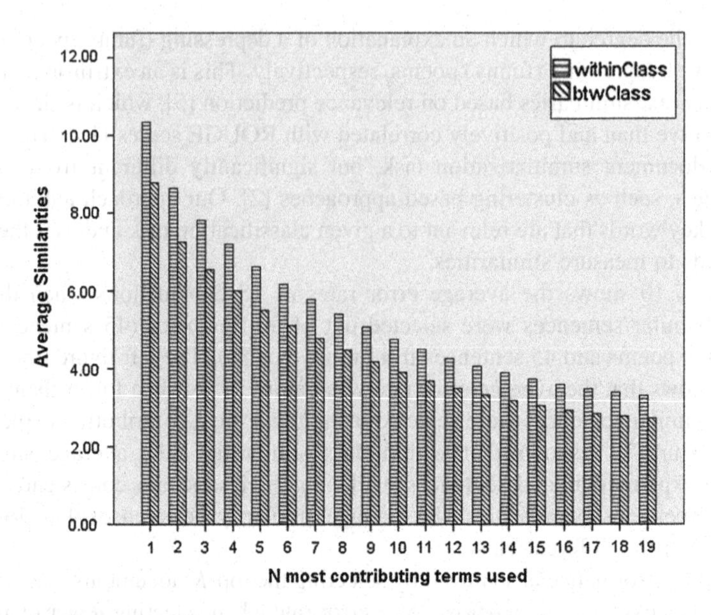

Fig. 7.11 Average similarity measures between explanations and poem sentences when the top-N most contributing terms are used to measure the similarities

7.6 Discussion and Future Work

Although feature selection and sensitivity analysis methods have been explored extensively in previous studies as to their ability to improve performance of machine learning algorithms [4, 11, 23, 25], the problem of generating explanations for each case has received much less attention. Decision tree classifiers [20] and other rule extraction methods [10, 17, 18, 21] can generate an explanation for each case, similar to our method, but do not have the explanation-term consistency or the explanation-term accuracy properties of our method. Similar rule extraction methods also are lacking in that no feature relevance information (e.g., contributions of each explanation terms) is provided.

This is the first report of a novel approach to generating consistent informative features for each separate case directly from SVM models and input data: consistent top-*N* features for each case as an explanation. This is also the first report of a novel approach to generating high-quality textual explanation for psychological classification: the selected features are used to generate textual explanations (sets of basic sentences) using semantic similarity measures. Other novel features include: (1) dynamic centroid identification in the context of SVM to identify reference points; and (2) selecting informative features for each case by combining both contributions and sensitivity.

We have shown that the explanations are consistent, accurate, display a high level of fidelity, and can generate text summaries with error rates below 35 %.

Furthermore, we have shown that the approach can be applied to imbalanced data by adjusting SVM hyperplanes and centroids using ROC curves. This approach can be easily extended to non-linear classifiers, for example, by combining with K-NN to identify support vectors that can be used as explanation reference points.

To improve the comprehensibility of explanations, the input text is parsed into basic-sentences and scored using a common sense database called ConceptNet. We believe that this approach overcomes the subjective nature of measuring comprehensibility. Considerable further research is required. The approach of extracting pieces of knowledge using machine learning in explaining psychiatric assessments has the potential to improve the usability of machine learning techniques in the medical and security domains. This approach can be further expanded by using alternative feature representations of text data sets, such as concept terms or semantic terms. There is massive potential for incorporating these sophisticated information extraction technologies within psychiatry and in medicine more generally.

References

1. Afifi, N., Diederich, J., Shanableh, T.: Computational methods for the detection of facial palsy. J. Telemedicine Telecare **12**(SUPPL. 3), 3–7 (2006)
2. Aliguliyev, R.M.: Clustering techniques and discrete particle swarm optimization algorithm for multi-document summarization. Comput. Intell. **26**(4), 420–448 (2010)
3. Andrews, R., Diederich, J., Tickle, A.B.: Survey and critique of techniques for extracting rules from trained artificial neural networks. Knowl.-Based Syst. **8**(6), 373–389 (1995)
4. Blum, A.L., Langley, P.: Selection of relevant features and examples in machine learning. Artif. Intell. **97**(1–2), 245–271 (1997). doi:10.1016/s0004-3702(97)00063-5
5. Dorr, B.J., Monz, C., President, S., Schwartz, R., Zajic, D.: A methodology for extrinsic evaluation of text summarization: Does rouge correlate?. In: Proceedings of the ACL 2005. pp. 1–8
6. Cawsey, A.: Explanation and interaction: the computer generation of explanatory dialogues. MIT Press, USA (1993)
7. Cortes, C., Vladimir, V.: Support-vector networks. Mach. Learn. **20**(3), 273–297 (1995)
8. Diederich, J.: Rule extraction from support vector machines: An introduction. Stud. Comput. Intell. **80** (2008)
9. DSM-IV: Diagnostic and statistical manual of mental disorders. American Psychiatric Association (1994)
10. Féraud, R., Clérot, F.: A methodology to explain neural network classification. Neural Networks **15**(2), 237–246 (2002)
11. Guyon, I., Elisseeff, A.: An introduction to variable and feature selection. J Mach Learn Res **3**, 1157–1182 (2003)
12. ICD10: International Statistical Classification of Disease and Related Health. World Health Organization, Geneva (1992)
13. Joachims, T.: Making Large-Scale SVM Learning Practical. Advances in Kernel Methods—Support Vector Learning. MIT-Press, NY (1999)
14. Morik, K., Brockhausen, P., Joachims, T.: Combining statistical learning with a knowledge-based approach—A case study in intensive care monitoring. In: Proceedings of the 16th International Conference on Machine Learning, Morgan Kaufmann Publishers, USA (1999)

15. Lin, C.-Y.: Rouge: A package for automatic evaluation of summaries. In: Proceedings of ACL workshop on Text Summarization Branches Out (2004)
16. Liu, H., Push, S.: Conceptnet: A practical commonsense reasoning toolkit. BT Technol. J. **22**, 211–226 (2004)
17. Menkovski, V., Christou, I.T., Efremidis, S.: Oblique decision trees using embedded support vector machines in classifier ensembles (2008)
18. Mitra, S., Hayashi, Y.: Neuro-fuzzy rule generation: survey in soft computing framework. IEEE Trans. Neural Networks **11**(3), 748–768 (2000)
19. Thagard, P., Little, A.: Models of Scientific Explanation. Cambridge University Press, Cambridge (2007)
20. Quinlan, J.R.: Induction of decision trees. Mach. Learn. **1**(1), 81–106 (1986)
21. Setiono, R., Liu, H.: A connectionist approach to generating oblique decision trees. IEEE Trans. Syst. Man Cybern. B Cybern. **29**(3), 440–444 (1999)
22. Tickle, A.B., Andrews, R., Golea, M., Diederich, J.: The truth will come to light: directions and challenges in extracting the knowledge embedded within trained artificial neural networks. IEEE Trans. Neural Networks **9**(6), 1057–1068 (1998)
23. Yan, J., Liu, N., Yan, S., Yang, Q., Fan, W., Wei, W., Chen, Z.: Trace-oriented feature analysis for large-scale text data dimension reduction. IEEE Trans. Knowl. Data Eng. **23**(7), 1103–1117 (2011). doi:10.1109/tkde.2010.34
24. Yang, Y: A study on thresholding strategies for text categorization. In: Proceedings of the 24th Annual International ACM SIGIR Conference on Research and Development in Information Retrieval, New Orleans, LA, 9–13 September 2001, pp. 137–145 (2001)
25. Yu, L., Liu, H.: Efficient feature selection via analysis of relevance and redundancy. J Mach Learn Res **5**, 1205–1224 (2004)

Chapter 8
An Alternative Method of Analysis in the Absence of Control Group

Felin, Joachim Diederich and Insu Song

8.1 Introduction

Control groups have played an important part in experimental psychology. There are, however, situations where control groups are hard to find or finding an appropriate one would be costly. In clinical settings, such as hospitals and private practices, data available for research are usually obtained from patients with mental illnesses or defects. In order to draw reasonable conclusions, however, control groups are often seen to be necessary as comparisons. Finding "healthy" controls in hospitals and private practices is not easily done given practitioners' lack of resources and time. It would, therefore, be advantageous in situations like these to have an alternative method of analysis that allows practitioners to conduct a valid study even when control groups are not available. Although such a method of analysis may appear foreign in the field of psychology, it is not so in the machine learning community.

Felin
School of Business and IT, James Cook University Australia, Brisbane, Australia
e-mail: felin@my.jcu.edu.au

J. Diederich (✉)
School of Information Technology and Electrical Engineering,
The University of Queensland, Brisbane Q4072, Australia
e-mail: j.diederich@uq.edu.au

I. Song
School of Business and IT, James Cook University, Singapore Campus,
Singapore 574421, Singapore
e-mail: insu.song@jcu.edu.au

M. Lech et al. (eds.), *Mental Health Informatics*,
Studies in Computational Intelligence 491, DOI: 10.1007/978-3-642-38550-6_8,

8.2 Background

8.2.1 Support Vector Machine

Researchers in the machine learning community have been using a popular method, called Support Vector Machine (SVM), for data analysis and classification. SVM was developed from statistical learning theory by Vapnik and colleagues [10]. It is called a "supervised" machine learning method because the data entered into the programs are labelled. In other words, the machine learns to distinguish one category from the other based on labelled examples [16]. When new data are entered, the machine uses the knowledge from the previous examples it has learned in order to classify the new data into categories. Each of the data entered is represented as a dot (vector) in the input space. A maximum margin classifier, such as SVM, separates the data by finding the best boundary decision through an algorithm. The boundary decision, or the hyperplane, maximises the margin between the nearest points to it on each side or support vectors [10, 21]. Sometimes, this hyperplane is in the form of a simple straight line, although, in most cases, it is non-linear. When the hyperplane is non-linear, an appropriate algorithm function or a kernel can be chosen to map the input space (where data are entered) into a feature space [18].

The method described above is for a regular two-class SVM. It requires the input of both positive and negative examples. In other words, data from both target group and control group are needed. In order to overcome the problem posited in the example earlier, a one-class SVM can be used, so named because it utilises data from only one class of the population, the target group. This can be done with different methods, and one such method is the Schölkopf methodology. It starts off in a similar manner to two-class SVM, with each data point represented by a vector on the input space, except that all the data are obtained from one group only. Here, the origin is treated as the only member of the second class. Then, from the origin, a circle is intermittently drawn to include other points to form the second class [19]. Thus, one starts from the origin and moves farther out in a circular pattern to finally stop at a point determined by an algorithm. In other words, the origin and the data close to it are treated as anomalies and, therefore, belong to a different group from the rest of the data. The principle of finding a boundary decision that maximises the margin still applies [25].

8.2.2 Applications and Performance of SVM in Different Areas of Research

As a classification tool, SVM has also been used in many different areas of research outside of the machine learning community, from text classification [14] to cancer cell detection [11]. When compared with other popular machine learning method, SVM was found to perform better at text classification [14]. SVM is also useful in research areas outside of the machine learning community. For example, SVM has been used to identify seizures from non-seizures in newborn babies, achieving a good detection rate of 89.2 % with one false seizure detection per hour [22]. In the field of clinical psychology, SVM has been used to diagnose mental illness by analysing transcribed interviews of patients with schizophrenia. Ex-Ray, which utilises SVM to analyse data, managed to attain a classification accuracy of 77 % in categorising schizophrenics from non-schizophrenics [7].

Like two-class SVM, one-class SVM has also been shown to have good classification accuracy in different areas. It was used to predict protein–protein interaction with an accuracy of about 80 % and detect asbestos in building material with an accuracy of 88 % [17]. When compared with other classifier methods, such as k-means and MLP, one-class SVM was found to have better classification accuracy in diagnosing abnormal ECG [24].

8.3 Comparing SVM to TLC and CLANG in Diagnosing Schizophrenic Speech

In order to examine the viability of SVM as an alternative method of analysis in clinical psychology, this chapter examines the performance of SVM and one-class SVM in diagnosing schizophrenic speech. Although two-class SVM has previously been used in analysing schizophrenic speech [7, 23], to the knowledge of the authors, no study has been done to examine the viability of one-class SVM in the proposed method. Schizophrenia diagnosis has been a contentious issue since its birth. From Krapelin to Bleuler, to the development of the Diagnostic and Statistical Manual of Mental Disorder (DSM), the concept of schizophrenia has changed and so has its diagnostic criteria. Presently, DSM-IV is the most widely used tool to diagnose mental illnesses, including schizophrenia. One of the symptoms of schizophrenia according to DSM-IV is disorganised speech. As a negative symptom of schizophrenia, disorganised speech is difficult to diagnose. Moller [20] suggested that this is because negative symptoms are less obvious than positive symptoms, such as hallucinations. Even the definition and nature of disorganised speech are contentious. Some view it as a product of disorganised thought, while others argue that it is the result of language deficits [5, 15]. How it is defined is important, since it affects the underlying defect measured in the assessments [8]. Disorganised speech has also often been referred to as formal thought disorder. Its characteristics include making up words, incomprehensible speech, and incoherence [15]. Schizophrenic patients often reply to questions in an irrelevant manner or their replies to spontaneous speech are brief, and when the replies are long enough, they convey little information [8]. Due to its unclear processes, there are a wide variety of assessments designed to evaluate disorganised speech. This study will look at two of these assessments, the Thought, Language and Communication (TLC) scale and the Clinical Language Disorder Rating Scale (CLANG).

TLC was developed by Andreasen [2]. It consists of 18 items and was found to have good interrater reliability [2, 3], and one study found a measure of interrater reliability of 0.87 [4]. The authors tried to ensure good reliability by describing thought disorder as language behaviour that can be openly observed and, therefore, assessed. Patients' speech was evaluated using the 18 items provided in the scale after interview. Another measure that assesses disorganised speech is CLANG, which consists of three subscales and 17 items. It was validated with participants from the Hong Kong Chinese population and was found to have a global interrater reliability of 0.88 for the whole scale and 0.93, 0.83, 0.88 for the three subscales [6].

8.3.1 Hypotheses

In order to test the effectiveness of SVM and one-class SVM, this paper compares them with TLC and CLANG in diagnosing schizophrenic speech. It was, therefore, hypothesised that SVM would be just as good at diagnosing schizophrenic speech as TLC and CLANG. Secondly, it was also hypothesised that one-class SVM would give similar performance to two-class SVM in diagnosing schizophrenic speech. It was thought that people with higher educational qualifications, such as university students or university graduates, would have better command of language. Since language deficit is an integral part of schizophrenia diagnosis, this study used participants in the control condition with similar educational backgrounds to those of the schizophrenia patients. Hence, it was predicted that the new control group in this study would be a better match to the schizophrenia group than the one found in Tilaka's study [23].

8.3.2 Method

8.3.2.1 Participants

Participants were recruited from advertisements and email by the first author. The control group in this study consisted of 11 females and one male, with ages ranging from 23 to 64 years old (M = 43.8. SD = 15.2). The 27 participants comprising the schizophrenia group were obtained from the data collected by Tilaka and colleagues, with 13 males and 14 females, age ranging from 21 to 62 years old (M = 43.9, SD = 10.5). The control group in that study consisted of 11 females and 16 males, with age ranging from 18 to 37 years old (M = 22.6, SD = 4.8)13. Table 8.1 summarises the characteristics of the participants for the three groups. It shows that compared to the Tilaka control group, the participants in the new control group were better matched to the schizophrenia group in terms of age, years of formal education and the language they most often used at home.

Table 8.1 Comparison of participants' characteristics

	New control group (n = 12)	Schizophrenia group (n = 27)	Tilaka control group (n = 27)
Age range (years)	23–64	21–62	18–37
Mean	43.8	43.9	22.6
Standard deviation	15.2	10.5	4.8
Years of education (%)			
>13	0	0	7
11–13	33.3	37	93
7–10	58.3	40	0
1–6	8.33	23	0
Language often used at home (%)			
English	25	26	86
Other	75	74	14

8.3.2.2 Materials

A list of questions was provided to guide the interviews. It was the same list that was used in the Tilaka study [23]. All interviews were recorded using voice recorders and a computer software program as back ups. Gift vouchers worth $5 each were presented to acknowledge participation.

8.3.2.3 TLC

This study also used TLC and CLANG to evaluate schizophrenia speech. TLC consists of 18 items: poverty of speech, poverty of content, pressure of speech, distractible speech, tangentially, derailment, incoherence, illogicality, clanging, neologisms, word approximations, circumstantiality, loss of goal, perseveration, echolalia, blocking, stilted speech, and self-reference. Each of the 18 items is rated on a 5-point Likert scale (0–4) or 4-point Likert scale (0–3), depending on the individual items, ranging from no TLC disorder, to mild, moderate, severe and extreme TLC disorder [2].

8.3.2.4 CLANG

CLANG, on the other hand, has three subscales (semantic, syntactic, and production) and 17 items (excess phonetic association, abnormal syntactic structure, excessive syntactic constraints, lack of normal semantic association, referential failures, discourse failure, excessive level of details, lack of details, aprosodic speech, abnormal prosody, pragmatic disorder, disfluency, dysarthria, poverty of speech, pressure of speech, neologisms, and paraphasic error). It is rated on a 4-point Likert scale, ranging from normal (0), mild [1], moderate [2], and severe [3, 6].

8.3.2.5 SVM

SVM analysis was performed using Ex-Ray. Ex-Ray is a computer program that uses SVM, a maximum margin classifier, to analyse data. An expert in the area performed the analysis. Features of the transcript were extracted. In this case, the order and context of the words was insignificant. Each word in the transcribed interviews was represented as a vector in the input space. The value of the vector was obtained from the frequency of the word in the transcript. The resulting output was classification of speech as either schizophrenic or nonschizophrenic [7].

8.3.2.6 Procedure

Before the study commenced, ethical clearance was obtained from the James Cook University Human Research Ethics Committee. Data from 27 schizophrenia patients and 27 control groups were obtained from the study done by Tilaka and colleagues with their permission. The 12 participants in the control group were approached by the first author who briefly described the study and gave each participant an Information Sheet with more details. Upon agreement, participants then signed the Informed Consent Form. This was followed by a 20-minute interview in which participants were asked simple questions designed to keep them talking. All interviews were recorded using a voice recorder and a computer software application as back-ups. Participants were informed of the necessity to audio-tape the interviews and gave their consent by ticking a box in the Informed Consent Form. At the end of the interview, the participants were thanked for their participations and rewarded with $5 Starbucks vouchers.

The 12 interviews were then transcribed by the interviewer for SVM analysis and rated using TLC and CLANG (audio interviews) by another person with a degree in Psychology (Honours), so as to avoid bias. The rater was unaware of the group to which the participants belonged. Prior to doing the rating, the rater had familiarised herself with the rating guidelines provided in their article by the authors of the scales [2, 6]. Ratings were made for each of the items before a global rating was produced. One of the interviews went on for about 28 min; so, the rater was advised to omit the last 6 min or so from the rating process.

8.3.3 Results

Receiver Operating Characteristic (ROC) curve was used to analyse the accuracy rate of each measure, and z-score analysis was done to test for significant differences. A ROC curve shows the trade off between false positive rate or sensitivity (X-axis) and true positive rate or 1-specificity (Y-axis). It is often used in medicine for diagnostic testing. False positive occurs when data are classified as positive when in actuality, they are negative. False positive rate is obtained by incorrectly

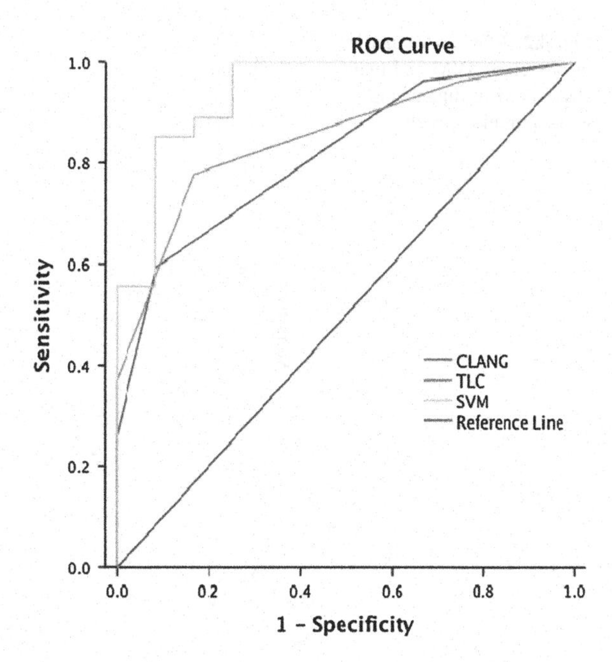

Fig. 8.1 ROC curve analysis of TLC, CLANG and SVM in diagnosing schizophrenic speech

classified negatives divided by total negatives. True positive, on the other hand, occurs when positive data are classified as positive. True positive rate is calculated from correctly classified positives divided by total positives. The point (0, 1) signifies 100 % correct classification, while a line in the middle that divides the graph equally (reference line) is representative of randomly guessing the classification [9]. The Area Under the Curve (AUC) value lies between 0 to 1 and is representative of the probability of accurate classification [12]. The closer the value is to 1, the better the measurement. A value of 0.5 (reference line) represents random guessing.

Figure 8.1 shows the ROC curve analysis of the three measures. It was found that TLC, CLANG, and Ex-Ray had Area Under the Curve (AUC) values of 0.849, 0.816, and 0.941, respectively. This was much higher than what would be the result of random guessing. In order to test if the difference in the AUC values was statistically significant, a z-score analysis was performed, using the following formula provided by Hanley and McNeil [13]:

$$z = \frac{A_1 - A_2}{\sqrt{SE_1^2 + SE_2^2 - 2rSE_1SE_2}} \tag{8.1}$$

where, A = area under the curve, r = correlation between A1 and A2 and SE = standard error. A z-score analysis showed that there was no significant difference between SVM and TLC in diagnosing schizophrenic speech, $z = -1.18$, $p > 0.05$. Similarly, there was also no significant difference between SVM and CLANG in diagnosing schizophrenic speech, $z = -1.45$, $p > 0.05$.

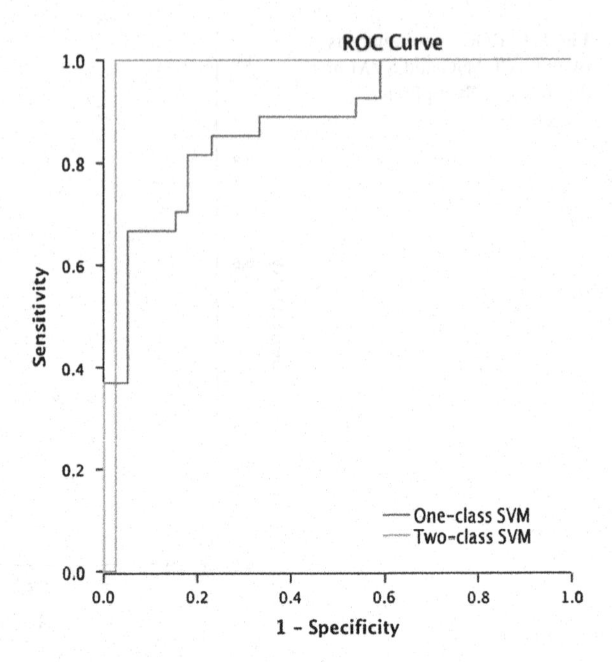

Fig. 8.2 ROC curve analysis of one-class SVM and two-class SVM in diagnosing schizophrenic speech

Figure 8.2 shows the ROC curve analysis of one-class and two-class SVM in differentiating between schizophrenics and non-schizophrenics. AUC values of one-class SVM and two-class SVM were found to be 0.875 and 0.974 respectively. There was, however, no significant difference between one-class SVM and two-class SVM in diagnosing schizophrenic speech, $z = -1.33$, $p > 0.05$.

Lastly, it was also found that there was no difference between the new control group and the one found in Tilaka's study, $z = 0.632$, $p > 0.05$.

8.4 Discussion

The results support the hypothesis that SVM is as good as TLC and CLANG in diagnosing schizophrenic speech. The second hypothesis, that one-class SVM is comparable to two-class SVM, was also supported. However, compared to the Tilaka control group, the new control group was not a better match to the schizophrenic group, since there was no significant difference between them.

The results show that SVM was as good as TLC and CLANG in diagnosing schizophrenic speech. This was to be expected, given the performance of SVM in other classification tasks mentioned in the beginning of the paper. Diederich [10], for example, found that SVM had a classification accuracy of 77 % in differentiating schizophrenics from non-schizophrenics. This result might prove to be useful in aiding clinicians in making diagnosis in mental health. Although TLC and CLANG were shown to be good measures of disorganised speech, they are still subject to the raters' judgments. An objective measure would erase the problem of bias and any possible influence of race, culture, and gender in the measurements. While the expertise of clinicians is still necessary to make a complete diagnosis—the diagnosis of schizophrenia, for example, is not based on disorganised speech only—SVM can aid in the making of that decision. That is not to say that SVM is without its drawbacks. In order to perform the SVM analysis, one needs to know the correct parameters to enter into the system. This might require the help of an expert or someone familiar with the system. Also, SVM does not take into account the context and order of words, even though this might affect diagnosis. Moreover, since analysis is done by computers, factors such as prosody and articulation difficulties, which are taken into consideration in TLC and CLANG, are not included in SVM.

Having established that SVM with data from schizophrenia and control groups was able to diagnose schizophrenic speech well, the study then compared two-class SVM with one-class SVM. The results show that one-class SVM was as good as two-class SVM in diagnosing schizophrenics based on speech. In other words, one-class SVM is a viable option as a method of analysis when control groups are not available. It is a feasible solution to the problem posited in the introduction above. This was in no way an attempt to remove control groups from their place in psychology or to undermine their importance, but an effort to provide researchers with an effective alternative should the need arise.

Lastly, the study also found that there was no significant difference between the new control group and Tilaka's, suggesting that the former was not a better match for the schizophrenia group. It might be that characteristics of the participants did not affect the result. It might also be the effect of the small sample size, since the sample size for the new control group was considerably smaller than for the older one. Therefore, while such characteristics as educational qualification might make a difference, the smaller sample size might hamper this effect, leading to a non-significant result. In fact, this was one of the limitations of the study, since getting participants with lower educational qualifications who spoke basic English proved to be challenging.

There are also other limitations to this study. Since the research used data from a previous study by Tilaka and colleagues [1], the interviews of participants in the schizophrenic and control groups were done by different people. Although the interviewers used the same list of questions provided, there might have been differences in style. Using data of schizophrenia patients from another study was unavoidable in this case due to restrictions, such as time and access in interviewing schizophrenic patients. Another limitation of the study lies in the inexperience of the independent rater in using TLC and CLANG. Although the authors of the scales provided guidelines, it would have been better if the rater was an experienced clinician familiar with characteristics of disorganised speech. These limitations, however, do not completely take away the result that SVM is a viable research tool and that one-class SVM can be an efficient alternative method of analysis. Future research should, therefore, be done incorporating improvements to compensate for these limitations, in order to confirm the results of this study. Future research can also look to expand this study by investigating the use of SVM in diagnosing other mental illnesses.

8.5 Conclusion

In conclusion, this study has demonstrated that SVM was as good as other measurements, such as TLC and CLANG, in diagnosing disorganised speech. It has also shown that in the absence of control groups, one-class SVM can be a viable option. The control group in this study, however, was not a better match than the previous one found in Tilaka. It is hoped that the availability of an alternative method of analysis without compromising results will help researchers and clinicians to better understand schizophrenia and other mental illnesses.

References

1. Tilaka, A.D., Diederich, J., Song, I., Teoh, A.: Automated Method for Diagnosing Speech and Language Dysfunction in Schizophrenia Mental Health Informatics. Springer, Berlin (2011)
2. Andreasen, N.C.: Scale for the assessment of thought, language, and communication (TLC). Schizophr. Bull. **12**(3), 473–482 (1986)
3. Andreasen, N.C., Grove, W.M.: Thought, language, and communication in schizophrenia: Diagnosis and prognosis. Schizophr. Bull. **12**(3), 348–359 (1986). doi:10.1093/schbul/12.3.348
4. Andreou, C., Bozikas, V.P., Papouliakos, I., Kosmidis, M.H., Garyfallos, G., Karavatos, A., Nimatoudis, I.: Factor structure of the Greek translation of the scale for the assessment of thought, language and communication. Aust. N. Z. J. Psychiatry **42**(7), 636–642 (2008)
5. Barrera, A., McKenna, P.J., Berrios, G.E.: Formal thought disorder in schizophrenia: An executive or a semantic deficit? Anglais **35**(1), 121–132 (2005)
6. Chen, E.Y.H., Lam, L.C.W., Kan, C.S., Chan, C.K.Y., Kwok, C.L., Nguyen, D.G.H., Chen, R.Y.L.: Language disorganisation in schizophrenia: Validation and assessment with a new clinical rating instrument. Hong Kong J. Psychiatry **6**(1), 4–13 (1996)
7. Diederich, J., Al-Ajmi, A., Yellowlees, P.: Ex-ray: Data mining and mental health. Appl. Soft Comput. J. **7**(3), 923–928 (2007)
8. Docherty, N.M.: Cognitive impairments and disordered speech in schizophrenia: Thought disorder, disorganization, and communication failure perspectives. J. Abnorm. Psychol. **114**(2), 269–278 (2005)
9. Fawcett, T.: An introduction to ROC analysis. Pattern Recogn. Lett. **27**(8), 861–874 (2006)
10. Furey, T.S., Cristianini, N., Duffy, N., Bednarski, D.W., Schummer, M., Haussler, D.: Support vector machine classification and validation of cancer tissue samples using microarray expression data. Bioinformatics **16**(10), 906–914 (2000)
11. Guan, P., Huang, D., He, M., Zhou, B.: Lung cancer gene expression database analysis incorporating prior knowledge with support vector machine-based classification method. J. Exp. Clin. Cancer Res. **28**(1), 103 (2009)
12. Hanley, J.A., McNeil, B.J.: The meaning and use of the area under a receiver operating characteristic (ROC) curve. Radiology **143**(1), 29–36 (1982)

13. Hanley, J.A., McNeil, B.J.: A method of comparing the areas under receiver operating characteristic curves derived from the same cases. Radiology **148**(3), 839–843 (1983)
14. Joachims, T.: Making large-scale SVM learning practical advances in Kernel methods: Support vector learning. MIT-Press, Cambridge (1999)
15. Kerns, J.G., Berenbaum, H.: Cognitive impairments associated with formal thought disorder in people with schizophrenia. J. Abnorm. Psychol. **111**(2), 211–224 (2002)
16. Kotsiantis, S.B.: Supervised machine learning: A review of classification techniques. Informatica **31**(3), 249–268 (2007)
17. Kuba, H., Hotta, K., Takahashi, H., Köppen, M., Kasabov, N., Coghill, G.: Automatic particle detection and counting by one-class SVM from microscope image In: Advances in Neuro-Information Processing, Lecture Notes in Computer Science, vol 5507, pp. 361–368. Springer, Berlin, Heidelberg (2009)
18. LaConte, S., Strother, S., Cherkassky, V., Anderson, J., Hu, X.: Support vector machines for temporal classification of block design fMRI data. NeuroImage **26**(2), 317–329 (2005)
19. Manevitz, L., Yousef, M.: One-class document classification via neural networks. Neurocomputing **70**(7–9), 1466–1481 (2007)
20. Moller, H.-J.: Clinical evaluation of negative symptoms in schizophrenia. European Psychiatry **22**(6), 380–386 (2007)
21. Shen, H., Wang, L., Liu, Y., Hu, D.: Discriminative analysis of resting-state functional connectivity patterns of schizophrenia using low dimensional embedding of fMRI. NeuroImage **49**(4), 3110–3121 (2010)
22. Temko, A., Thomas, E., Marnane, W., Lightbody, G., Boylan, G.: EEG-based neonatal seizure detection with support vector machines. Clin. Neurophysiol. **122**(3), 463–473 (2010)
23. Tilaka, A.D.: A comparison of observer-rated scales with an automated method for speech disorder in schizophrenia. 4th year thesis, James Cook University, Singapore (2010)
24. Woo, S.-M., Lee, H.-J., Kang, B.-J., Ban, S.-W.: ECG signal monitoring using one-class support vector machine. In: Proceedings of the 9th WSEAS International Conference on Applications of Electrical Engineering, Penang, Malaysia, World Scientific and Engineering Academy and Society (WSEAS), pp. 132–137 (2010)
25. Zhang, R., Zhang, S., Muthuraman, S., Jiang, J.: One class support vector machine for anomaly detection in the communication network performance data. In: Proceedings of the 5th conference on Applied electromagnetics, wireless and optical communications, Tenerife, Canary Islands, Spain, World Scientific and Engineering Academy and Society (WSEAS) (2007)

Chapter 9
Stress and Emotion Recognition Using Acoustic Speech Analysis

Margaret Lech and Ling He

9.1 Stress and Emotion

Both stress and emotion represent psycho-physiological states involving characteristic somatic and autonomic responses [38]. Stress is a psychological and biological term characterized by loss of ability to appropriately respond to difficult emotional and physical conditions that can be either real or imagined. Stress is characterized by subjective strain, dysfunctional physiological activity, and deterioration of performance [14, 67]. Typical stress symptoms include fast heart rate, increased adrenaline production, difficulty to cope with relatively simple tasks, feeling of strain and exhaustion and inability to concentrate. Stress may be induced by external factors such as workload, noise, vibration or sleep loss or by internal factors such as fatigue [63]. Existing stress detection and classification research uses most frequently stress categories based on different levels of difficulties that a given person has to deal with [63].

Emotion comprises of complex psychological and physiological phenomena including person's state of mind and the way an individual interacts with the environment. Generally, emotion involves: physiological arousal, expressive behaviors, and conscious experience [19]. Emotion is closely related to the state called mood. Unlike emotion which is a short-term (minutes–hours) psycho-physiological state, mood is a relatively long lasting emotional state (hours–weeks). In contrast to simple emotions, moods are less specific, less intense, and less likely to be triggered by a particular stimulus or event [50].

M. Lech (✉)
School of Electrical and Computer Engineering, RMIT University,
Melbourne 3001, Australia
e-mail: margaret.lech@rmit.edu.au

L. He
Department of Medical Informatics and Engineering, School of Electrical Engineering and Information, Sichuan University, Chengdu, China

M. Lech et al. (eds.), *Mental Health Informatics*,
Studies in Computational Intelligence 491, DOI: 10.1007/978-3-642-38550-6_9,

The importance of emotional state and stress level analysis has been well recognized as a key factor in the Mental Status Examination. Most common, prototypical emotion models postulate that humans evolved to experience a limited number of prototypical emotions (e.g. happiness, anger, fear, sadness, etc.). Each discrete emotion is assumed to be an effect of a specific pattern of peripheral physiological response associated with a dedicated central nervous system representation [29, 49]. The more complex emotional experiences can then be understood as an effect of weighted integration of different brain regions to generate a range of emotional valence.

Dynamics of emotions and the individual abilities to cope with different emotional states provide important cues in the diagnosis of mental disorders such as depression, near suicidal state and schizophrenia. The Diagnostic and Statistical Manual Disorder criteria for major depressive episode for example, include both affective and somatic symptoms, but greater importance is placed on the affective symptoms. An individual cannot meet the criteria for major depressive episode without admitting to experience prolonged episodes of sadness, reduced pleasure or interest in formerly pleasurable activities (2002, [29]).

Classical methods of diagnosis of mental disorders such as depression or schizophrenia are predominantly based on interviews with patients and their families as well as patient's responses to diagnostic questionnaires. The main disadvantage of these methods is their subjective nature, as well as the fact that they rely on the honesty and motivation of a patient to participate in the diagnostic process. Sometimes people suffering from mental ill-health are not willing or able to participate in such examinations. There are also reports pointing to the misunderstanding of the items in questinarries due to the complexity of wording. The computational methods of speech analysis examined in this chapter eliminates these drawbacks and provide a potential for an objective assessment of patient's emotional state.

Experiment described in this Chapter describe a new computational methodology allowing to asses patien't emotional state and stress level in an objective way. The methodology calculates a set of acoustic parameters (features) from the speech signal of a person being examined and provides diagnosis throught the classification process which determines the diagnostic class (type of emotion or stress level) to which the speech signal belongs.

9.2 How Stress and Emotion are Expressed in Speech?

The speech signal plays an essential role in human communication. Apart from conveying linguistic information between speakers, it also carries a large paralinguistic content including vital information about speakers' emotions, personalities, attitudes, feelings, levels of stress and current mental states [60]. As a biological signal, speech contains medical-diagnostic as well as psychological-behavioral information. In comparison with other biological signals, such as for example ecg or eeg, the diagnostic potential of speech signals has been very much under-utilized.

One of the reasons for this under-utilization is a combination of high complexity and a wide bandwidth, which makes speech analysis relatively more complex than analysis of other more often used bio-signals.

9.3 Rationale for Stress and Emotion Classification in Speech

The validity of an automatic stress and emotion detection in speech is based on the assumption that the stress or emotional state of a person affects the acoustic qualities of speech, and therefore the presence (or absence) of stress or emotion can be detected through an analysis of changes in the acoustical properties of speech. Moreover, a comparative analysis of acoustic characteristics of speech can provide information about the stress level or type of emotion expressed through speech.

9.3.1 Physiological Basis

Physiological bases for stress and emotion detection in speech result from a number of studies [58, 59, 66, 67] conducted since the 1980s. These studies are showing that the effect of emotion on speech is due to tonic activation in the somatic nervous system and sympathetic as well as parasympathetic activation of the autonomic nervous system (ANS). For example, the temporal rate of articulation and the frequency range of vowels can be modified by changes in the timing of the muscle movements controlling the motion amplitudes of the articulatory structures. These muscles are driven by the limbic control system. Direct sympathetic and parasympathetic effects controlled by the limbic system can indirectly influence speech production by introducing changes in respiration and phonation. These could affect the fundamental frequency of vocal cords vibration (pitch) by causing changes in subglottal air pressure and vocal cord tension. Other ANS-caused effects such as mucus secretion may significantly alter speech characteristics during intense emotional arousal.

Psychomotor disturbances appear to be the unique and defining symptoms of mood disorders. There is evidence that symptoms of psychomotor agitation or retardation may actually precede the full onset of a depressive episode and that these symptoms may be used to detect and monitor mental illness [13].

9.3.2 *Acoustic Properties of Speech as Indicators of Stress or Emotion*

Emotional speech recognition aims to automatically identify the emotional or physical state of a person from his or her voice. The emotional state of a speaker produces what is called the emotional aspect of speech. Although, the emotional aspect of speech does not alter its linguistic contents, it is an important factor in human communication because it provides feedback information about physiological and mental state of a speaker.

9.4 Previous Work on Emotion Recognition in Speech

The concept of an automatic emotion recognition was introduced in mid-1980s when a number of authors suggested the use of statistical properties of speech in automatic emotion recognition [66]. In the early 1990s, progress in the computer technology made it possible to design new, advanced feature extraction and classification algorithms. Computers became capable of processing large number of data provided by hours of audio-visual recordings within practical computational times. These improvements opened ways to practical implementations of new important applications of the speech technology including speech and speaker recognition and more recently, stress and emotion recognition.

9.4.1 *Speech Data used in Previous Studies*

The value and quality of numerical simulations of stress and emotion recognition in speech depend on how representative are the data sets used to generate models of emotions. Generations of truly representative data sets has proven to be very difficult and therefore, only very few high quality data sets are available at present.

The majority of studies use acted speech where, actors or randomly chosen participants are reading the same text or a list of words with different emotions. The classification results based on acted emotions are generally high. For example, Ref.[74] reported an average correct classification rate of 89 % for four classes (neutral, angry, loud and Lombard) from the SUSAS Simulated Stress domain and TEO-critical bands (TEO-CB) features. Wagner et al. [69], reported average classification rates of 75 % when using prosodic acoustic features and the EPSaT corpus comprising recordings of professional actors reading short dates and numbers with 10 different emotional states: content, encouraging, friendly, happy, interested, angry, anxious, bored, frustrated, and sad.

In most cases, natural speech recordings with spontaneously generated emotions show lower classification rates than speech with acted emotions. For example, Ref. [40] used the natural speech corpus HMIHY containing 5,690 complete human–computer dialogues. This corpus was developed at AT & T Research Labs using a system that enables AT & T customers to interact verbally with an automated agent over the phone. Seven emotional labels: positive/neutral, somewhat frustrated, very frustrated, somewhat angry, very angry, somewhat other negative, very other negative were classified using acoustic, prosodic, lexical, pragmatic, and contextual features. The classification accuracy ranged from 73 to 79 %. [74] reported classification rates of about 98 % while using a part of the SUSAS corpus containing two classes; actual stress and neutral speech. These results were produced using TEO-CB features. In the later study, [69] reported classification results using the German Aibo emotion corpus containing spontaneous emotional speech collected from 51 children (31 girls/20 boys) interacting with Sony's robot dog Aibo. The emotional states used in the classification process where angry, emphatic (as a pre-stage to anger), motherese (or baby-talk) and neutral. The MFCC features were classified using the SVM and HMM methods. The results ranged from 43.5 to 56.5 %. As indicated in the above few examples, the difficulty of drawing definite conclusions arises from the fact that numbers of classes and class definitions vary between different data sets. The emotional arousal is not normalized and often not specified across different data. There is also an issue of affect subjectivity which adds additional complexity to the process of generating emotional speech corpora.

9.4.2 Studies using Classical Features: Fundamental Frequency F_0, Formants, Energy and Rhythm

Classical features including fundamental frequency, formants, energy and rhythm, were widely exploited in stress and emotion recognition, because they were related to the arousal level of emotions. It was observed that, the prosodic features of speech produced under stress and emotion vary from the features under neutral condition. The most often occurring changes include changes in the utterance duration, decrease or increase of pitch, shift of formants and different levels of energy. For instance [71], have shown that anger is characterized by higher level of energy and pitch, compare to other four emotions: disgust, fear, joy and sadness. It was also shown that male speakers express anger with a slower speech rate than a female under the similar conditions [37]. Liscombe et al. [39], extracted 10 statistical analyzed prosodic features from energy, formants, pitch and the ratio of voiced frames to identify the non-negative (positive and neutral) and negative emotions. Similar feature sets were applied in [4, 8, 17, 25, 28, 32, 36, 75] to identify different kinds of emotions.

Generally, the statistic prosodic features did not achieve high affection recognition accuracy. This could be partially attributed to the difficulty to calculate accurate values of the prosodic features, as well as the difficulty to estimate parameters based on the speaker and text independent basis. For example, a widely known autocorrelation method for pitch estimation was shown to be very sensitive to the presence of noise leading to the interference from the first formant. The formants are most often calculated using linear prediction (LP) analysis. Like in the case of the fundamental frequency, the most often occurring problem related to the LP formants estimation is the false identification due to the noise. The rate of speech could potentially provide information of different emotions, but only assuming speaker dependency. Since the speech rate is strongly speaker-dependent, it generally does not provide consistent results in speaker-independent emotion classification. For instance, some speakers prefer express anger with an increasing speaking rhythm, though the others reduced the rate. These shortcomings as well as the fact that there are no universal consensus due to the speaker or textual dependency, limit the use of prosodic features (pitch, formants and rhythm) as efficient stress and emotion discriminates in speech. Due to the key importance of the feature extraction to the stress and emotion recognition, recent research efforts are predominantly focused on finding the right type of features and a large number of new approaches to the feature extraction have been proposed.

9.4.3 Studies Using Mel-Frequency Cepstral Coefficients

The Mel Frequency Cepstral Coefficients (MFCC) used widely in speech and speaker recognition provide signal characteristics based on the human auditory perception and usually lead to improved performance compare to features that don't take into account these characteristics. It has been therefore argued that feature extraction based on human auditory perception could also provide superior results in the cases of stress and emotion recognition. The MFCCs have been applied to the stress and emotion classification in speech [17, 28, 32, 33, 43, 75] leading to relatively moderate results.

New et al. [51, 52], applied the MFCCs to differentiate between six types of emotions (anger, disgust, fear, joy, sadness and surprise). The classification accuracy for six types of emotions using MFCC feature was 59 %, which was better than the linear coefficients linear prediction cepstral coefficients (LPCC) which achieved 56.1 % but not as good as 78 % of accuracy achieved by the proposed short time log frequency power coefficients.

Iliev et al. [27] applied MFCCs features of different orders to the glottal waveform and to speech signal to classify four emotions: happy, angry, sad, and neutral. The results indicated that the best performance was provided by the MFCC of order six for both glottal and speech signals, with the classification accuracy around 60 %. Clave et al. [8], applied feature vectors including pitch, jitter, shimmer, formants and MFCCs to detect fear-type emotions occurring during abnormal situations. The SAFE corpus was developed in this work, based on the fiction movies. The corpus contained recordings of both normal and abnormal situation in order to classify fear and neutral emotions. Despite the diversity of the data, the system obtained promising result with the correct recognition rate around 70 %. Yildirim et al. [72] used MFCCs features to detect three emotions (frustrated, polite and neutral) in children during spontaneous dialog interactions with computer characters. It was observed that MFCC features achieved the highest average correct classification rates, ranging from 66.4 to 70.6 % across genders and age groups, compared to other acoustic features: pitch frequency, root mean square energy, voicing and zero-crossing-rate. Zhou et al. [74] applied MFCC to do the pairwise stress classification using simulated (neutral, angry, loud and Lombard) and actual (neutral and actual) domain of SUSAS (Speech Under Simulated and Actual Stress) database. The results indicated that the proposed TEO based features achieved better recognition accuracy than the MFCC and pitch.

In general, most of the existing studies showed that the MFCCs achieve only moderate rates of correct emotion classification in speech.

9.4.4 Studies using TEO Based Features

Another important type of features proposed for emotion recognition by Zhou et al. [74] provides sensitivity to the number of additional harmonics and cross-harmonics in speech signal occurring due to additional sound sources generated by a non-linear air flow in the vocal tract. It is assumed that in the emotional state of stressed speech, the fast nonlinear air flow generates vortices located near the false vocal folds. The feature extraction method described in Ref. [74] uses the area under the normalized Teager energy (TEO) autocorrelation envelope. The correct classification rates for two classes neutral and stress were around 90 % which was higher than rates achieved using the fundamental frequency F_0 and MFCC. Similar results were obtained in Ref. [15], where the TEO features were used to classify four emotions (happy, sad, angry and neutral) in Mandarin speech. The results demonstrated superior performance of the TEO features when compared to the MFCC features. New et al. [51, 52], applied Teager energy operator (TEO) nonlinear frequency domain LFPC features (NFD-LFPC) and TEO nonlinear time domain LFPC features (NTD-LFPC). These features were tested using five stress levels. The results showed that the NFD-LFPC gave 86 % of the correct classification rates, while the NTD-LFPC provided 76 %. In the work by Torabi et al. [68], a combination of TEO, pitch and LFPC features was tested in simulated stress classification providing on average about 89 % of the correct classification rates. In Ref. [42], the TEO based features showed excellent performance in the detection of early symptoms of major depression in adolescent. The classification accuracy for female participants was 79 % and for male participants 87 %.

At present, the TEO based features appear to provide the highest correct classification rates for stress and emotion recognition in speed.

9.4.5 Studies Using Glottal Features

Several glottal features were studied as potential cues for emotion differentiation. It has been demonstrated that the glottal features show strong correlation with the emotional speech characteristics [20].

Moore et al. [47, 48] investigated the role of glottal features in the detection of the clinical depression, which is a mood or emotion disorder. The classification was based on the following glottal features: glottal timing (closed and open instants of glottis), glottal ratios (ratio of closing phase to opening phase, ratio of open phase to the total cycle, ratio of closed phase to the total cycle) and glottal shimmer. The glottal features showed very good performance when used in combination with prosodic features (fundamental frequency and formants) providing 89 % of correct classification rates for males and 92 % for females. Ozdas et al. [53] tested the slope of the glottal flow spectrum and achieved good accuracy of 85 % for the classification into depressed and near-term suicidal patients. Iliev et al. [26], applied glottal features representing glottal symmetry to classify happiness, anger and sadness, the classification performance varied between 48.96 and 82.29 % depending on the type of emotion. Low et al. [42], applied glottal time and frequency domain parameters to detect early symptoms of clinical depression in adolescents. The classification accuracy was up to 63 % for female and 72 % for male participants.

In general, the glottal features appear to provide relatively high classification rates however not as high as the rates provided by the TEO features.

9.4.6 Studies Investigating the Impact of Different Frequency Bands on Stress and Emotion Discrimination

Feature extraction based on limited frequency band could provide very useful data reduction increasing computational efficiency. Elimination of frequency bands that do not provide important emotion-characteristic information could also lead to improved classification rates. The majority of investigators placed high significance on the low frequency bands (0–1.5 k Hz) [5, 13, 66] and low significance on the high frequency bands. Although in Ref. [51, 52], the opposite was suggested. Recently, Hansen et al. [18] proposed a robust stressed detection method using weighted frequency sub-bands. A weighting scheme for all frequency bands was proposed with weights adaptively adjusted for individual speakers.

9.4.7 Shortcomings of Existing Studies

Majority of reviewed here works investigated only a limited number of specific features, The speech data bases and the emotional labels varied from study to study making a direct comparison very difficult. The experiments described in the following sections test and compare the performance of a large number of features. All features were tested in a consistent way using the same two classifiers and the same data sets representing natural, not acted speech.

9.5 Stress and Emotion Classification Experiments

9.5.1 Speech Data

The quality of data-driven stress and emotion recognition methods depends heavily on the data sets used to generate mathematical models of emotions, and the reliability of the subjective annotation method [49]. The process of generation of truly representative data sets has proven to be very difficult due to factors such as proper experimental design, environmental validity, ethics approvals, as well as the accuracy of the annotation process [9]. As a result, only very few high quality emotional speech data sets are available for research.

Two data sets containing natural (not acted) speech were used in this study: the Speech Under Simulated and Actual Stress (SUSAS) data and the Oregon Research Institute (ORI) data. The SUSAS data provided natural speech samples representing different stress levels, whereas the ORI data contained natural speech samples representing five different emotions.

The Speech Under Simulated and Actual Stress (SUSAS) database is a well-known and frequently used collection of audio samples used in automatic stress and emotion recognition studies [14, 63]. The database comprises speech recordings made under a range of acted and actual stress. Details of the recording process and the validation procedures can be found in Ref. [19]. The SUSAS data contains sections that provide natural vocal expressions under different stress levels and therefore offer high environmental validity. Only speech samples recorded under actual stress conditions (SUAS) selected from the Dual Tracking Task domain of the SUSAS database were used in this study. The Dual Tracking Task domain contains speech recordings from pilots performing tasks which addressed the pilot's two key goals: flight control and target acquisition. The task difficulty was controlled by time constraints for completion, increased resource competition or motivation. To facilitate the collection of pilot's speech, randomized words from a fixed list of 35 words were displayed on the screen and the pilots were instructed to read them while performing the tasks. The data was collected from 7 speakers (3 female and 4 male) under three different stress levels: high level stress, low level stress and neutral. Speech data selected for processing contained the total of 3,179 speech recordings, including 1,202 and 1,276 recordings representing high- and low-level stress, respectively, and 701 recordings representing neutral speech. All speakers had a general USA-English accent.

The second database used in this study was obtained from the Oregon Research Institute (ORI) in the USA. The speech was retrieved from a sound track of video recordings collected for the purpose of behavioral studies within the family [10]. It contains recordings of parents' speech produced during problem-solving conversations with their adolescents. The family discussed how to resolve two topics of disagreement, identified prior to the recording session. The conversations were conducted in a quiet laboratory room with family members seated a few feet apart as would be typical for a discussion between familiars. Lapel wireless microphones (model: Audio Technica ATW-831-w-a300) were placed on the participant's shirts at the chest level. Although, adolescent participants were fitted with other sensors measuring physiological signals such as electrocardiograph (ECG), impedance cardiogram (ICG), skin conductance, and respiratory and blood pressure, they did not impede speech behavior. The recordings used in this study a subset of the ORI data including 71 adult speakers (27 female and 44 male), all having a general USA-English accent. The data was annotated in real time by trained research assistants using the Living in Family Environments (LIFE) coding system [41] providing a second-by-second emotional labeling based on voice as well as facial expressions and body movements cues. Tested recordings represented five emotions: angry, anxious, dysphoric, neutral and happy. Each emotion was represented by 200 utterances (100 male and 100 female), and each utterance was of an average length of 2.3 s. The ORI data offered high environmental validity and psychophysiological accuracy; the data set was relatively large compared to the SUSAS data, and the speech recordings contain spontaneous speech sentences which are not limited to a fixed text or list of words. The main disadvantage of the ORI corpora was in its restricted availability.

9.5.2 Classification Method

The stress and emotion recognition experiments were based on the typical pattern recognition approach illustrated in Fig. 9.1. During the supervised training stage, emotion models were produced using a set of speech samples representing known emotional classes. These models were then applied in the testing stage to determine the unknown emotional classes of the test samples. The sampling rate of the ORI data was reduced to 8 kHz to match the only available sampling rate of the SUSAS data. Thus the analyzed speech had a narrow bandwidth of 4 kHz. The characteristic features were derived on a frame-by-frame basis using a frame length of 256 samples (12.5 ms) with 192-point (75 %) overlap.

Each emotional class was divided into 80 % of recordings to be used in the training stage, and the remaining 20 % to be used in the testing stage. The training and testing sets were kept mutually exclusive i.e. data used in training was not

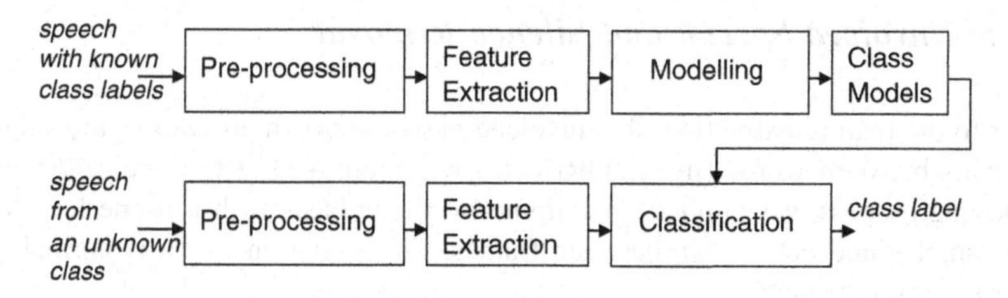

Fig. 9.1 Flowchart of the training and classification process

used in testing. For each feature-classifier combination, the classification process was cross-validated 15 times, each time with different training and testing data sets. The training and testing sets were changed for each test repetition using the standard stratified 5-fold cross validation cycle [12, 61] repeated 3 times, and each time with a different randomly chosen initial order of the data samples. The average percentage of the identification accuracy (APIA %) [57] was then calculated using:

$$APAI\,\% = \frac{1}{N_r}\frac{N_C}{N_T} \times 100\,\% \tag{9.1}$$

where N_C is the number of test inputs correctly identified, N_T is the total number of test inputs, and $N_r = 15$ is the number of repeated algorithm executions.

9.5.3 Pre-processing

In the pre-processing stage the amplitudes of speech samples were normalized into the range $\langle -1; +1 \rangle$. After the removal of noise and unvoiced/silence intervals, the voiced speech frames were concatenated and used in the two-stage processing illustrated in Fig. 9.1.

9.5.4 De-Noising

Both the SUSAS and ORI databases were recorded in real-life noisy conditions. To reduce the background noise, a wavelet-based method developed by Donoho [11] was used. Speech frames containing N samples with standard deviation σ, were decomposed using the wavelet transform (WT) with the mother wavelet db2 up to the second level, and the universal threshold given as $\sigma\sqrt{2\log(N)}$ was applied to each wavelet sub-band to remove components of amplitudes less than the threshold value. The signal was then reconstructed using the inverse wavelet transform.

9.5.5 Unvoiced Speech and Silence Removal

Prior to the feature extraction, the unvoiced parts of speech, as well as the silence intervals between words (in the ORI data) were removed. The unvoiced/silence removing process was applied on a frame-by-frame basis with a frame length of 256 samples and no overlap between frames. The signal energy was normalized for each frame using:

$$\bar{E}[k] = (E[k] - \tilde{E}[k])/std[E] \quad (9.2)$$

where k denotes the frame number, E[k] is the mean value of energy for a given frame and std(E) is the corresponding standard deviation. Speech samples with energy E[k] less than an experimentally chosen threshold of zero were removed and the remaining speech samples were concatenated and used in the feature extraction process. The concatenated voiced speech was analyzed using short-time frames.

9.5.6 Feature Extraction

The characteristic features were derived on the frame-by-frame basis using a frame length of 256 samples, with 196-point (75 %) overlap [56].

A wide range of different features were generated and their performance was compared using the same speech data samples and two types of classifiers. The features were divided into three groups.

The first group of features included classical prosodic, spectral and glottal parameters typically used to describe the linear source-filter model of speech production [55]. The second group included parameters representing area under the normalized TEO autocorrelation enveloped calculated using different frequency band sub-division methods. As indicated in Ref. [74], these parameters were related to the acoustic phenomena caused by the supra-glottal vortices assumed by the non-linear model of speech production postulated by experimental studies [64, 65]. Finally, the third group included parameters representing spectral energy. These parameters were also related to the non-linear model of speech production however, this group was specifically designed to observe the acoustic effects of intra-glottal vortices recently discovered during laryngological experiments [34, 35].

9.5.7 Modeling and Classification

Two well established methods of data modeling and classification were tested: the Gaussian Mixture Model (GMM) [55] and the k-Nearest Neighbors (KNN) [16]. In all tests involving the GMM classifier, five Gaussian mixtures were used to model each emotional or stress-level class. The classification tests had speaker, text and gender independent character.

9.5.8 Stress and Emotion Recognition Experiment Based on the Classical Prosodic, Spectral and Glottal Features

Most frequently used in stress and emotion classification features [9, 21, 63] include the fundamental frequency (F_0), formants, MFCC and glottal parameters. These parameters are based on the traditional understanding of how voiced speech is produced given by the source-filter (SF) model proposed in 1950 by Fant. The SF model assumes that the air flow through the vocal folds and vocal tract has a unidirectional and laminar character. The vibration of vocal folds provides a periodic signal known as the glottal wave. The glottal wave is then passed through the vocal tract cavities that act as a filter. One vibration cycle of the glottal folds includes the opening and closing phases in which the vocal folds are moving apart or together, respectively. The number of cycles per second determines the fundamental frequency F_0 of the glottal vibration. The glottal wave is modulated by the vocal tract filter configuration with resonant frequencies known as formants. The SF model assumes that there is only a single sound source (vibrating vocal folds) generating a harmonic series with the fundamental frequency (F_0) in speech signals.

9.5.8.1 Prosodic Features: Fundamental Frequency and Formants

The fundamental frequency (F_0) of the vocal fold vibration was estimated for each voiced frame of the speech signal using a modified autocorrelation method described in Ref. [7]. The first three formant frequencies were estimated as the resonant frequencies of the vocal tract filter using linear predictive (LP) analysis [73].

9.5.8.2 Spectral Features; Mel-frequency Cepstral Coefficients

The mel-frequency cepstral coefficients (MFCC) are widely used acoustic features for speech modeling and recognition [55, 63, 74]. The MFCC are the cosine transform coefficients calculated for the log power spectrum mapped onto the mel-frequency scale, which closely approximates the human auditory system's response. The first 12 coefficients of the discrete cosine transform (DCT) applied to the mel log powers provided the MFCC features corresponding to a given frame.

9.5.8.3 Glottal Features

Glottal features included 17 glottal time domain (GT) and 4 glottal frequency domain (GF) parameters defined in [2, 3, 70] and calculated using the TTK Aparat Glottal Inverse Filtering Toolbox [1, 2]. The GT features described the dynamic range of the glottal wave and timing between various stages of the glottal cycle, whereas the GF features provided ratios between amplitudes of harmonic components.

9.5.8.4 Classification Results Based on Prosodic, Spectral and Glottal Features

As illustrated in Table 9.1 and the classical feature parameters (F_0, formants, MFCC, GT and GF) derived from the classical speech production model provided an average classification accuracy ranging from 42 to 65 % for stress and from 20 to 52 % for emotions. In the case of emotions, the GMM classifier provided consistently better performance than the KNN classifier. However, in the case of emotions there was no clear consistency allowing determining which classifier was the most efficient.

9.5.9 Stress and Emotion Recognition Experiments Using Features Derived from the Teager Energy Operator

A significant number of recent studies pointed to the relatively high performance of the acoustic parameters derived from the Teager Energy Operator (TEO) in stress [22, 63], emotion [23], anger [14], clinical depression recognition [42] and language identification [24]. For example, in the depression recognition described in [42], the accuracy was 72–86 % for the TEO features compared to 66–73 % for the glottal parameters, 59–62 % for the prosodic parameters and 51–69 % for the spectral features. In Ref. [74] the TEO features provided up to 98 % average accuracy in stress recognition against MFCC providing 97 % and F_0 providing 89 %. In anger recognition, [18] reported results with TEO combined with MFCC and log energy features providing 83 % and MFCC combined with log energy providing 81 % of the average accuracy. One of the possible explanations for the

Table 9.1 APIA % for stress and emotion classification using classical features: F0, formants, MFCC, GT and GF

Dataset	F0		Formants		MFCC		GT		GF	
	GMM	KNN	GMM	KNN	GMM	KNN	GMM	KNN	GMM	KNN
Stress	50	44	52	62	59	65	60	51	48	42
Emotion	38	31	52	45	49	40	36	36	35	29

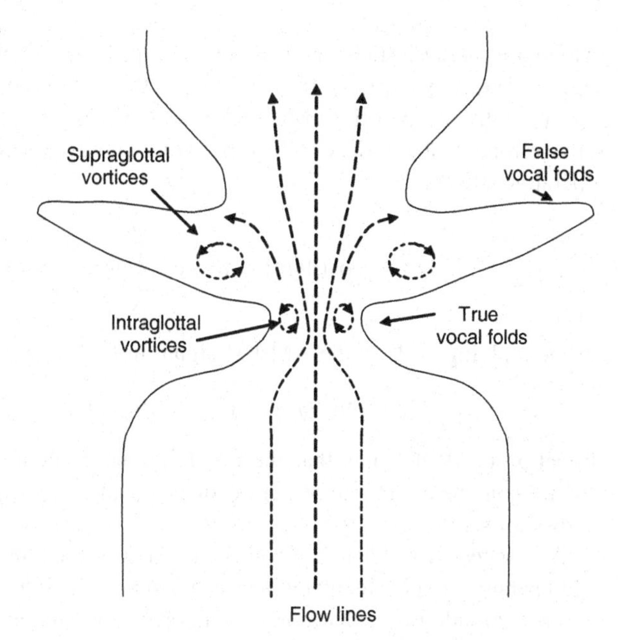

Fig. 9.2 Nonlinear model of the glottal flow formation

consistently high performance of the TEO features is that the TEO parameter represents cross-energy of a signal with itself [44, 45], and therefore it can detect transient occurrence of additional harmonics. As indicated in Ref. [74], these transient harmonic components may be generated by the supraglottal vortices formed during the opening stage of the vocal folds (see Fig. 9.2). The nonlinear air flow that forms the supraglottal vortices can generate sound when interacting with each other or when colliding with the hard surfaces of the vocal tract [6, 54, 52]. It is likely that under stress or emotion, different characteristic patterns of these mechanisms related to different types of emotions or stress levels can be produced. Following this assumption, a number of TEO-based parameters representing modified versions of the area under the normalized autocorrelation envelope (TEO-Auto-Env) introduced by Zhou et al. [74] were defined and applied to the stress and emotion classification in speech.

9.5.9.1 Features Based on the Teager Energy Operator

Speech signals could be regarded as an effect of amplitude and frequency modulation of separate oscillatory waves and modeled as a combination of several amplitude and frequency modulated (AM-FM) oscillatory components [30, 31,44, 45] given as:

$$\bar{E}[k] = (E[k] - \tilde{E}[k])/std[E] \tag{9.3}$$

where a[n] is the instantaneous amplitude, q[k] is the modulating signal, ω_c is the source frequency (carrier), $0 < \omega_h < \omega_c$ is the maximum frequency deviation, and θ is a constant phase offset. Maragos et al. [44, 45] proposed the following discrete time estimate of the speech instantaneous energy known as the Teager energy operator (TEO):

$$x[n] = a[n]\cos(\Phi[n]) = a[n]\cos\left(\omega_c n + \omega_h \int_0^n q[k]dk + \theta\right) \tag{9.4}$$

when applying (9.4) to the AM-FM signal in (9.3), the TEO can be expressed as:

$$\Psi(x[n]) = x^2[n] - x[n+1]x[n-1]. \tag{9.5}$$

Equation (9.5) indicates that the the TEO energy contour follows instantaneous changes in the harmonic structure of a signal instead of averaging the energy across all samples.

As suggested in [74], if the speech signal is broken into small bands and the TEO parameters are calculated for each band, it is easier to observe the presence or absence of additional harmonic components within each band. Moreover, the speech analysis becomes more robust if the characteristic features are derived not directly from the TEO but from the normalized TEO autocorrelation function given as:

$$R_{\Psi(x)}[k] = \frac{1}{2M+1}\sum_{n=-M}^{M} \Psi(x[n])\Psi(x[n+k]) \tag{9.6}$$

where M is the number of samples within the analyzed speech frame.

As illustrated in Fig. 9.3, the TEO based features were calculated on a frame-by frame basis within relatively narrow frequency bands. Depending on the bandwidth sub-division m, the following TEO based features were defined:

- *TEO-CB*—the area under the normalized TEO autocorrelation envelope calculated for the speech signal within 16 logarithmically increasing (Fig. 9.4) Critical Bands (CB) reflecting characteristics of the human auditory system [46]. The filtering was based on the band pass Gabor filters as described in Ref. [74].
- *TEO-DWT*—the area under the normalized TEO autocorrelation envelope calculated for the speech signal within 5 octave bands of the Discrete Wavelet Transform decomposition (Fig. 9.4). This scale uses a relatively small number of frequency bands which leads to the spectral resolution rapidly decreasing towards the high frequencies.
- *TEO-WP*—the area under the normalized TEO autocorrelation envelope calculated for the speech signal within 8 octave bands of the Wavelet Packet (WP) decomposition (Fig. 9.4). In the WP analysis the signal was passed through twice the number of filters used in the DWT analysis, providing additional high frequency bands.

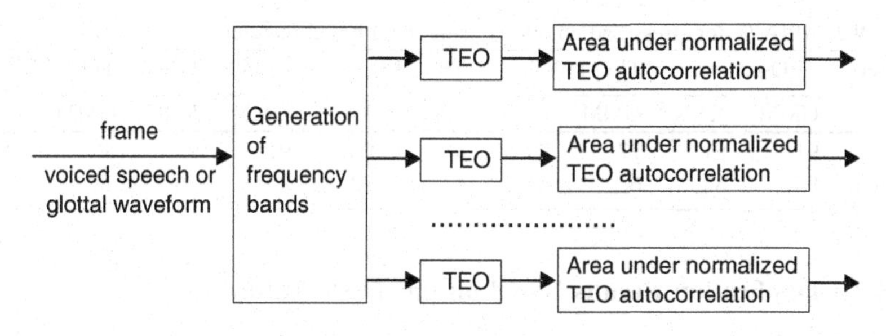

Fig. 9.3 Flowchart of the TEO based feature extraction process

No	Critical Bands Filters			Discrete Wavelet Transform			Wavelet Packet			Perceptual Wavelet Packet		
	Lower	Upper	Bandwidth	Lower	Upper	Bandwidth	Lower	Upper	Bandwidth	Lower	Upper	Bandwidth
1	100	200	100	0	250	250	0	500	500	0	125	125
2	200	300	100	250	500	250	500	1000	500	125	250	125
3	300	400	100	500	1000	500	1000	1500	500	250	375	125
4	400	510	110	1000	2000	1000	1500	2000	500	375	500	125
5	510	630	120	2000	4000	2000	2000	2500	500	500	625	125
6	630	770	140				2500	3000	500	625	750	125
7	770	920	150				3000	3500	500	750	875	125
8	920	1080	160				3500	4000	500	875	1000	125
9	1080	1270	190							1000	1250	250
10	1270	1480	210							1250	1500	250
11	1480	1720	240							1500	1750	250
12	1720	2000	280							1750	2000	250
13	2000	2320	320							2000	2250	250
14	2320	2700	380							2250	2500	250
15	2700	3150	450							2500	3000	500
16	3150	3700	550							3000	3500	500
17										3500	4000	500

Fig. 9.4 Frequency bands used in TEO features

- *TEO-PWP-S*—the area under the normalized TEO autocorrelation envelope calculated for the speech signal within 17 dyadic bands of the Perceptual Wavelet Packet (PWP) decomposition chosen to closely approximate the Critical Bands (Fig. 9.4). Selections of bands approximating the Critical Bands helped to reflect the human auditory characteristics. Compare to the CB, the PWP decomposition provided frequency bands with improved frequency resolution at the high frequency range.
- *TEO-PWP-G*—the area under the normalized TEO autocorrelation envelope calculated for the glottal time waveform within 17 dyadic bands of the PWP decomposition (Fig. 9.4). These features use the same bands as TEO-PWP, however the decomposition is applied to the glottal waveform rather than speech.

In all wavelet based features the mother wavelet db2 was used. The frequency responses of the db2 filters showed very good flatness of the frequency response within the pass-bands and provided higher computational efficiency compared to the band pass Gabor filters suggested in Ref. [74].

Table 9.2 APIA % for stress and emotions using TEO based features

Dataset	TEO-CB		TEO-DWT		TEO-WP		TEO-PWP-S		TEO-PWP-G	
	GMM	KNN	GMM	KNN	GMM	KNN	GMM	KNN	GMM	KNN
Stress	91	91	77	79	88	90	91	93	86	90
Emotion	85	85	62	63	67	72	85	86	78	80

9.5.9.2 Classification Results Based on the TEO Features

Table 9.2 shows that the TEO-PWP-S features calculated for the speech signals within 17 perceptual wavelet packet bands provided the best classification accuracy for both stress and emotions. The TEO-PWP-S features were very close in performance to the TEO-CB parameters and the difference between them was found to be statistically insignificant. The third best performance was given by TEO-PWP-G. All of these three types of futures take into account human auditory characteristic, which confirms the importance of these characteristics in vocal stress and emotion recognition.

9.6 Conclusions

Classification results generated by both classifiers, GMM and KNN were very close and followed similar trends. The *t* test (paired two sample for means) showed that the difference between means for GMM and KNN across all tested feature extraction methods was not statistically significant ($p = 0.28$, $df = 15$, Pearson correlation = 0.96) for the stress data from the SUAS corpora, and statistically significant ($p = 0.04$, $df = 15$, Pearson correlation = 0.96) for the emotional data from the ORI data base. In the statistically significant cases, the GMM classifier provided higher average classification values than the KNN classifier.

The classification experiments based on the classical features lead to relatively low classification accuracy ranging from 42 to 65 % for stress and 29–52 % for emotions. Features assuming the existence of nonlinear vortex formation, on the other hand, lead to significantly better performance. Depending on the sub-band selection, and type of classifier, the TEO based features assumed to be sensitive to the acoustic consequences of the supraglottal vortices provided average classification accuracy for stress within 77–91 % and for emotions within 62–86 %.

These results support the idea that the changes in acoustic speech characteristic caused by nonlinear mechanisms occurring during the speech formation can be provide vital cues for determining a mental or emotional state of a speaker. Further theoretical and experimental studies are needed to verify these conclusions.

References

1. Airas, M.: TKK Aparat: An environment for voice inverse filtering and parameterization. Logopedics Phoniatrics Vocology **33**(1), 49–64 (2008)
2. Airas, M., Pulakka, H., Bäckström, T., Alku, P.: A toolkit for voice inverse filtering and parametrisation. In: Proceedings of the 9th European Conference on Speech Communication and Technology (Interspeech'2005—Eurospeech): 2145–2148, Lisbon, Portugal, 4–8 Sept 2005
3. Alku, P.: Glottal wave analysis with pitch synchronous iterative adaptive inverse filtering. Speech Commun. **11**(2–3), 109–118 (1992)
4. Ang, J., Dhillon, R., Krupski, A.: Prosody-based automatic detection of annoyance and frustration in human-computer dialog. In: Proceedings of the International Conference on Spoken Language Processing, ICSLP 2002, Colorado (2002)
5. Banse, R., Scherer, K.R.: Acoustic profiles in vocal emotion expression. J. Pers. Soc. Psychol. **70**(3), 614–636 (1996)
6. Barney, A., Shadle, C.H., Davies, P.O.A.L.: Fluid flow in a dynamic mechanical model of the vocal folds and tract. J. Acoust. Soc. Am. **105**(1), 444–455 (1999)
7. Boersma, P.: Accurate short-term analysis of the fundamental frequency and the harmonics-to-noise ratio of a sampled sound. IFA Proc. **17**, 97–110 (1993)
8. Clavel, C., Vasilescu, I., Devillers, L., Richard, G., Ehrette, T.: Fear-type emotion recognition for future audio-based surveillance systems. Speech Commun. **50**(6), 487–503 (2008)
9. Cowie, R., Douglas-Cowie, E., Tsapatsoulis, N., Votsis, G., Kollias, S., Fellenz, W., Taylor, J.G.: Emotion recognition in human-computer interaction. IEEE Signal Process. Mag. **18**(1), 32–80 (2001)
10. Davis, B., Sheeber, L., Hops, H., Tildesley, E.: Adolescent responses to depressive parental behaviors in problem-solving interactions. J. Abnorm. Child Psychol. **28**(5), 451–465 (2000)
11. Donoho, D.L.: Denoising by soft thresholding. IEEE Trans. Inf. Theory **41**(3), 613–627 (1995)
12. Efron, B., Tibshirani, R.J.: An Introduction to the Bootstrap. Chapman & Hall/CRC, New York (1993)
13. France, D.J., Shiavi, R.G., Silverman, S., Silverman, M., Wilkes, M.: Acoustical properties of speech as indicators of depression and suicidal risk. Biomed. Eng. IEEE Trans. **47**(7), 829–837 (2000)
14. Gaillard, A.W.K., Wientjes, C.J.E.: Mental load and work stress as two types of energy mobilization. Work Stress **8**(2), 141–152 (1994)
15. Gao, H., Chen, S, Su, G.: Emotion classification of Mandarin speech based on TEO nonlinear features. In: Eighth ACIS International Conference on Software Engineering, Artificial Intelligence, Networking, and Parallel/Distributed Computing, SNPD 2007 (2007)
16. Gersho, A.: Vector quantization and signal compression. Kluwer Academic Publishers, Dordrecht (1992)
17. Grimm, M., Kroschel, K., Mower, E., Narayanan, S.: Primitives-based evaluation and estimation of emotions in speech. Speech Commun. **49**(10–11), 787–800 (2007)
18. Hansen, J.H.L., Wooil, K., Rahurkar, M., Ruzanski, E., Meyerhoff, J.: Robust emotional stressed speech detection. EURASIP J. Adv. Signal Process. **2011**, Article ID 906789 (2011)
19. Hansen, J.H.L., Bou-Ghazale, S.: Getting started with SUSAS: A speech under simulated and actual stress database. EUROSPEECH-1997, 1743–1746 (1997)
20. He, L., Lech, M., Allen, N.: On the importance of glottal flow spectral energy for the recognition of emotions in speech. Interspeech 2010, Makuhari, Japan, 26–30 Sept 2010
21. He, L., Lech, M., Maddage, N., Memon, S., Allen, N.: Emotion recognition in spontaneous speech within work and family environments. iCBBE 2009, June 2009 in Beijing, China (2009)

22. He, L., Lech, M., Maddage, N., Allen, N.: Emotion recognition in speech of parents of depressed adolescents. iCBBE 2009, Beijing, China, 11–13 June 2009
23. He, L., Lech, M., Maddage, N., Memon, S., Allen, N.: Stress and emotion recognition using Log-Gabor filter analysis of speech spectrograms. ACII 2009, Amsterdam, Sept 2009
24. Hemant, A.P., Basu, T.K.: Identifying perceptually similar languages using Teager energy based cepstrum. Eng. Lett. **16**(1), 2008 (2008)
25. Huber, R., Batliner, A., Buckow, J., Noth, E., Warnke, V., Niemann, H.: Recognition of emotion in a realistic dialogue scenario. In: Proceedings of the International Conference on Spoken Language, ICSLP 2000, Beijing, (2000)
26. Iliev, A.I., Scordilis, M.S.: Emotion recognition in speech using inter-sentence Glottal statistics. In: Systems, Signals and Image Processing, 2008. IWSSIP 2008. 15th International Conference (2008)
27. Iliev, A.I., Scordilis, M.S., Papa, J.P., Falcão, A.X.: Spoken emotion recognition through optimum-path forest classification using glottal features. Comput. Speech Lang. **24**(3), 445–460 (2010)
28. Iliou, T., Anagnostopoulos, C.N.: Comparison of different classifiers for emotion recognition. In: 13th Panhellenic Conference on Informatics, PCI '09 (2009)
29. Ingram, R. (ed.): The International Encyclopedia of Depression, Springer, New York (2009)
30. Kaiser, J.F.: On a simple algorithm to calculate the 'energy' of a signal. Proc. Int. Conf. Acoust. Speech Signal Process. **1**, 381–384 (1990)
31. Kaiser, J.F.: Some useful properties of Teager's energy operator. Proc. Int. Conf. Acoust. Speech Signal Process. **3**, 149–152 (1993)
32. Kim, E.H., Hyun, K.H., Kim, S.H., Kwak, Y.K.: Improved emotion recognition with a novel speaker-independent feature. IEEE/ASME Trans. Mechatronics **14**(3), 317–325 (2009)
33. Kim, E.H., Hyun, K.H., Kim, S.H., Kwak, Y.K.: Speech emotion recognition separately from voiced and unvoiced sound for emotional interaction robot. In: International Conference on Control, Automation and Systems, ICCAS 2008 (2008)
34. Khosla, S., Murugappan, S., Gutmark, E.: What can vortices tell us about vocal vibration and voice production. Curr. Opin. Otholaryngology Head Neck Surg. **16**, 183–187 (2008)
35. Khosla, S., Murugappan, S., Paniello, R., Ying, J., Gutmark, E.: Role of vortices in voice production: Norma versus asymmetric tension. Larygoscope **119**, 216–221 (2009)
36. Lee, C.M., Yildirim, S., Bulut, M., Kazemzadeh, A., Busso, C.: Emotion recognition based on phoneme classes. In: Proceedings of the International Conference on Spoken Language Processing, ICSLP 2004, Korea (2004)
37. Iida, A., Campbell, N., Iga, S., Higuchi, F., Yasumura, M.: A speech synthesis system with emotion for assisting communication. In: Proceedings of ISCA Workshop on Speech and Emotion, Belfast, vol. 1, 167–172 (2000)
38. Leslie, S., Greenberg, J.D.S.: Emotion in psychotherapy: Affect, cognition, and the process of change. Guilford Press, New York (1987)
39. Liscombe, J., Riccardi, G., Hakkani-Tur, D.: Using context to improve emotion detection in spoken dialog systems. Interspeech **2005**, 1845–1848 (2005)
40. Liscombe, J.: Detecting emotion in speech: Experiments in ThreeDomains. In: Proceedings of HLT/NAACL 2006, New York (2006)
41. Longoria, N., Sheeber, L., Davis, B.: Living in family environments (LIFE) Coding. A reference manual for coders. Oregon Research Institute (2006)
42. Low, L.S.A., Maddage, N., Lech, M., Sheeber, L.B., Allen, N.B.: Detection of clinical depression in adolescents speech during family interactions. IEEE Trans. Biomed. Eng. **58**(3), 574–586 (2011)
43. Low, L.S.A., Lech, M., Maddage, N.C., Allen, N.: Mel frequency cepstral feature and Gaussian mixtures for modeling clinical depression in adolescents. In: Proceedings on IEEE International Conference on Cognitive Informatics, ICCI '09 (2009)
44. Maragos, P., Kaiser, J.F., Quatieri, T.: On amplitude and frequency demodulation using energy operators. Signal Process. IEEE Trans. **41**(4), 1532–1550 (1993)

45. Maragos, P., Kaiser, J.F., Quatieri, T.: Energy separation in signal modulations with application to speech analysis. IEEE Trans. Signal Process. **41**(10), 3024–3051 (1993)
46. Moore, B.: An introduction to the psychology of hearing. Academic Press, San Diego (2001)
47. Moore, E.I.I., Clements, M.A., Peifer, J.W., Weisser, L.: Critical analysis of the impact of glottal features in the classification of clinical depression in speech. IEEE Trans. Biomed. Eng. **55**(1), 96–107 (2008)
48. Moore, E.I.I., Clements, M., Peifer, J., Weisser, L.: Comparing objective feature statistics of speech for classifying clinical depression. In: 26th Annual International Conference of the IEEE Engineering in Medicine and Biology Society, IEMBS '04 (2004)
49. Murphy, F.C., Nimmo-Smith, L., Lawrence, L.D.: Functional neuroanatomy of emotions: A meta-analysis Cognitive. Affect. Behav. Neurosci. **2002**, 207–233 (2002)
50. Myers, D.G.: Theories of emotion. Psychology, 7th edn. Worth Publishers, New York (2004)
51. New, T.L., Foo, S.W., DeSilva, L.C.: Speech emotion recognition using hidden Markov models. Speech Commun. **41**(4), 603–623 (2003)
52. New, T.L., Foo, S.W., DeSilva, L.C.: Classification of stress in speech using linear and nonlinear features. In: IEEE International Conference on Acoustics, Speech, and Signal Processing (2003)
53. Ozdas, A., Shiavi, R.G., Silverman, S.E., Silverman, M.K., Wilkes, D.M.: Investigation of vocal jitter and glottal flow spectrum as possible cues for depression and near-term suicidal risk. Biomed. Eng. IEEE Trans. **51**(9), 1530–1540 (2004)
54. Pulakka, H.: Analysis of human voice production using inverse filtering, highspeed imaging, and electroglottography. Master's thesis, Helsinki University of Technology, Espoo, Finland (2005)
55. Quatieri, T.: Speech Signal Processing. Prentice Hall, Englewood Cliffs (2002)
56. Rabiner, L.R., Schafer, R.W.: Digital Processing of Speech Signals (Signal Processing Series), Prentice-Hall, Englewood Cliffs (1978)
57. Reynolds, D., Rose, R.: Robust text-independent speaker identification using Gaussian mixture speaker models. IEEE Trans. Speech Audio Process. **3**(1), 72–83 (1995)
58. Scherer, K., Zei, B.: Vocal indicators of affective disorders. Psychother. Psychosom. **49**, 179–186 (1998)
59. Scherer, K.: Expression of emotion in voice and music. J. Voice **9**(3), 235–248 (1995)
60. Scherer, K.R.: Vocal communication of emotion: A review of research paradigms. Speech Commun. **40**, 227–256 (2003)
61. Schuller, B., Batliner, A., Seppi, D., Steidl, S., Vogt, T., Wagner, J., Devillers, L., Vidrascu, L., Amir, N., Kessous, L., Aharonson, V.: The relevance of feature type for the automatic classification of emotional user states: Low level descriptors and functionals. In: Proceedings of Interspeech, pp. 2253–2256 (2007)
62. Shinwari, D., Scherer, K.R., Afjey, A., Dewitt, K.: Flow visualization in a model of the glottis with a symmetric and oblique angle. JASA **113**, 487–497 (2003)
63. Steeneken, H.J.M., Hansen, J.H.L.: Speech under stress conditions: overview of the effect on speech production and on system performance. In: Proceedings., 1999 IEEE International Conference on Acoustics, Speech, and Signal Processing ICASSP '99 (1999)
64. Teager, H.: Some observations on oral air flow during phonation. Acoust. IEEE Trans. Speech Signal Process. **28**(5), 599–601 (1980)
65. Teager, H.M., Teager, S.: Evidence for nonlinear production mechanisms in the vocal tract. In: NATO Advanced Study Inst. On Speech Production and Speech Modeling, Bonas, France, vol. 55, pp. 241–261. Kluwer Academic Publishers, Boston (1989)
66. Tolkmitt, F.J., Scherer, K.R.: Effect of experimentally induced stress on vocal parameters. J. Exp. Psychol. Hum. Percept. Perform. **12**(3), 302–313 (1986)
67. Thayer, R.E.: The biopsychology of mood and arousal. Oxford University Press, New York (1989)
68. Torabi, S., Almas Ganj, F., Mohammadian, A.: Semi-supervised classification of speaker's psychological stress. In: Biomedical Engineering Conference, CIBEC 2008. Cairo International (2008)

69. Wagner, J., Vogt, T., André, E.: A systematic comparison of different HMM designs for emotion recognition from acted and spontaneous speech. Lecture Notes in Computer Science, Affective Computing and Intelligent Interaction, Springer, Berlin, Heidelberg (2007)
70. Veeneman, D., BeMent, S.: Automatic glottal inverse filtering from speech and electroglottographic signals. IEEE Trans. Acoust. Speech Signal Process. **33**(2), 369–377 (1985)
71. Ververidis, D.K., Kotropoulos, C.: Emotional speech recognition: Resources, features, and methods. Speech Commun. **48**, 1162–1181 (2006)
72. Yildirim, S., Narayanan, S., Potamianos, A.: Detecting emotional state of a child in a conversational computer game. Comput. Speech Lang. **25**(1), 29–44 (2011)
73. Zhao, W., Zhang, C., Frankel, S.H., Mongeaue, L.: Computational aeroacoustics of phonation, part 1: computational methods and sound generation mechanisms. J. Acoust. Soc. Am. **112**, 2134–2146 (2002)
74. Zhou, G., Hansen, J.H.L., Kaiser, J.F.: Nonlinear feature based classification of speech under stress. Speech Audio Process. IEEE Trans. **9**(3), 201–216 (2001)
75. Zhou, J., Wang, G., Yang, Y., Chen, P.: Speech emotion recognition based on rough set and SVM. In: IEEE International Conference on Cognitive Informatics. ICCI 2006 (2006)

Chapter 10
Detection and Prediction of Clinical Depression

Margaret Lech, Lu-Shih Low and Kuan Ee Ooi

10.1 Depression as a Major Public Health Problem

The emotional health of individuals has a significant impact on national health and economic outcomes [1]. Emotional disorders, such as anxiety and depression, are amongst the most common and disabling illnesses of any type observed in the Worldwide community, and have been recognised as some of the major public health issues.

Depression is one of the most common psychological disorders in the community. At the beginning of the 21st century, the World Health Organization estimated that 121 million people in the world suffer from clinical depression [2]. Moreover, depression is estimated to become the second-greatest burden of disease in the world by the year 2020. Existing diagnostic and treatment resources are very limited and likely to remain this way in the foreseeable future. Therefore, it is particularly important to look for new preventative measures that reduce the impact of depression on humanity.

Depressive disorders seriously affect social, emotional, educational and vocational outcomes. It is also the most common precursor of suicide. It is estimated that up to one in eight individuals will require treatment for depressive illness in their lifetime [1, 3]. The prevalence of depression, the world's fourth most serious health threat in 1990, is expected to rise steadily [4].

Depression and anxiety account for most of the economic, social and personal costs of mental disorders. Depression greatly impairs a person's ability to function physically, socially, and at work. In adolescents depression may be associated with loss of energy and social withdrawal but may also result in disruptive behaviours or substance use (drugs and alcohol). In the longer term, depression can reduce social and vocational opportunities for young people as a result of early school dropout and sporadic employment opportunities.

M. Lech (✉) · L.-S. Low · K. E. Ooi
School of Electrical and Computer Engineering, RMIT University, Melbourne, Australia
e-mail: margare.lech@rmit.edu.au

M. Lech et al. (eds.), *Mental Health Informatics*,
Studies in Computational Intelligence 491, DOI: 10.1007/978-3-642-38550-6_10,

10.2 Depression in Adolescents

Yearly depression prevalence rates have reached 15 % in inner-city community samples of women. This is around double that found in men. The onset of depression is most likely at age 17, with Major Depression (MD) being the most common form. An early intervention preventing the onset of clinical depression would provide a very important method for reducing the burden of the disease. Efficient depression prediction methods are therefore needed to determine the risk for an onset in young individuals. A report from the Institute of Medicine of the United States in 1994 [5], strongly indicates the need to increase research on preventive methods in order to reduce the incidence (that is, the number of new cases) of mental disorders in the population. One of the goals for the prevention research is the clear identification of groups at high imminent risk for the disorder.

Depression appears at different stages of the life cycle and it is one of the most common mental health problems in adolescents. Adolescents are usually defined as aged 13–20 years. It is estimated that a depressive episode affects between 14–30 % of young females and 13–17 % of males [6, 7]. Depression also occurs in children younger than 13 years of age, but becomes progressively more prevalent after puberty and reaches adult levels in the late teens. During the early stages depression is often unrecognised and under-treated [8] leading to many undesirable social, health, education and employment issues.

Early diagnosis of depression is extremely useful and can mean a minimal disturbance of typical functioning and development of social and academic skills. Unfortunately children often are not be able or not willing to express verbally their feelings and thus help with an early diagnosis. The conventional diagnosis of depression in adolescents is often based on observations of behavioural patterns, and interviews with parents and teachers. This process is time consuming and the illness is usually recognised when in advanced stages.

Current diagnostic methods are qualitative and largely based on the personal skills, experience and intuitive judgment of a mental health practitioner. The number of highly skilled professionals is limited, and their availability is restricted to major towns and health centres. As a result, each year, thousands of cases of depression are not being diagnosed and left untreated, leading to potential suicides. These problems are of particular concern in the rural areas of many countries where the number of suicides amongst young people is alarmingly large.

An automatic speech analysis in diagnosis of depression is currently an important subject of ongoing research. It can provide an efficient and reliable mass screening methodology for detection of depression in adolescents and such addressing the huge prevalence of the depression problem in adolescents.

10.3 Speech Acoustics as Correlates of Depression

Utilizing a subjective assessment [6], conducted a pilot study of severely depressed patients and found that listeners could perceive noticeable differences in prosodic characteristics of speech such as pitch, loudness, speaking rate, and articulation in depressed patients before and after treatment.

This observation led to numerous studies searching for acoustic correlates of depression [7, 9–13]. The most often investigated parameters included prosodic parameters such as fundamental frequency (F0), formants, jitter, shimmer, intensity of the speech signal, and speech rate. Other commonly used speech parameters include cepstral features (i.e. mel frequency cepstral coefficients), spectral features (i.e. power spectral density) and glottal features. The Teager energy operator (TEO), which measures the number of additional harmonics due to the nonlinear airflow in the vocal tract that produces the speech signal [14] also, attracted attention of researchers.

There is strong evidence that these parameters could be used to discriminate between non-depressed and depressed adult patients, and possibly between different stages of depressive disorder [15–18].

Acoustic speech parameters can be applied in the process of depression diagnosis and also as indicators of effectiveness of various treatments for depression.

Due to significant differences between adult and adolescent speech [8] studies specifically designed to investigate the effects of depression on speech in adolescents are needed. The following sections review previous work and show how to design diagnostic algorithms aiming to detect onset of depression and assess the risk of depression in adolescents.

10.4 Physiological Basis for Speech Based Diagnosis

Studies conducted since the 1980s [11, 17], gathered considerable evidence that emotional arousal produces changes in speech production by affecting respiratory, phonatory, and articulatory processes. This is largely due to the fact that emotional arousal activates the somatic nervous system and the sympathetic and parasympathetic autonomic nervous system (ANS). For example, the temporal rate of articulation and the frequency range of vowels can be modified by changes in the timing of the muscle movements controlling the motion amplitudes of the articulatory structures. These muscles are driven by the limbic control system. The sympathetic and parasympathetic effects controlled by the limbic system can influence speech production by introducing changes in respiration and phonation. Resulting changes in subglottal air pressure and vocal cord tension could have an effect on the fundamental frequency of vocal cord vibration (F_0). Other ANS-dependent effects such as mucus secretion may alter speech characteristics during intense emotional arousal. There is an evidence that psychomotor disturbances are particularly distinctive symptoms of mood disorders. Symptoms of psychomotor agitation or retardation may actually precede the full onset of a depressive episode and thus provide early indication of high risk for mental illness [5].

10.5 Studies Related to Speech Based Diagnosis of Depression

Psychiatrists and clinical psychologists have long used the subjectively perceived characteristics of patients' voices as indicators of their mental states but until recently no objective measures were available [7].

The use of acoustical properties of speech as objective indicators of depression and suicidal risk has been studied since the mid-1980's. Since depression and suicidality manifest themselves through certain emotional changes, the automatic classification of depression is closely related to the studies of emotion recognition in speech.

Depressed speech has often been characterised as dull, monotone, monoloud, lifeless, and "metallic" [19]. Patients with severe depression tend to speak slowly and with longer pauses [7, 20]. These perceptual qualities have been associated with acoustical fluctuations involving fundamental frequency (F_0), amplitude modulation (AM), formant structure, power distribution, shimmer, jitter and speech rate.

The level of correlation built to recognize complex relationships between speech parameters and depression has customarily been assessed using multivariate analyses [17, 21, 22].

Darby [23], described a pilot study in which 13 depressed patients were evaluated before and after treatment with antidepressant medication. Patients were rated on scales for severity of depression and speech deviations. Scores on "depressed voice" most consistently distinguished depressed participants. In [24], the rate of change of voice fundamental frequency (F_0) due to depression was measured. A total of 16 patients were tested during depressive episodes and then after recovery. It was shown the standard deviation of the rate of F_0 change and the relative occurrence of silent intervals are strongly correlated with the severity of depression. In Ref. [21], a sample of 30 depressive patients were investigated during the course of recovery from depression. The recovery process was assessed based on changes in symptoms and through changes in speaking behaviour and voice sound characteristics. The results revealed that the F_0 and energy contours displayed consistently high correlations with depressive symptoms. In Ref. [25], fluency of speech and prosody were rated and compared for 22 elderly depressed patients and an age-matched normal control group. It was concluded that depression was strongly correlated with speech acoustics. In Ref. [26] presented results of a major longitudinal study of depressive disorders conducted at the Max-Planck-Institute for Psychiatry, Munich. In the described experiments, 11 female and 5 male depressives were audio–video-recorded while speaking with clinical interviewers. For selected utterances during depressed and recovered mood states several voice and speech parameters were obtained, using digital analysis techniques. The results showed that an increase in speech rate and a decrease in pause duration are powerful indicators of mood improvement in the course of therapy (remission from depressive state). In female but not in male patients, a decrease in minimum fundamental frequency of the voice predicted the mood improvement.

One of the first fully automatic approaches to the classification of depression was introduced in [11, 27] when speech as a psychomotor symptom of depression and suicidality were investigated. Acoustical and statistical analyses were performed on clinically diagnosed populations to determine if the acoustical properties of speech change with depression severity, and if they can be used to classify the mental health condition of individual subjects. In the first stage of research, speech samples of three groups: control (10 female), dysthymic (17 female), and major depressed (21 female) patients were tested. In the second stage of research, acoustical properties of speech of normal (24 male), major depressed (21 male), and high-risk suicidal (22 male) patients were analysed. Features derived from the formants and from the Power Spectral Density (PSD) were found to be the best discriminators of class membership in both male and female patients. The Amplitude Modulation (AM) features emerged as strong class discriminators of the male participants. Features derived from F_0 were generally ineffective discriminators in both male and female groups.

Later reports [16, 17] investigated acoustic properties of speech for near-term suicidal risk assessment. Effects of suicidal state on the glottal (vocal cords) characteristics were investigated. Changes in vocal jitter and slope of the glottal flow spectrum were investigated as possible indicators of near-term suicidal state. Two-sample maximum likelihood (ML) classifier was used to examine whether vocal jitter and glottal spectral slope sensitivity could be used to perform pairwise differentiation between 10 non-depressed controls, 10 depressed patients and 10 near-term suicidal male patients. Speech samples of the non-depressed, depressed and suicidal patients were selected from audio recordings of clinical interviews, treatment sessions and suicide notes. The analysis was based on 30 s of continuous speech from each participant. It was found that the mean vocal jitter was a significant discriminator only between suicidal and non-depressed groups. The slope of the glottal source spectrum was found to be a significant discriminator between all three groups. Classification based on the combined feature set (jitter and glottal source spectrum) showed an improvement of the correct classification rate, reaching 85 % correct results for control versus suicidal classifications, 90 % for control versus depressed, and 75 % for depressed versus suicidal classifications. These studies strongly supported the hypothesized link between speech phonation, depression and near-suicidal risk.

More recent works on automatic depression recognition in speech continued searching for acoustic speech parameters that provide strong indication of depression [7, 14, 15, 17] while also looking at other factors such as the gender [13, 28] and age [13]. Depending on gender and the type of acoustic features used in the recognition process, the binary (depressed/non-depressed) classification accuracy has been reported to be as high as 80–90 %.

Some of the most significant works include [14, 15, 28] which describe an analysis of variation in prosodic feature statistics and glottal features of speech for patients suffering from a depressive disorder and uses these results in an automatic classification of speech into two classes: non-depressed and depressed. The classification based on glottal statistics [F_0, Energy Deviation Statistics (EDS) and Energy Median Statistics (EMS)] achieved accuracy ranging from 67 to 94 %. The classification results based on glottal features showed accuracy ranging from 87 to 100 %.

In the later study [22], the performance of prosodic, vocal tract and glottal features in the discrimination between 15 depressed patients (6 males and 9 females) and 18 healthy control people (9 males and 9 females) was examined. The speech corpus consisted of one recorded session from each participant reading a short story long enough to provide about 3 min of continuous speech. The feature selection strategy utilized the following combinations of feature groups: prosodic measures alone, prosodic and vocal tract measures and all three types together. It was found that the combination of prosodic and glottal parameters produced better overall discrimination than the combination of prosodic and vocal tract features. These studies provided strong indication that glottal descriptors are strongly correlated with the emotional and mental state of a speaker.

Majority of the depression recognition studies were restricted to small populations of patients. Also, the speech recordings made during patients' clinical interviews, treatment sessions or fixed text reading sessions were not representative of natural speech that normally occurs in family or work environments. Moreover, majority of studies investigated speech acoustics of adults. Since, the symptoms of depression often first appear during adolescence at a time when the voice is changing, in both males and females, specific studies of acoustic correlates of depression in adolescent populations are needed.

10.6 Acoustic Speech Classification for Diagnosis of Depression in Adolescents

In Ref. [13] described a study of depression diagnosis in adolescents based on a large clinical data base. Acoustic correlates of depression in a large sample of 139 adolescents including 68 clinically depressed (49 males and 19 females) and 71 healthy controls (44 males and 27 females) were investigated. The proposed depression detection methodology was tested using speech recordings made during three types of naturalistic interactions between adolescents and their parents. Each of the three interactions was conducted for 20 min, resulting in a total of 60 min of observational data (video recordings) for each family. The interactions can be briefly described as follows:

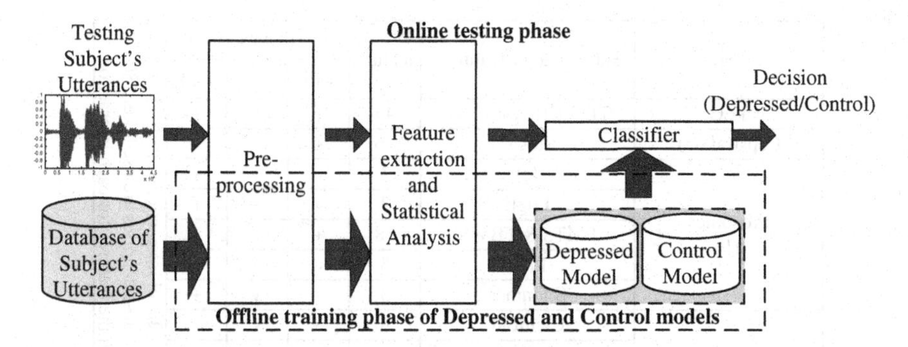

Fig. 10.1 Speech modeling and classification for depressed and healthy control adolescents

1. *Event planning interaction* (*EPI*) The family plans a vacation together and reminisces about a fun time they spent together in the past.
2. *Problem-solving interaction* (*PSI*) The family tries to resolve two topics of disagreement, identified based on a questionnaire completed by the adolescent and parents.
3. *Family consensus interaction* (*FCI*) This family discussion involves planning the writing of book chapters on the experience of growing up/raising a child that reflect the shared perspective of both the adolescents and their parents.

The general training and classification framework used to discriminate between the depressed and non-depressed speech samples is illustrated in Fig. 10.1. For each participant, 60 min of speech data broken down into 1 min's segments was analyzed.

For both the training and testing phases, detection of voiced frames using the linear predictive technique described in (27) was implemented by first segmenting the normalized speech segment into 25 ms frames with 50 % overlap between frames using a rectangular window. From these voiced frames, acoustic features were extracted and normalized within each subject. Statistical analyses were then carried out to discard any acoustic features that were statistically non-significant (marked with—in Fig. 10.2) in distinguishing the speech of depressed adolescents from that of control adolescents. Finally, using two different machine-learning techniques of Gaussian mixture model (GMM) and the support vector machine (SVM), the selected extracted acoustic features were modeled into their respective classes (depressed and control class).

Five groups of acoustic features were examined: Teager energy operator (TEO) features, cepstral (C), prosodic (P), spectral (S) and glottal (G) features. Acoustic features grouped into these categories are closely related to the physiological and perceptual components that characterize speech in the human speech production model. The feature categories of TEO which measures the non-linear airflow in the

Category	Sub-category features[a]	No. of feature coeff.	Significance (male)			Significance (female) – In all interactions of EPI, PSI and FCI, all the feature sub-categories are used; i.e. 186 coefficients from all the features for each interaction
			EPI	PSI	FCI	
TEO	TEO-CB-Auto-Env	45	+	+	+	
Cepstral (C)	MFCC	36	+	+	+	
Prosodics (P)	F0	3	-	+	+	
	LogE	3	+	+	+	
	FMTS & FBWS	18	+	+	+	
	Jitter	3	-	+	-	
	Shimmer	3	+	+	+	
Spectral (S)	Centroid	3	+	-	-	
	Flux	3	+	+	+	
	Entropy	3	+	+	+	
	Roll-off	3	+	+	+	
	PSD	27	+	+	+	
Glottal (G)	GLT	27	+	+	+	
	GLF	9	+	+	+	
	Total	186	180	183	180	

[a]All features include their delta (Δ) and delta-delta (Δ-Δ)

Fig. 10.2 MANOVA and ANOVA analysis on the sub-category features for both male and female adolescents (adapted from [13])

vocal tract and the glottal (G) characteristics which measures the glottal shape and pulse relates to the physiological components of the human speech production. Whereas, the feature categories of cepstral (C), prosodic (P) and spectral (S) are related to the perceptual aspect of speech. Figure 10.2 shows types of physical parameters falling into each of the five categories.

As illustrated in Figs. 10.3 and 10.4, the TEO based features clearly outperformed all other features and feature combinations, providing classification accuracy ranging between 81–87 % for males and 72–79 % for females. Close, but slightly less accurate, results were obtained by combining glottal features with prosodic and spectral features (67–69 % for males and 70–75 % for females).

Training/Testing Features		Overall Accuracy %					
		EPI		PSI		FCI	
		MALE	FEMALE	MALE	FEMALE	MALE	FEMALE
P		59.83	66.60	50.87	67.33	58.87	62.28
S		61.26	64.96	51.64	58.08	51.07	69.38
G		59.59	71.91	74.56	62.77	66.03	73.46
P + S		61.95	69.61	58.31	68.22	57.91	65.99
P	+ G	60.65	69.19	65.96	65.56	64.90	68.55
S	+ G	62.65	71.67	54.21	66.69	57.77	70.01
P + S	+ G	66.50	72.40	67.18	75.25	69.10	70.41

Fig. 10.3 Classification performance of prosodic, spectral and glottal features using SBCCA with 1 min test utterances (adapted from [13])

Training/Testing Features		Overall Accuracy increase (+) / decrease (-)					
		EPI		PSI		FCI	
		MALE	FEMALE	MALE	FEMALE	MALE	FEMALE
P	+ TEO	+21.60%	+2.43%	+31.35%	-0.92%	+25.13%	+4.61%
S	+ TEO	+17.32%	+0.82%	+27.83%	+4.30%	+29.29%	-5.08%
G	+ TEO	+22.41%	+7.07%	+6.80%	+4.73%	+13.37%	-5.90%
P + S	+ TEO	+15.67%	+1.19%	+11.35%	-6.34%	+19.17%	-0.79%
P + G	+ TEO	+19.00%	-0.90%	+17.68%	+7.14%	+15.75%	+0.62%
S + G	+ TEO	+16.93%	-0.30%	+24.83%	+2.65%	+19.99%	-2.38%
P + S + G	+ TEO	+13.75%	-2.01%	+14.47%	-0.38%	+10.59%	-0.76%

Fig. 10.4 Influence of TEO category in percentage accuracy improvement and their statistical significance when added to prosodic, spectral and glottal features (adapted from [13])

Training/ Testing Features: TEO	Event Planning Interaction (EPI)					
	Male			Female		
	Sensitivity	Specificity	Accuracy	Sensitivity	Specificity	Accuracy
	81.67	81.04	81.36	80.64	77.27	78.87
	Problem Solving Interaction (PSI)					
	Male			Female		
	Sensitivity	Specificity	Accuracy	Sensitivity	Specificity	Accuracy
	86.94	78.98	82.96	81.38	70.02	75.70
	Family Consensus Interaction (FCI)					
	Male			Female		
	Sensitivity	Specificity	Accuracy	Sensitivity	Specificity	Accuracy
	80.83	92.45	86.64	72.08	71.94	72.01

Fig. 10.5 TEO category classification performance (adapted from [13])

In all types of classification shown in Figs. 10.3 and 10.4, strong gender differences in the classification accuracy were observed.

Figure 10.5 These findings showed that depression can be detected based on naturalistic speech samples at an early stage of life. The detection accuracy strongly depends on ender and type of acoustic features, however the non-linear approach based on the TEO-based features provided the highest correlation with depression in the speech of both male and female adolescents.

It can be concluded that the detection of clinical depression still presents a challenging task due to the large number of potential genetic, psychological, social, cultural and environmental factors contributing to the development of this condition [29]. Future studies are needed to verify existing findings on larger databases representing diversity of populations, languages, genders, ages and types of depressive disorders. Further investigations into different linear and non-linear approaches for modeling depressive speech characteristics in order to improve discrimination between depressed and control subjects would also be beneficial.

10.7 Early Prediction of Depression Based on Acoustic Speech Analysis

Current approaches to depression risk assessment in children and adolescents are focused on identifying characteristics such as family history, early adversity, gender, age or socioeconomic status. These factors have been shown to provide higher likelihood of depression [30]. Numerous studies have undertaken the task of recognizing early behavioral and psychological signs and symptoms of the disorder that are not classified as full-blown symptoms [5, 30–32]. For example, adolescents of parents being treated for depression who score high in depression symptoms scales are at higher risk of developing clinical depression within the following year [33]. Similarly, women who are pregnant and have high depression symptoms levels are at high risk of developing pre- and post-partum depression [34]. Individuals with one or two short alleles of the serotonin transporter gene are more likely to develop a clinical depression when they are faced with stressful life events [35]. In Ref. [36], the concept of emotional inertia characterizing a specific type of psychological maladjustment showing high resistance to emotional changes was investigated. People with high emotional inertia are resistant to external influences and preserve their current emotional state for a long time. It was found that depressed individuals in particular tend to have higher levels of emotional inertia. In Ref. [37] emotional inertia was shown to predict the emergence of clinical depression in adolescents 2.5 years later.

Successful applications of the acoustic speech analysis in the detection of clinical depression [11, 13–17, 22, 28] brought up the possibility that subtle changes in speech acoustics could indicate risk for depression before the symptoms of depression can be recognized using standard diagnostic tests.

Experiments described in [38, 39] demonstrated for the first time that acoustic speech analysis and classification can be indeed used to determine very early signs of Major Depression in adolescents. The acoustic speech analysis was able to single out individuals at risk of depression as early as two years before they meet clinical diagnostic criteria for the full-blown disorder.

Using speech classification based on acoustic features the risk of developing depression was determined for adolescent individuals who have never experienced depression episodes and were diagnosed as non-depressed when the speech data was collected. The prediction results were validated through medical examinations conducted two years after the speech data was recorded.

Prior to the data collection a large sample of 2,479 potential participants representing Year Six primary school students (age range: 9–12 years) were screened using the Early Adolescent Temperament Questionnaire-Revised (EATQ-R). The screening procedure produced a risk-enriched and gender balanced sample of 245. Of this sample, 191 families with 94 female children and 97 male children agreed to participate in the first laboratory session at time T1. The age of children in this group was 12–13. During the first laboratory session, audio-visual recordings were made of adolescents while conducting discussions with their parents. The recordings captured images and speech from naturalistic discussions between parents and children. All participants had never suffered depression before, and were diagnosed as having no symptoms of depression at the time when the audiovisual recordings were made. Two years after the first stage, the second (follow-up) stage (T2) was conducted with the same participants as in the first stage. During this stage no video or audio recordings were taken but all adolescent participants were tested by psychologists using conventional diagnostic tests to determine their current state of mental health. The results showed that 15 participants (6 male and 9 female) suffered from the Major Depressive Disorder (MDD) and 3 participants (1 male and 2 female) had other mood disorders (OMD). The remaining adolescent participants had no symptoms of depression or other mood disorders.

Using the diagnostic information collected at T2, the speech recordings of adolescent participants made in stage T1 were divided into two classes: “At Risk” (AR) referring to adolescents who were non-depressed in T1 but developed MDD by T2, and “Not At Risk” (NAR) representing participants who were non-depressed in T1 and did not show any symptoms of depression at T2. At stage T2 of data collection, it became apparent that the initial recordings made at T1 contained data from only 15 AR participants. To match the population’s sizes for each class (AR and NAR), the speech dataset used in the prediction experiments included a total of 30 participants, 15 of which belonged to the AR class and 15 to the control, NAR class. From the gender point of view, the AR class included 6 male and 9 female adolescents. This ratio reflected the well know trend in depression epidemics with almost twice as many females as males likely to develop depression during adolescence. In order to match the gender ratio determined by the AR group, the control NAR class was also composed of 6 male and 9 female participants.

Figures 10.6 and 10.7 illustrate the overall framework of the basic single-channel prediction procedure commonly used in speech classification and recognition systems [11, 13, 14, 15, 16, 17, 27, 38, 39]. The procedure included two main stages: training stage (see Fig. 10.6) and classification and decision making stage (see Fig. 10.7). The training stage used a set of data with known classes to build statistical models of the AR and NAR classes. After the pre-processing, feature parameters characterizing the speech acoustics of each class were calculated. The probability density functions of these parameters were passed to the Gaussian Mixture Model (GMM) algorithm to build the Gaussian Mixture Models of the AR and NAR classes. Since four different types of acoustic speech parameters [glottal (G), prosodic (P), Teager energy operator (TEO) and spectral (S)] were calculated, four separate GMMs were built to represent each class (AR and NAR). These class models were then used in the classification stage.

The procedures involved in the classification and decision making process also included pre-processing and feature calculation followed by a relatively simple process of Bayesian classification [40] providing the final class estimate (prediction result).

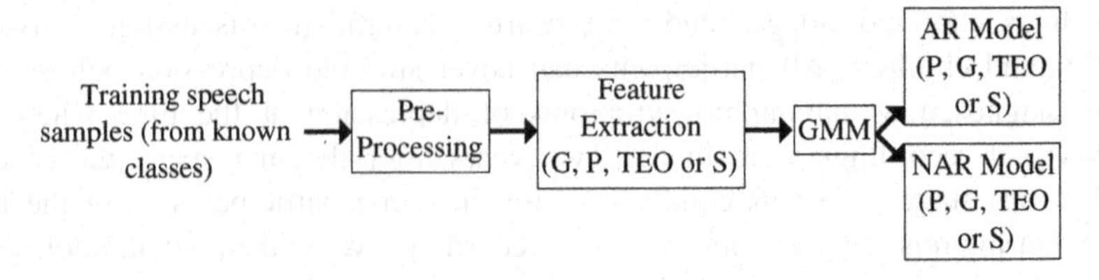

Fig. 10.6 An overview of the training stage of single-channel system generating AR and NAR models for a given type of features (G, P, TEO or S)

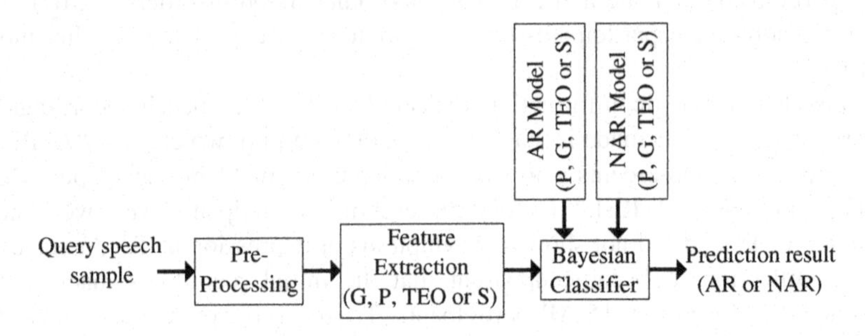

Fig. 10.7 An overview of a single-channel classification system

Individual contributions of four different types of acoustic parameters: prosodic, glottal, TEO and spectral to depression related changes of speech characteristics were investigated using a single-channel binary classification approach based on the training and classification systems illustrated in Figs. 10.6 and 10.7 respectively.

Figure 10.9 shows that, the single-channel methodology led to results only slightly higher than the guessing level for a binary classification. It was observed that single channel classification was effective in predicting depression with a desirable specificity to sensitivity ratio and accuracy higher than chance level only when using glottal or prosodic features.

The low efficiency, the single channel classification (based on a single type of features) led to the development of a multi-channel classification with a weighted classification decision procedure illustrated in Fig. 10.8. The values of the weight coefficients were determined using a supervised classification process. The higher was the channel accuracy, the higher was the weight value assigned to that channel. The final classification decision was made based on the sign of a weighted sum $r(x_i)$ of classification outcomes from each channel.

As illustrated in Fig. 10.9, the multi-channel method, which used a weighted combination of four features: prosodic, glottal, TEO and spectral provided significantly higher accuracy and more desirable specificity to sensitivity ratio than the single channel approach.

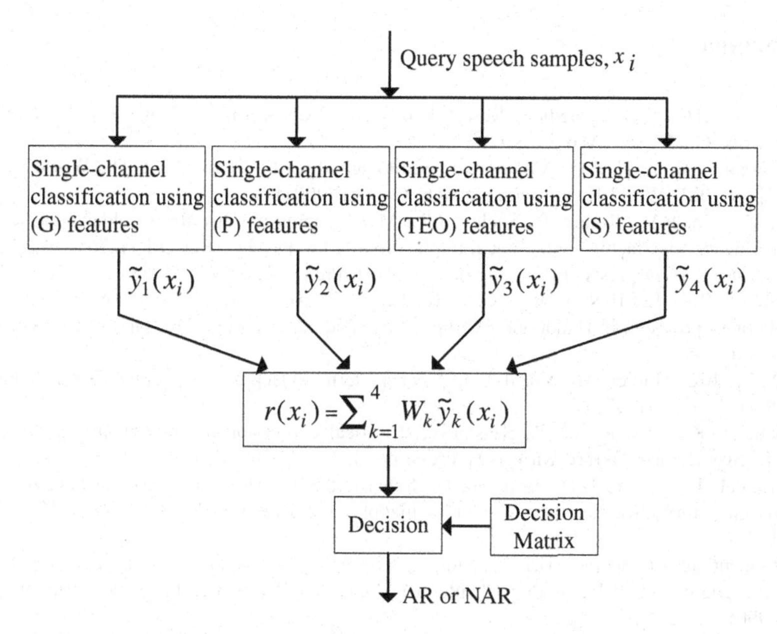

Fig. 10.8 The multi-channel classification system using weighted decision. *AR* denotes that the speaker is "at risk" of depression and *NAR* denotes that the speaker is "not at risk" of depression

Features		Sensitivity (%)	Specificity (%)	Accuracy (%)
Pure Guess		50.00	50.00	50.00
Single-Channel	Glottal	76.19	62.50	69.35
	Prosodic	73.21	52.98	63.10
	TEO	43.45	60.71	52.08
	Spectral	60.12	47.62	53.87
Multi-channel		78.57	66.96	72.77

Fig. 10.9 Depression prediction results for individual features (adapted from [41])

In the case of the person based approach with two separate sets of weights for the depressed and non-depressed individuals, the new multi-channel method provided a high accuracy level of 73 % and a desirable sensitivity to specificity ratio of 79/67 for predicting future depression.

The depression prediction methodology proposed in [41] offers an objective measure for the assessment of risk for depression. It is also a low cost and relatively easy to implement approach. The achieved sensitivity, specificity and accuracy values make it suitable for mass screening tests of large populations of adolescents (Fig. 10.9).

References

1. National Health and Medical Research Council: Depression in Young People: Clinical Practice Guidelines. AGPS (1997)
2. Communications N.M.H.: Mental and neurological disorders. Fact Sheet: The World Health Report 2001, World Health Organization, Geneva (2001)
3. Lewinsohn, P.M., Rohde, P., Seeley, J.R.: Major depressive disorder in older adolescents: prevalence, risk factors, and clinical implications. Clin. Psychol. Rev. **18**(7), 765–794 (1998)
4. Tongue, B.J.: Depression in young people. Aust. Prescr. **21**, 20–22 (1998)
5. Muñoz, R.F., Le, H.N., Clarke, G.N., Barrera, A.Z., Torres, L.D.: Preventing the Onset of Major Depression, in Handbook of Depression, 2nd edn, pp. 533–553. Guilford Press, New York (2008)
6. Darby, J.K., Hollien, H.: Vocal and speech patterns of depressive patients. Folia Phoniatr. **29**(4), 279–291 (1977)
7. Scherer, K.L., Johnstone, T., Klasmeyer, L. vocal expression of emotion in handbook of affective science. Oxford University Press, pp. 433–456 (2003)
8. Puschel, J., Stassen, H.H., Bomben, G., Schartfetter, D., Hell, D.: Speaking behavior and speech sound characteristics in acute schizophrenia (Elsevier). J. Psych. Res. **32**, 89–97 (1988)
9. Blumenthal S.J., Kupfer D.J.: Suicide over the life cycle: Risk factors, assessment and treatment of suicidal patients (Chapter 6). American Psychiatric Press, Washington, DC (1990)
10. Cavenar, J.O., Keith, H., Brodie, H., Weiner, R.D.: Signs and Symptoms in Psychiatry, pp. 227–249. Lippincott, Philadelphia (1983)
11. France D.J: Acoustical properties of speech as indicators of depression and suicidal risk., PhD Th., Vanderbilt University(1997)
12. Hollien, H., Green, R., Massey, K.: Longitudinal research on adolescent voice change in males. J. Acoust. Soc. Am. **96**(5), 2646–2654 (1994)
13. Low, L.S.A., Maddage, N.C., Lech, M., Sheeber, L., Allen, N.: Detection of clinical depression in adolescents' speech during family interactions. IEEE Trans. Biomed. Eng. **58**(3), 574–586 (2011)
14. Moore II, E., Clements, M., Peifer, J., Weisser, L.: Investigating the Role of Glottal Features in Classifying Clinical Depression. IEEE EMBS Cancun, Mexico, 2849–2852, 17–21 (2003), and Biology Society, IEMBS 26th Annual International Conference, vol. 1: 17–20 (2004)
15. Moore, II E., Clements, M., Peifer, J., Weisser, L.: Analysis of prosodic variation in speech for clinical depression. IEEE EMBS Cancun, Mexico, 2925–2928, 17–21 (2003)
16. Ozdas, A., Shiavi, R.G., Silverman, S.E., Silverman, M.K., Wilkes, D.M.: Investigation of vocal jitter and glottal flow spectrum as possible cues for depression and near-term suicidal risk. IEEE Trans. Biom. Eng. **51**(9), 1530–1540 (2004)
17. Ozdas, A.: Analysis of paralynguistic properties of speech for near-term sucidal risk assesment. PhD Th., Vanderb. University (2001)
18. Theodoridis, S., Koutroumbas, K.: Pattern Recognition, 1st edn. Academic Press, Massachusetts (1998)
19. Moses, P.: The Voice of Neurosis. Grune and Stratton, New York (1954)
20. Siegman, A.W.: The pacing of speech in depression. In: Masser, J.D. (ed.) Depression and Expressive Behaviour, pp. 83–102. Erlbaum, Hillsdale, NJ (1987)
21. Kuny, S., Stassen, H.H.: Speaking behaviour and voice sound characteristics in depressive patients during recovery. J. Psychiatr. Res. **27**(3), 289–307 (1993)
22. Moore II, E., Clements, M.A., Peifer, J.W., Weisser, L.: Critical analysis of the impact of glottal features in the classification of clinical depression in speech. IEEE Trans. Biomed. Eng. **55**(1), 96–107 (2008)
23. Darby, J.K.: Speech and voice parameters of depression: a pilot study. J. Comm. Disorder **17**(2), 75–85 (1984)

24. Nilsonne, Å., Sundberg, J., Ternstrom, S., Askenfelt, A.: Measuring the rate of change of voice fundamental frequency in fluent speech. J. Acous. Soc. Am. **83**(2), 716–728 (1998)
25. Alpert, M., Pouget, E.R., Silva, P.: Reflections of depression in acoustic measures of patient's speech. J. Aff. Dis. **66**, 59–69 (2001)
26. Ellgring, H., Scherer, K.R.: Vocal indicators of mood change in depression. J. Nonverbal Behav. **20**(2), 83–100 (1996). Springer Netherlands
27. France, D.J., Shiavi, R.G., Silverman, S., Silverman, M., Wilkes, D.M.: Acoustical properties of speech as indicators of depression and suicidal risk. IEEE Trans. Biomed. Eng. **47**(7), 829–837 (2000)
28. Moore, II E., Clements, M., Peifer, J., Weisser, L.: Comparing objective feature statistics of speech for classifying clinical depression. Engineering in Medicine and Biology Society, IEMBS 26th Annual International Conference, vol. 1, pp. 17–20 (2004)
29. Sheeber, L.B., Allen, N.B., Leve, C., Betsy, D.B., Shortt, J.W., Katz, L.F.: Dynamics of affective experience and behavior in depressed adolescents. J. Child Psychol. Psychiatry **50**(11), 1419–1427 (2009)
30. Muñoz, R.F., Barrera, A.Z., Torres, L.D.: Overview of depression prevention. In: Ingram, R.E. (ed.) International Encyclopedia of Depression, pp. 447–452. Springer Publishing (2009)
31. Mrazek, P., Haggerty, R.: Reducing Risk for Mental Disorders: Frontiers for Preventive Intervention Research. The National Academy Press, Washington, D.C. (1994)
32. Muñoz, R.F., Ying, Y.W.: The Prevention of Depression: Research and Practice. Johns Hopkins University Press, Baltimore (1993)
33. Garber, J., Clarke, G.N., Weersing, V.R.: Prevention of depression in at-risk adolescents: a randomized controlled trial. JAMA **301**, 2215–2224 (2003)
34. Henshaw, C., Elliott, S.: Screening for perinatal depression. Jessica Kingsley Publishers, London (2005)
35. Dorado, P., Peñas-Lledó, E.M., González, A.P., Cáceres, M.C., Cobaleda, J., Llerena, A.: Increased risk for major depression associated with the short allele of the serotonin transporter promoter region (5-HTTLPR-S) and the CYP2C9*3 allele. J. Fundam. Clin. Pharmacol. **21**, 451–453 (2007)
36. Kuppens, P., Allen, N., Sheeber, L.B.: Emotional inertia and psychological maladjustment. Psychol. Sci. **21**, 984–991 (2010)
37. Kuppens, P., Sheeber, L.B., Yap, M.B.H., et al.: Emotional inertia prospectively predicts the onset of depressive disorder in adolescents. Emotions **12**, 283–289 (2012)
38. Ooi, K.E.B., Lech, M., Allen, N.B.: Multi-channel weighted speech classification system for prediction of major depression in adolescents. IEEE Trans. Biomed. Eng. **60**(2):497–506 (2013)
39. Ooi, K.E.B., Low, L.S.A., Lech, M., Allen, N.: Early prediction of major depression in adolescents using glottal wave characteristics and Teager energy parameters, ICASSP 2012, March 25–30, Kyoto, Japan (2012)
40. Bernardo J.M., Smith A.F.M.: Bayesian Theory. Wiley Series in Probability and Statistics (2001)
41. Ooi, K.E.B., Low, L.S.A., Lech, M., Allen, N.B.: Prediction of clinical depression in adolescents using facial image analysis. Image Analysis for Multimedia Interactive Services, WIAMIS (2011)

Chapter 11
Automated Method for Diagnosing Speech and Language Dysfunction in Schizophrenia

Anne Debra Tilaka, Joachim Diederich, Insu Song and Ai Ni Teoh

11.1 Introduction

The year 2011 marked one hundred years since the introduction of the diagnostic category schizophrenia and for a century, speech and language dysfunction (SLD) has been strongly associated with schizophrenia. At a descriptive clinical level, thought disorder in schizophrenics can be divided into positive and negative symptoms [25]. Positive thought disorder includes, among other things, the use of neologisms (new unusual words), incoherence, derailment (the speaker is losing track) and glossomania (association chaining, which may also occur in mania). Negative thought disorder means poverty of speech (e.g., reduced vocabulary) and correlates with other, non-linguistic negative symptoms (e.g., flat affect). SLD occurs in other mental health disorders as well, for instance, in mania and depression [17]. This study, however, focuses on schizophrenia, since incoherent speech and language is among the main symptoms of the disorder [17, 25].

A. D. Tilaka (✉)
School of Arts and Social Sciences, James Cook University, Singapore 574421, Singapore
e-mail: debradass@yahoo.com.sg

J. Diederich
School of Information Technology and Electrical Engineering, The University of Queensland, Brisbane, QLD 4072, Australia
e-mail: j.diederich@uq.edu.au

I. Song
School of Business/IT, James Cook University, Singapore Campus, Singapore 574421, Singapore
e-mail: insu.song@jcu.edu.au

A. N. Teoh
North Dakota State University, Fargo, ND 58102, USA

M. Lech et al. (eds.), *Mental Health Informatics*,
Studies in Computational Intelligence 491, DOI: 10.1007/978-3-642-38550-6_11,

11.1.1 The Importance of Speech and Language Disorders for the Assessment of Schizophrenia

There are speech and language differences between individuals affected by schizophrenia and non-psychotic subjects. Firstly, several studies demonstrated that schizophrenic patients communicate less compared to normal subjects [3, 15, 16, 23, 26]. Qualitatively, schizophrenic SLD includes two features which are commonly referred to as 'poverty of speech' (lack of speech or reduced vocabulary) and 'poverty of content' (lack of variety) [3, 11]. Schizophrenic SLD persists longitudinally, occurring in about 80–90 % of patients during the acute stages of hospitalization [22, 33, 37], and prevailing in about 39 % of the patients during the post-acute stages [3, 6, 22, 38].

Since SLD is associated with cognitive impairments [13, 18], it is regarded as a reliable clinical marker of a psychotic disorder, as it can be directly observed [10, 37]. SLD is also considered as an early vulnerability indicator of schizophrenia, since its presence in children and adolescents is a significant predictor of adult psychosis [4, 27, 31, 32]. Unlike positive SLD (e.g., derailment, incoherence), it is the negative type (poverty of speech and content) that is indicative of a poor prognosis [3, 5, 21, 24, 28]. Reliable and valid measures of SLD are critical for research and clinical practice.

11.1.2 Speech and Language Disorder Measures

11.1.2.1 Thought, Language and Communication Scale

Common measures of SLD are observer-rated scales, as they provide for a broad assessment of symptoms. The most widely used instrument is the Thought, Language and Communication scale (TLC) [2, 21, 28, 36] which is based on a phenomenological approach [28]. It consists of 18 items: poverty of speech, poverty of content, pressure of speech, distractibility, tangentiality, loss of goal, derailment, circumstantiality, illogicality, incoherence, neologisms, word-approximations, stilted-speech, clanging, preservation, echolalia, blocking and self-reference.

TLC was validated by demonstrating that schizophrenics obtained greater SLD an normal participants [1, 2]. Furthermore, compared with other clinical groups (mania and depression), schizophrenic patients consistently scored high over extended periods of time [1, 2]. Other TLC studies have produced similar results [3, 5, 11, 36, 37]. Among the 18 TLC items, schizophrenics normally obtain high scores on 'poverty of speech' and 'poverty of content'. These findings have been replicated numerous times [3, 5, 11, 33, 36, 37].

TLC has also been used for diagnostic purposes. The scale achieved an overall accuracy of 84 % in correctly determining schizophrenia and mania with a class validation rate of 80 % (83 % in a replication study) [3]. Although non-psychotic participants were included, the study did not provide classification rates for this group [1]. Cuesta and Peralta found that the TLC scale was able to differentiate between patients affected by schizophrenia or mania with an accuracy of approximately 80 % [11].

Many of the diagnostic studies that used TLC focused on comparing schizophrenia with mania and did not necessarily include non-clinical participants. An exception was the study by Berenbaum et al. [5] who refined the TLC scale. When the authors compared schizophrenics with non-psychotic participants, accuracy rates were a mere 64 % indicating that the original TLC was performing better. Overall, the vast majority of studies demonstrated that TLC has good discriminative and predictive properties.

11.1.2.2 Clinical Language Disorder Ratings Scale

The Clinical Language Disorders Rating Scale (CLANG) utilises a linguistic approach and is structured according to linguistic levels: syntax, semantics and production. The majority of the 17 items are described in linguistic terms (excess phonetic-association, abnormal syntactic-structure, excessive syntactic-constraints, lacking semantic-association, referential failures, discourse failures, excessive details, lacking details, prosodic speech, abnormal prosody, pragmatic disorder, dysfluency, dysarthria, and paraphasic error), except for three that include phenomenological terms (poverty of speech, pressure of speech, and neologisms). Generally, speech refers to motor production and language refers to content. For CLANG, transcripts of audio-recorded speech are used, and in this sense, this study is both on speech as well as on language.

CLANG was first validated with a sample of 204 Hong Kong Chinese schizophrenic patients [10]. Another study involved British participants. In the study, schizophrenic patients obtained higher SLD scores compared to normal participants [9]. In comparison to other clinical groups (mania and depression), schizophrenic subjects obtained the highest SLD scores [8]. Qualitatively, over half of CLANG's items can be linked with TLC items, which contributes to its convergent validity [10]. Furthermore, CLANG's production factor (poverty of speech, lack of details and aprosody) correlates with TLC's poverty of speech and poverty of content. Schizophrenics scored highest on the CLANG item 'lack of details', which parallels TLC's 'poverty of content' [8].

When CLANG was used for prediction (in this case differentiating schizophrenia from depression), it achieved an overall accuracy of 76 % [8]. In another study, CLANG achieved a perfect accuracy of 100 % in correctly identifying non-clinical participants, and 70 % accuracy in identifying schizophrenic participants in a mixed group of normal and various clinical subjects (psychosis) [9]. The authors conclude that, when other clinical groups are combined with schizophrenic participants, accuracy rates are compromised. Although studies using CLANG are limited, the scale has shown good performance when discriminating between normal and psychotic participants, and moderately good performance when differentiating between participants with other psychotic disorders.

11.1.2.3 Strengths and Weaknesses of the Scales

Observer-rated scales have been instrumental in SLD research and are in widespread clinical use. The main advantage is their simplicity with concise definitions and instructions for raters [1, 10]. TLC is straight forward to use [19], while CLANG requires a basic understanding of general linguistic concepts [10]. Both scales have Likert scores, offer flexible scoring with separate items, have subsections, and include total scores [10, 19]. Statistically, both TLC [3, 5, 7, 11, 33, 36, 37] and CLANG [8–10] have good reliability and validity. Furthermore, observer scales, if applied live, have the advantage of face-to-face interactions that allow better interpretation of speech, because of the accompanying non-verbal expressions [1].

Nevertheless, observer-rated scales suffer from shortcomings. Subjectivity can bias the assessment, as the result of different levels of expertise, background, and training, or cultural and personal factors come into play [29]. For example, one study that employed six psychiatrists with different levels of training resulted in widely distributed scores [5]. Cultural background can also impact evaluations. In one study, American psychiatrists mistakenly identified some of the colloquialisms of the British participants as indicators of language impairments [5].

In clinical practice, it is difficult to ascertain if high inter-rater reliability among raters really exists, while research practice requires standardized training and testing procedures [10, 16, 19] that provide this information. However, even in a research setting, poor inter-rater reliability on certain items is not always identified, especially if items occur infrequently [3, 12, 20].

According to a Canadian survey, many psychiatrists do not use scales because they are apprehensive about their usefulness [30]. The standard practice is to conduct a Mental Status Examination (MSE) [35] and consult the DSM-IV-TR [17]. Although the MSE and DSM can be criticized for lacking detailed Likert-like ratings [35], they remain practical in clinical settings, where time constraints are paramount.

Notwithstanding the strengths of scales, their weaknesses warrant an investigation into other methods of evaluating SLD. One possibility is to look beyond manual methods towards automated techniques.

11.1.3 Advantages of Automated Measures

It is now possible for automated methods to offer benefits similar to those of standardized observer-rated scales. Fully automated programmes are user-friendly, since they remove the labour of scoring and the generation of reports that are interpretative in nature [34]. The greatest advantage of automated methods is the objectivity they provide, which contrasts with the inherent subjectivity of scales [34].

Since automated programmes offer time and cost saving advantages [34], mental health professionals may welcome the idea of using such measures in everyday practice. Unlike clinicians who need substantial time and training to gain experience in assessing SLD efficiently, automated programmes use "machine learning" to mimic experienced clinical decision making processes [14].

11.1.3.1 Ex-Ray

Mental health practitioners, consciously and unconsciously, analyse the language of their patients, identify patterns and use this information for clinical assessment, or classification, using DSM IV or ICD10. Machine learning techniques can be applied in psychiatry to analyse data, including speech and language. This chapter investigates a novel approach to psychiatric classification and diagnostic screening that utilises widely available data. This computational approach is compared to observer rated scales.

This study uses a computational method called Ex-Ray [14] which uses a particular machine learning technique: Support Vector Machines (SVMs). SVMs are a class of algorithms which are well-suited to learning classification and regression tasks. SVMs have also been used for ranking problems, e.g., a ranking with regard to the severity of a disorder. SVMs have been utilised in a wide variety of tasks, including text and image classification as well as bio-medical applications. SVMs utilise kernels to work in a high-dimensional feature space. In binary classification tasks, the margin between the two classes is maximized in order to find the best possible separation. An SVM algorithm finds an optimal decision boundary in the multi-dimensional feature space by finding a hyperplane, which has maximum distance from prototypical samples, called "support vectors." The learned hyperplane is then used as a decision boundary of the SVM classifier.

11.1.4 Objective and Hypotheses

Since the computational method offers similar advantages as observer-rated scales and overcomes some of their weaknesses, the objective of this study is to compare Ex-Ray with TLC and CLANG in its ability to determine SLD. As an automated and objective instrument not affected by subjectivity and inter-rater issues, the computational method should achieve a higher classification accuracy than the observer-rated scales on a sample of randomised schizophrenic and normal speech samples.

The minor hypotheses of this study are that each of the measures (TLC, CLANG and Ex-Ray) will be able to correctly separate schizophrenic from normal participants by use of speech samples. The main hypothesis is that Ex-Ray will have the same performance as the scales or even outperform these in terms of accuracy and quality of receiver operating characteristic (ROC) curves.

11.2 Method

11.2.1 Participants

A total of fifty-four subjects (n = 27 schizophrenics; n = 27 controls) participated in this study. Schizophrenic subjects were recruited from two centres of the Singapore Association of Mental Health (SAMH) by a supervisor who was unaware of the purpose of the study. These participants were at the post-acute stage of the DSM-IV-TR4 diagnosis without other comorbid issues and were taking neuroleptics.

Non-psychotic participants were recruited from a batch of first year psychology students of James Cook University Australia (Singapore campus). The exclusion criteria were: no recent history of mental illness, depression, substance abuse or alcohol intoxication. Normal participants were rewarded with one course credit point to fulfil part of the requirements for some core psychology modules, while schizophrenia participants were rewarded with a cash token of two Singapore dollars.

The age of schizophrenic participants ranged from 21 to 62 (M = 43.9, SD = 10.5), with 13 males and 14 females. The ethnic composition of the sample was 81 % Chinese, 12 % Indians and 7 % Malays (reflecting the demographics of Singapore). All the participants could converse in English, even though at home, the majority (74 %) spoke other languages (e.g., Chinese, Tamil and Malay) and a minority (26 %) spoke mostly English. The age of the non-psychotic participants ranged from 18 to 37 (M = 22.6, SD = 4.8), with 11 males and 16 females. Among them, 78 % were Chinese, 19 % were Indians and 4 % were Malays. All participants were conversant in the English language, with the majority (86 %) speaking English at home, while the rest (14 %) used mainly other languages.

11.2.2 Apparatus

Ex-Ray performed well in a preliminary SLD study [14], achieving a 77 % accuracy in distinguishing schizophrenics from normal participants. TLC consists of 18 phenomenological items, each to be rated on a 5-point Likert scale (0 = no more than one instance of SLD, 1 = mild SLD, 2 = moderate SLD, 3 = severe SLD, and 4 = extreme SLD). As stated above, TLC has good psychometric properties with high inter-rater reliability ($k > 0.80$) for common items such as poverty of speech and content and a high intra-class correlation coefficient that ranged from 0.78 to 0.85 in previous studies [8, 24]. CLANG has 17 linguistic items to be rated on a 4-point Likert scale (0 = normal speech, 1 = mild SLD, 2 = moderate SLD, and 3 = severe, pervasive SLD). CLANG has high internal reliability for the subscales (the entire scale's alpha coefficient is 0.76) with an intra-class correlation of 0.88 for the full scale [18]. Convergent validity was established with the Brief Psychiatric Rating Scale (BPRS) [18] and the Schneiderian First-Rank Symptom (SFRS) [9], while criterion validity was established with TLC [18].

11.2.3 Procedure

Ethical clearance was obtained from the James Cook University (JCU) Human Research Ethics Committee.

11.2.3.1 Interview

After obtaining informed consent, an unstructured interview was conducted with each participant. Interviews were approximately 20 min in length, conducted in English and audio recorded. A list of open-ended questions had been prepared earlier by referring to the manuals of TLC and CLANG to guide the interview. The interviews with schizophrenic participants were carried out in a Singapore Association of Mental Health room with a clinician present, while the interviews with non-clinical participants took place in a JCU research lab.

There were two teams of interviewers (Team A and B), each comprised of two persons. The interviewers were not blind to the purpose of the study. As there were two locations, participants from one SAMH centre were interviewed by Team A, while those in the other centre were interviewed by Team B. In each of the locations, half of the schizophrenic participants were interviewed by the first interviewer, while the other half of the participants were interviewed by the second person. The normal participants were divided into two groups and interviewed in a similar manner by the two teams that had conducted the schizophrenic group interviews.

11.2.3.2 TLC and CLANG Scoring

The content of each interview was independently scored by two raters on every item of TLC and CLANG scales. A global score was also given for each scale based on the overall content of the interview. Prior to conducting the ratings, a practice session was held to facilitate the understanding of items and to discuss potential discrepancies in rating behaviour. All audio recorded samples were de-identified and randomized. To ensure blind ratings, interviews conducted by Team A were rated by Team B and vice versa. Half of these samples were rated with TLC first followed by the CLANG; the remainder were rated in reverse order. The two global ratings awarded by the raters for each participant were averaged into one rating per participant and scale.

11.2.3.3 Ex-Ray Learning

Speech samples were manually transcribed by the interviewers. The transcripts were handed to an Ex-Ray programmer for analysis. The transcripts were segmented into words, each word was stemmed, and functional words (such as "to" and "the") were removed. The words were ranked according to document frequency, and words with less than two occurrences were removed. The selected words were then used as attributes, and thus each transcript was represented as a vector of the frequencies of words.

In Ex-Ray, the input features are normalized frequencies of words. Recordings of interviews are transcribed into text documents and each document is segmented into a list of words. Words in the whole corpora are ranked and infrequent words are discarded. The normalized frequency (normalized to the length of documents) of each word in the ranked list of words are then used as input features of each document. That is, an input feature $\mathbf{x} = (v_1, \ldots, v_d) \in \Re^d$ is a d-dimensional vector and each feature value v_i is a normalized frequency of a word:

$$v_i = \text{Frequency of the } i\text{th Word / The Length of Document} \tag{11.1}$$

where the length of document is the L2-Norm of word frequencies in a document. The task is then to find a function $f : \mathbf{x} \rightarrow D$ by use of SVM learning that maps the input feature vector $\mathbf{x} \in \Re^d$ to a class label $D \in \{+1, -1\}$.

11.2.3.4 Statistical Analysis

The data from all participants was included in the statistical analysis. Data analyses were performed using the Predictive Analytics Software (PASW Statistics, v.18) with alpha level set at 0.05. Only averaged global scores of TLC and CLANG were used for analysis. For the assessment of group membership, participants were identified as schizophrenics if they scored 1 or more on the averaged global score of each scale, or as control if they scored less than 1.

Standardised global ratings were calculated for TLC (M = 0.95, SLD = 1.14), CLANG (M = 0.79, SLD = 0.95), and Ex-Ray (M = −0.06, SLD = 0.97), because of the different Likert scores in the two observation scales. Cronbach's alphas were computed on the averaged global scores of TLC and CLANG for inter-rater reliability within Team A and Team B, respectively.

In order to obtain the classification accuracy of each measure, (ROC) curve analyses were conducted. Finally, to test for differences between the ROC curves of Ex-Ray and TLC, as well as between Ex-Ray and CLANG, z-score analysis was performed by manually calculating the critical ratio z.

11.3 Results

11.3.1 Differences in Word Frequencies Between the Subject and Control Groups

The mean relative-frequency of unique words in each transcript differed significantly between the subject and control groups (see Figs. 11.1, 11.2, 11.3). The mean relative-frequency $\mu 1$ of the control group was larger than the mean relative-frequency $\mu 2$ of the schizophrenia group (N1 = 27, N2 = 27, $\mu 1 = 0.3172$, $\mu 2 = 0.2720$, SE1 = 0.0160, SE2 = 0.0088, μ diff = 0.045, SE_diff = 0.0182, t = 2.469, df = 40.6, $p < 0.009$).

In addition, there was a difference in the number of new words added to the overall corpus with each 100 word segment. The average number of new words added to the control group corpus was consistently larger than the average number of new words added to the subject group corpus in 22 of the 100-word segments (N = 22, μ diff = 2.78, SE_diff = 0.327, t = 8.60, df = 21, $p < 0.002$).

Since the transcripts obtained from the schizophrenia and control groups differed in length, blocks of 100 word segments were formed by use of the transcripts

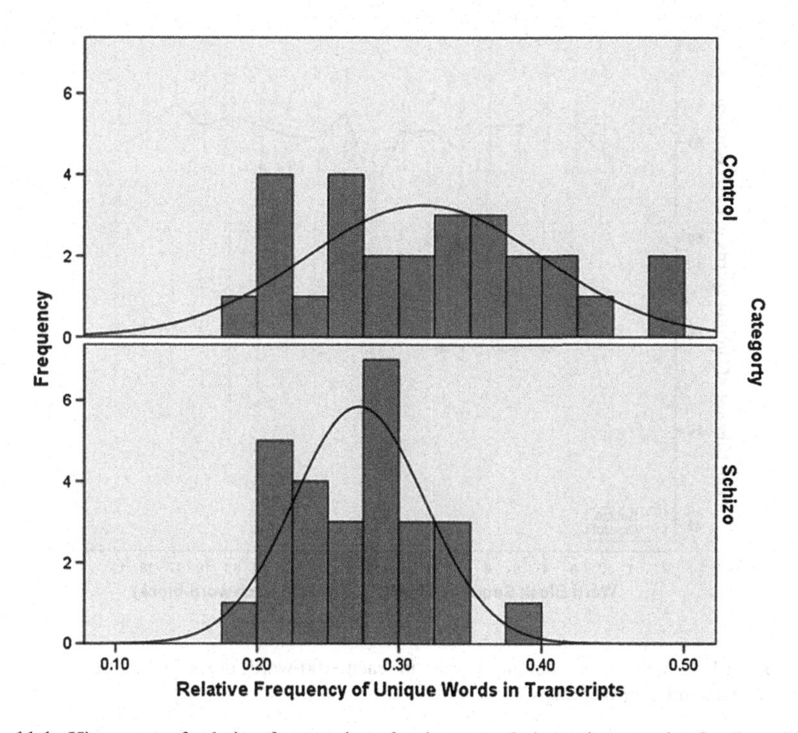

Fig. 11.1 Histogram of relative frequencies of unique words in each transcript for the subject (schizophrenia) and control groups

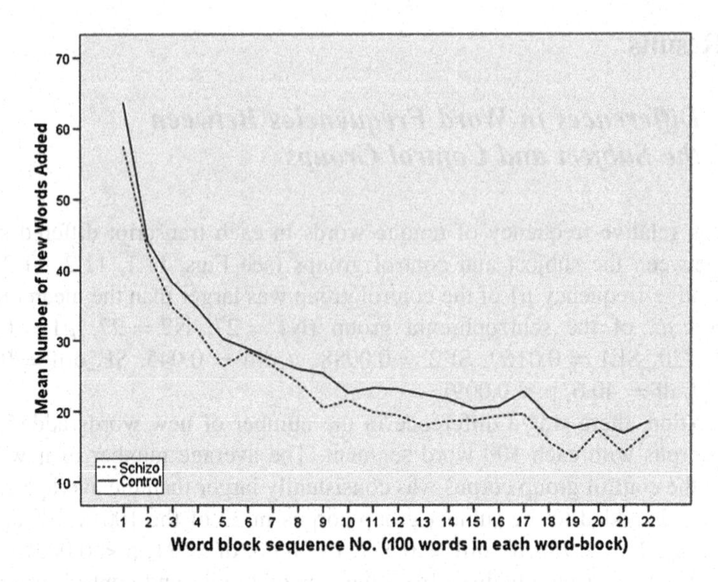

Fig. 11.2 Mean number of new words added to the corpus with each 100-word block (schizophrenia and control groups)

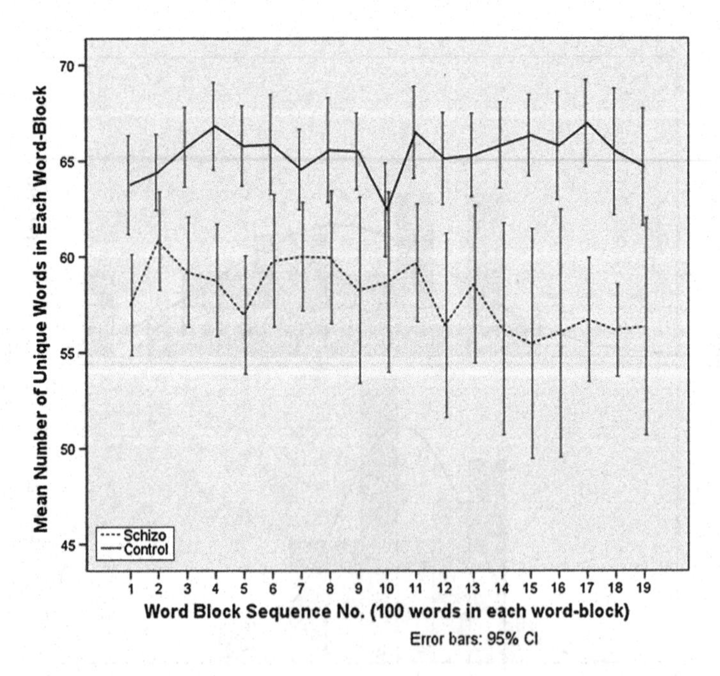

Fig. 11.3 Mean number of unique words in each 100-word block of transcripts for the schizophrenia and control groups

from both groups. The mean number of unique words in each 100 word segment again differed significantly between the subject and control groups (N1 = 43, N2 = 22, $\mu 1 = 63.9$, $\mu 2 = 57.8$, SE1 = 0.486, SE2 = 0.394, μ_diff = 6.07, SE_diff = 0.737, t = 8.24, df = 63, $p < 0.001$).

11.3.2 Ex-Ray Versus TLC and CLANG

The Cronbach's alpha inter-rater reliability for TLC for Team A and Team B was 0.85 and 0.95, respectively, while that of CLANG was 0.84 and 0.96 for Team A and Team B.

Thus, the first hypothesis which stated that TLC would correctly discriminate between schizophrenic and normal participants was supported, as ROC analysis revealed a high value for area under the curve (AUC) for TLC that was not due to chance (AUC = 0.98, SE = 0.02, $p < 0.001$). The ROC curve (see Fig. 11.4) had a sensitivity of 0.96, specificity of 0.96, and an optimal cut-off point of −0.62. This indicates that TLC differentiated between schizophrenic and normal participants with a high accuracy of 98 %. It correctly identified 96 % of the schizophrenics, and 96 % of the normal participants.

The second hypothesis stated that CLANG would correctly classify schizophrenic and normal participants. This hypothesis was also supported with a high AUC value (AUC = 0.97, SE = 0.02, $p < 0.001$), a sensitivity of 0.96, a specificity of 0.96 at an optimal cut-off point of −0.56. CLANG differentiated between schizophrenic and non-clinical participants with an accuracy of 97 %, and it correctly predicted 96 % of schizophrenic patients and 96 % of normal participants.

In line with the third hypothesis that Ex-Ray would correctly classify schizophrenic and non-clinical participants, the AUC value was significantly higher than

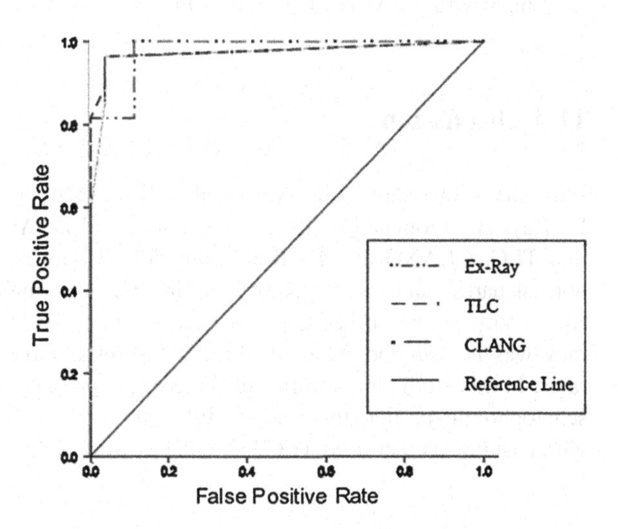

Fig. 11.4 Receiver operating characteristic *curves* of the thought, language and communication (TLC) scale, the clinical language disorder rating (CLANG) scale, and Ex-Ray

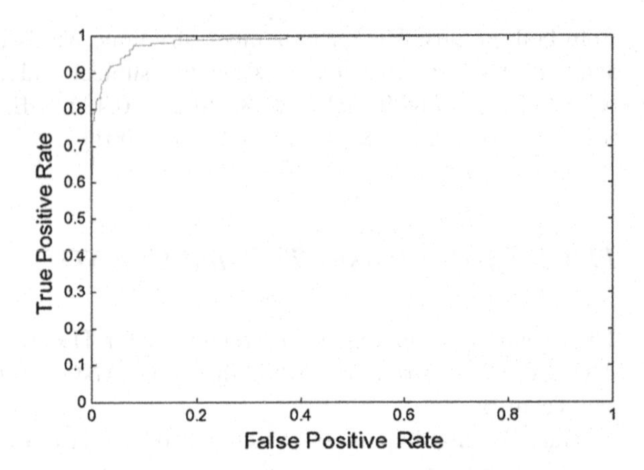

Fig. 11.5 ROC *curve* for Ex-Ray only if 100-word blocks are used

0.5 (AUC = 0.98, SE = 0.01, $p < 0.001$), with a sensitivity of 0.89, specificity of 0.89 and an optimal cut-off point of −0.13. As expected, Ex-Ray discriminated between schizophrenics and normal participants with an accuracy of 98 %. In addition, it correctly recognised 89 % of the schizophrenic cases and 89 % of non-psychotic participants.

It was also hypothesized that Ex-Ray would outperform both the TLC and CLANG scales in differentiating between schizophrenics and non-clinical participants. Contrary to this hypothesis, z-score analysis showed that the accuracy rate of Ex-Ray did not differ significantly from that of TLC, as the obtained z-score (0.08) was less than the critical value at alpha level of 0.05 (one-tailed). Similarly, with an obtained z score (0.25) that is less than the critical value, Ex-Ray did not differ significantly from CLANG in its accuracy.

Ex-Ray, however, performed at a very high level. If blocks of 100 words were used for classification instead of entire transcripts, the classification accuracy was very high with an AUC of 0.98 (see Fig. 11.5).

11.4 Discussion

This study compared observer-rated scales, such as TLC and CLANG, with Ex-Ray, an automated method for evaluating SLD. All minor hypotheses stating that TLC, CLANG and Ex-Ray could differentiate between schizophrenics and normal participants were confirmed. However, the main hypothesis that Ex-Ray would surpass the performance of observer-rated scales with its predictive accuracy was not supported, as all three measures obtained similarly high accuracy rates. In this study, the abilities of these observer-rated scales to correctly identify schizophrenic participants and to differentiate them from controls is consistent with past efforts that used TLC [3, 5, 11] as well as those that used CLANG [8, 9].

For Ex-Ray, the high classification rates obtained indicate that it has diagnostic value as a SLD measure, comparable to the performance of observer-rated scales.

Why did the computational method perform so well? The difference in unique words used (Figs. 11.1, 11.2, 11.3) is evidence for poverty of speech (and possibly poverty of content) in the schizophrenic group. Since there is a significant difference in the vocabulary used by both groups, SVMs that take word frequencies as input ("bag of words") can easily determine a decision boundary between both groups. Further analyses of the data may also reveal positive symptoms in the speech samples obtained from the schizophrenics, which would make the classification task even easier.

There are several explanations why Ex-Ray did not surpass the performance of the observer-rated scales, despite being a more objective measure. Firstly, there was an unexpectedly high inter-rater reliability among the raters (Cronbach's alpha was 0.90 on both the scales). This value is higher than those reported in previous studies [3, 10]. The scales' high inter-rater reliability and classification accuracy may be attributed to the small sample, compared to past studies [3, 10]. Next, as the ratings were not conducted live, the raters had more time to refer to manuals to determine scores. Since the interviews allowed for open-ended responses, some participants mentioned coming to 'school' or to the 'centre'. Indirectly, this may have provided information about the clinical background of the participants. Also, all raters were trained together and had similar background and experience as psychology students.

Ex-Ray correctly identified 89 % of the schizophrenic and non-clinical participants. This equates to incorrect classifications of 11 % for each group, which is higher than the incorrect classifications (4 %) obtained by both the scales. The higher number of classification errors by Ex-Ray can be partially explained by cultural language differences. The speech samples that Ex-Ray used came from a majority of participants who were Chinese (80 %), followed by Indians and Malays (6 %). English spoken by the Singaporean sample is peppered with ethnic words to describe local food, songs, and movies. Such words were elicited due to the nature of the questions. The human raters were familiar with most of the local "lingo" and relied on their judgment and background to decide if an expression was, indeed, an instance of a SLD. Obviously, Ex-Ray has no access to this kind of background knowledge.

In a follow-up study with a different control group, which matched the schizophrenic group in terms of ethnicity, socio-economic status and educational background, the Ex-Ray performance was confirmed with an overall accuracy that matched the results in this study. It is, therefore, a valid conclusion that support vector machines perform very well on this type classification task.

Acknowledgments The authors wish to thank all those involved in the data collection: Lynette Tham, Esther Hong, and Sabrina Yeo, and all the mental health professionals at the Singapore Mental Health Association, as well as the participants in this study. Thank you also to Margaret Lech, Adam Vogel, and Susan Wright for providing comments on earlier versions of this document.

References

1. Andreasen, N.C.: Thought, language, and communication disorders: i. Clinical assessment, definition of terms, and evaluation of their reliability. Arch. Gen. Psychiatry **36**(12), 1315–1321 (1979). doi:10.1001/archpsyc.1979.01780120045006
2. Andreasen, N.C.: Scale for the assessment of thought, language, and communication (TLC). Schizophr. Bull. **12**(3), 473–482 (1986)
3. Andreasen, N.C., Grove, W.M.: Thought, language, and communication in schizophrenia: Diagnosis and prognosis. Schizophr. Bull. **12**(3), 348–359 (1986). doi:10.1093/schbul/12.3.348
4. Bearden, C.E., Rosso, I.M., Hollister, J.M., Sanchez, L.E., Hadley, T., Cannon, T.D.: A prospective cohort study of childhood behavioural deviance and language abnormalities as predictors of adult schizophrenia. Schizophr. Bull. **26**(2), 395–410 (2000)
5. Berenbaum, H., Oltmanns, T.F., Gottesman, I.I.: Formal thought disorder in schizophrenics and their twins. J. Abnorm. Psychol. **94**(1), 3–16 (1985)
6. Breier, A., Berg, P.H.: The psychosis of schizophrenia. Biol. Psychiatry **46**, 361–364 (2003)
7. Buchanan, R.W., Strauss, M.E., Breier, A., Kirkpatrick, B., Carpenter, W.T.J.: Attentional impairments in deficit and nondeficit forms of schizophrenia. Am. J. Psychiatry **154**(3), 363–370 (1997)
8. Ceccherini-Nelli, A., Crow, T.J.: Disintegration of the Components of Language as the Path to a Revision of Bleuler's and Schneider's Concepts of Schizophrenia, vol. 182 (2003) First published. doi:10.1192/bjp.02.211
9. Ceccherini-Nelli, A., Turpin-Crowther, K., Crow, T.J.: Schneider's first rank symptoms and continuous performance disturbance as indices of dysconnectivity of left- and right-hemispheric components of language in schizophrenia. Schizophr. Res. **90**(1), 203–213 (2007)
10. Chen, E.Y.H., Lam, L.C.W., Kan, C.S., Chan, C.K.Y., Kwok, C.L., Nguyen, D.G.H., Chen, R.Y.L.: Language disorganisation in schizophrenia: Validation and assessment with a new clinical rating instrument. Hong Kong J. Psychiatry **6**(1), 4–13 (1996)
11. Cuesta, M.J., Peralta, V.: Does formal thought disorder differ among patients with schizophrenic, schizophreniform and manic schizoaffective disorders? Schizophr. Res. **10**(2), 151–158 (1993)
12. Cuesta, M.J., Peralta, V.: Thought disorder in schizophrenia. Testing models through confirmatory factor analysis. Eur. Arch. Psychiatry Clin. Neurosci. **249**(2), 55–61 (1999)
13. DeLisi, L.E.: Speech Disorder in Schizophrenia: Review of the Literature and Exploration of its Relation to the Uniquely Human Capacity for Language, vol. 27 (2001) First published
14. Diederich, J., Al-Ajmi, A., Yellowlees, P.: Ex-ray: Data mining and mental health. Appl. Soft Comput. J. **7**(3), 923–928 (2007)
15. Docherty, N.M., Cohen, A.S., Nienow, T.M., Dinzeo, T.J., Dangelmaier, R.E.: Stability of formal thought disorder and referential communication disturbances in schizophrenia. J. Abnorm. Psychol. **112**(3), 469–475 (2003)
16. Docherty, N.M., DeRosa, M., Andreasen, N.C.: Communication Disturbances in Schizophrenia and Mania, vol. 53 (1996) First published. doi:10.1001/archpsyc.1996.01830040094014
17. DSM-IV-T.R.: Diagnostic and Statistical Manual of Mental Disorders, Text Revision, 4th edn. American Psychiatric Association
18. Elvevag, B., Foltz, P.W., Rosenstein, M., DeLisi, L.E.: An automated method to analyze language use in patients with schizophrenia and their first-degree relatives. J. Neurolinguistics **23**(3), 270–284 (2009)
19. Elvevag, B., Foltz, P.W., Weinberger, D.R., Goldberg, T.E.: Quantifying incoherence in speech: An automated methodology and novel application to schizophrenia. Schizophr. Res. **93**(1–3), 304–316 (2007)

20. Faber, R., et al.: Comparison of schizophrenic patients with formal thought disorder and neurologically impaired patients with aphasia. Am. J. Psychiatry **140**(10), 1348–1351 (1983)
21. Fraser, W.I., King, K.M., Thomas, P., Kendell, R.E.: The Diagnosis of Schizophrenia by Language Analysis, vol. 148 (1986) First published. doi:10.1192/bjp.148.3.275
22. Harrow, M., Marengo, J.T.: Schizophrenic Thought Disorder at Followup: Its Persistence and Prognostic Significance, vol. 12 (1986) First published. doi:10.1093/schbul/12.3.373
23. Holzman, P.S., Shenton, M.E., Solovay, M.R.: Quality of thought disorder in differential diagnosis. Schizophrenia bulletin; schizophrenia. Bulletin **12**(3), 360–372 (1986)
24. Jampala, V.C., Taylor, M.A., Abrams, R.: The diagnostic implications of formal thought disorder in mania and schizophrenia: A reassessment. Am. J. Psychiatry **146**(4), 459–463 (1989)
25. Kuperberg, G.R.: Language in schizophrenia. Part I. An introduction. Lang. Linguist. Compass **4**(8), 576–589 (2010)
26. Liddle, P.F., Ngan, E.T.C., Caissie, S.L., Anderson, C.M., Bates, A.T., Quested, D.J., White, R., Weg, R.: Thought and Language Index: An Instrument for Assessing Thought and Language in Schizophrenia, vol. 181 (2002) First published. doi:10.1192/bjp.181.4.326
27. Makowski, D., Waternaux, C., Lajonchere, C.M., Dicker, R., Smoke, N., Koplewicz, H., Min, D., Mendell, N.R., Levy, D.L.: Thought disorder in ado-escent-onset schizophrenia. Schizophr. Res. **23**(2), 147–165 (1997)
28. McKenna, P., Oh, T.M.: Schizophrenic Speech: Making Sense of Bathroots and Ponds that Fall in Doorways. Cambridge University Press, Cambridge (2005)
29. Myers, D.: Social Psychology, 9th edn. McGraw-Hill International Edition, New York (2008)
30. Oluboka, O., Stewart, S., Haslam, D., Wodlinger, J., Adams, S.: The Use of Rating Scales by Canadian Psychiatrists: Qualitative and Quantitative Evidence. http://www.priory.com/psychiatry/Rating_Scales_Canadian_Psychiatry.htm. http://www.priory.com/psychiatry/Rating_Scales_Canadian_Psychiatry.htm. Accessed 10 Jan 2010
31. Ott, S.L., Roberts, S., Rock, D., Allen, J., Erlenmeyer-Kimling, L.: Positive and negative thought disorder and psychopathology in childhood among subjects with adulthood schizophrenia. Schizophr. Res. **58**(2), 231–239 (2002)
32. Parnas, J., Schulsinger, F., Schulsinger, H., Mednick, S.A., Teasdale, T.W.: Behavioral Precursors of Schizophrenia Spectrum: A Prospective Study, vol. 39 (1982) First published. doi:10.1001/archpsyc.1982.04290060020005
33. Peralta, V., Cuesta, M.J., de Leon, J.: Formal thought disorder in schizophrenia: A factor analytic study. Compr. Psychiatry **33**(2), 105–110 (1992)
34. Roid, G.H., Johnson, W.B.: Computer assisted psychological assessment. In: Rey-nolds, C.R. (ed.) Comprehensive Clinical Psychology 3 (1998)
35. Sadock, B.J., Sadock, V.A.: Synopsis of Psychiatry: Behavioural Sciences in Clinical Psychiatry, 9th edn. Lippincott Williams & Wilkins, Philadelphia (2003)
36. Simpson, D.M., Davis, G.C.: Measuring thought disorder with clinical rating scales in schizophrenic and nonschizophrenic patients. Psychiatry Res. **15**(4), 313–318 (1985)
37. Taylor, M.A., Reed, R., Berenbaum, S.A.: Patterns of speech disorders in schizophrenia and mania. J. Nerv. Mental Dis. **182**(6), 319–326 (1994)
38. Wykes, T., Leff, J.: Disordered speech: Differences between manics and schizophrenics. Brain Lang. **15**(1), 117–124 (1982)

Chapter 12
Suicide Risk Analysis

Carol Choo, Joachim Diederich, Insu Song and Roger Ho

12.1 Suicide Risk Assessment

The treatment of suicidal clients includes a comprehensive risk assessment that takes into account demographics, past history, and current assessment [28]. The assessment also includes a review of psychiatric, medical, and family histories. A history of affective illness, schizophrenia, substance abuse, and past suicidal behaviour is associated with increased suicide risk. Hopelessness, severe anxiety or dysphoria, experience of psychological disintegration, failure, despair, impulsivity, and active substance abuse are related to suicide risk.

Suicide assessment typically considers long standing risk factors, such as mental illness or history of previous attempts and the current state of the individual. Chronic risk factors, such as age and sex, are static and enduring, but warning signs are episodic and variable, such as thoughts of suicide [25]. Warning signs include precipitant events, intense affective states, such as severe anxiety and agitation, and behaviours, such as speech or action suggesting suicide or communicating intent, deterioration in social or occupational functioning, and increased substance abuse [6, 19]. Suicide risk is increased with combinations of

C. Choo (✉)
School of Engineering, Health, Science and Environment, Charles Darwin University, Darwin, Australia
e-mail: Carol.Choo@cdu.edu.au

J. Diederich
School of Information Technology and Electrical Engineering, The University of Queensland, Brisbane, QLD 4072, Australia
e-mail: j.diederich@uq.edu.au

I. Song
Singapore Campus, Singapore 574421, Singapore
e-mail: insu.song@jcu.edu.au

R. Ho
Department of Psychological Medicine, National University Hospital, Singapore, Singapore
e-mail: pcmrhcm@nus.edu.sg

M. Lech et al. (eds.), *Mental Health Informatics*,
Studies in Computational Intelligence 491, DOI: 10.1007/978-3-642-38550-6_12,

factors, for example, substantially higher risks occur among those who have a history of suicide attempts, and with a psychiatric diagnosis, such as mood disorder and schizophrenia [4, 21]. Some of the risk factors are "time-related", suicide within a year of presentation of major depressive disorder is predicted by panic attacks, insomnia, severe anxiety, diminished concentration, alcohol use, and anhedonia, whereas suicide more than a year after assessment is related to more severe hopelessness, suicidal ideation, and a history of prior attempts [11]. When researchers tried to use the commonly recognized suicide risk factors to predict suicide, it was found that their predictive power was poor with low clinical utility. Pokorny [24] tried to use the 20 best predictors of suicide to identify the 67 subjects who committed suicide in a sample of 4,800 American veterans. The predictors included diagnosis of depression or schizophrenia, history of suicide attempts or having been placed on suicide caution, overt evidence of depression on the basis of a clinical examination, insomnia, and guilt feelings. It was found that statistical analysis yielded 1,206 false-positive identifications and had limited usage in a clinical capacity. Goldney and Spence [12] also found that the predictive ability of six clinical features of suicide was poor. These clinical features included presence of depression or schizophrenia, history of previous admissions and involuntary admissions, substance abuse, and attempted suicide. Even in high risk patients with affective disorders, it was found that the prediction of suicide using the suicide risk factors was poor. The risk factors used were number of prior attempts, presence of a bipolar disorder, gender, and outcome at discharge [13].

Instruments to predict repeated attempted suicide have also been devised, such as the Edinburgh Risk of Repetition Scale [16]. However, when used in a different setting, there was only a modest ability to predict the repetition of suicide attempts [8, 15] used a statistical model to identify repeat suicide attempters using demographic and sociological variables. These potential predictors included age, gender, civil status, level of education, previous history of attempts, method of attempts, history of and concurrent usage of substances and alcohol with the attempt, history of physical and psychosocial harm caused by alcohol, and recent changes in domestic circumstances. The model predicted 96 % of suicide repeaters and 81 % of non-repeaters, but the authors cautioned about extending the usage of the model to other settings.

12.2 Repeated Suicide Attempts

The above literature review shows that a history of suicide attempts is an important risk factor for eventual suicide, and it is an important piece of data to obtain in suicide risk assessment, but there is a lack of in-depth research in repeated suicide in Asia. Studies have shown that socio-demographic factors associated with repeated suicide include age group of 25–49 years old, being divorced, being unemployed, and from a lower social class. Psychiatric and psychosocial characteristics include higher levels of depression, hopelessness, powerlessness, presence of substance abuse, personality disorder, unstable living conditions, a criminal record, psychiatric treatment, and a history of traumatic life events, including broken homes and family violence [2, 16, 27]. The clinical picture of repeated attempters that has emerged shows emotional dysregulation, severe clinical features, and elevated suicide risk factors [2]. The repeated attempters were described as hostile, angry, and irritable, with severe interpersonal conflicts, poor social support, and dysfunctional interpersonal problem solving. Compared to those who attempted suicide for the first time, the prevalence of psychiatric disorders among the repeat attempters was higher, with greater breadth of Axis I diagnoses, with comorbid mood, anxiety, and alcohol abuse disorders. They also presented with more prominent borderline personality overlay in terms of Axis II pathology [26]. Compared with single-episode attempters, repeat attempters showed more symptom chronicity, worse coping histories, more frequent histories of substance abuse and suicidal behaviour in the family, higher suicide lethality and depression scores, greater likelihood of inpatient admission, and worse prognosis [17].

Aggressive youths were also more likely to have repetitive suicidal behaviour [23]. Youths who attempted suicide more than once had more chronic emotional distress, higher likelihood of personality disorder, more school problems, life stress, anger and dysphoria, and more serious suicide intent than the single-attempters [5].

12.3 Cluster Analysis and Data Mining in Suicide Research

Data mining has been used in many health related areas to explore large amounts of data. In the current study, data mining techniques was used in an exploratory study of suicide attempters in Singapore in order to attempt to identify clinically useful and heuristically relevant clusters that could inform future research in suicide assessment and intervention. Data mining is the process of extracting useful information, patterns, and trends often previously unknown from large quantities of data [29]. The useful outcomes include classification, where the entities are grouped into meaning subclasses, and data dependency analysis, where relationships or associations between the items are detected [18]. Clustering techniques have been used to extract task-relevant diagnostic categories from psychiatric reports and have potential for use in screening, diagnosis, and classification in psychiatry and medicine [9]. Data mining techniques have been used for data exploration of the records of mentally ill patients to improve service delivery [14] to identify anomalies in data, and to compare the care given to mental health patients [1]. Data mining has also been used to extract information and patterns from client concerns in adolescent mental health services [22], and from clinical mental health cases for decision support [10]. An additional use has been to facilitate information retrieval from psychiatric documents [30].

In order to study the taxonomy of suicide and identify characteristics that are heuristically useful for informing further research in suicide risk assessment and intervention strategies, cluster analysis has been used to analyze suicide data.

Astudy was done on information obtained from Medical Examiner's files on male youth suicides in Canada from 1980 to 1986 [3]. Most variables were measured on a dichotomous basis, such that the clustering of individuals was based on low but statistically significant negative autocorrelations. K-means cluster analysis was performed which used centroid linkage analysis to define groups of cases which were as similar as possible on the variables within the cluster, and as dissimilar as possible to the cases in the other clusters. Thus, six types or clusters of suicide in young males were identified. The largest group, Cluster A, consisted of males aged 20–24 years old, without psychiatric disturbance, with a history of illegal drug use, and a precipitant of interpersonal crisis, such as breakup with a girlfriend or partner. The second cluster, Cluster B, consisted of psychotics and chronic depressives, with prior suicide attempts. The third group, Cluster C, had experienced alcohol abuse and chronic unemployment. Cluster D consisted of indigenous people living on reserves, with extreme poverty, and isolation from social services or health centres. Cluster E was characterized by physical illness and inability to work. Individuals in Cluster F had histories of a disruptive childhood and parental separation, suicide attempts, unstable interpersonal relationships, and criminal activity. The results of the Canadian study have implications for targeted interventions for the different clusters identified.

Classification of suicides can assist clinicians in the identification of patients with future suicidal risks and in the planning of appropriate suicide interventions for identified risk clusters. In a study done in Hong Kong, hierarchical cluster analysis extracted two subgroups in terms of expressed suicide intent and deliberation assessed by the Beck Suicide Intent Scale, SIS [7]. The first cluster extracted was associated with charcoal burning suicide, absence of psychiatric illness, indebtedness, better problem-solving ability, chronic stress, and higher SIS scores. The second cluster extracted was associated with jumping from a height, psychotic disorders, psychiatric treatment, acute stress, and lower SIS scores.

12.4 The Current Study

This study is based on an archival retrospective review of medical records and psychiatric reports of patients who were admitted for a suicide attempt from 2004 to 2006 at the National University Hospital (NUH) in Singapore. All cases of attempted suicide were seen by medical officers in the emergency department. The patients were then referred to the Consultation Liaison (CL) team for assessment and management. The assessment was conducted by a medical officer under the supervision of a consultant psychiatrist, and the interview took approximately 20 min. At the time of the evaluation, the medical officer made a formal psychiatric and/or medical diagnosis using their medical judgement, based on DSM-IV criteria. After assessment, a management plan was recommended (e.g., discharge, transfer to NUH psychiatric ward, transfer to Institute of Mental Health, or refer for psychiatric follow up).

Table 12.1 Demographic characteristics of suicide attempters

		Frequency	Percentage (%)
Gender			
	Female	461	69.2
	Male	205	30.8
Ethnicity			
	Chinese	425	63.8
	Indian	105	15.8
	Malay	100	15.0
	Other	36	5.4
Method of attempt			
	Overdose	577	78.5
	Cutting	21	3.1
	Jumping	9	1.3
	Stabbing	6	0.9
	Hanging	1	0.1
	Combined overdose and cutting	83	12.4

12.4.1 Participants

For this study, all case records of patients seen in NUH following a suicide attempt between January 2004 to December 2006 were reviewed. The ethnic breakdown of the suicide attempters was 63.8 % Chinese, 15.8 % Indian, 15 % Malay, and 5.4 % of other ethnicities (e.g., Eurasian). Ages ranged from 10 to 85 years old ($M = 29.7$, $SD = 16.1$). The highest rates for both genders were found in those aged between 15 to 24 years old. Of the 666 patients admitted to NUH for a suicide attempt from January 2004 to December 2006, 461 of the patients were female, and 205 were male. Overdoes accounted for 78.5 % of the suicide attempts (Table 12.1).

There were 39 patients with a previous formal psychiatric/medical diagnosis at the time of evaluation. Of those, 41 % had been diagnosed with depression, 18 % with substance abuse, 10 % with adjustment disorder, 8 % with schizophrenia and borderline personality disorder respectively, 5 % with chronic medical illness, and 3 % each with acute stress reaction, bipolar disorder, post traumatic stress disorder, and alcohol abuse, respectively. In this sample of suicide attempters, 94 % did not have a formal diagnosis prior to evaluation.

12.4.2 Data Mining and Cluster Analysis: Methods and Results of Data Analysis

As part of an exploratory study to identify patterns in the risk and protective factors for suicide attempters, and to reveal characteristics that are heuristically useful and clinically relevant to inform further research, cluster analysis was used to analyze the data. Textual data were examined using data mining methods. Text mining techniques were used to analyze the medical notes and psychiatric reports of the suicide attempters. Categorical data, such as diagnosis, numerical data, such as age, and textual data extracted from the psychiatric reports were used to identify patterns and frequent substructures, such as multiple admissions, and stressors. Clustering algorithms were used to segment the textual, numerical, and categorical data collected from psychiatric assessments and medical notes into relatively homogeneous areas. Two step cluster analysis was performed based on linkage analysis, where the outcome was to make associations between various cases and to define groups of cases which were as similar as possible on the variables and as dissimilar to the cases in the other clusters as possible. The entities between the clusters had more distinct features, while those within the same cluster had closer proximity.

There are several steps involved in data mining, which include preparing and organizing the data for mining, selecting tools, carrying out the mining, and pruning the results for further analysis. The present study employed the data mining task of clustering and affinity grouping. In contrast with classification, clustering does not group entities based on predefined attributes, but from analysis of the data, using a directed bottom-up approach [29]. The information obtained from the medical notes and assessment reports was of a textual form, but the data were not structured and formatted in the way that could be used for cluster analysis. The data had to be prepared and pre-processed. The details of the steps are described below.

The textual data were first prepared and put in the right format, whereby the raw textual data from medical reports were subjected to pre-processing techniques. In the first analysis, the textual data in the patients' medical records from various databases were collated for each patient. A separate vocabulary file was generated, whereby the terms were ranked according to their frequency of occurrence in the reports. Each report was converted into a bag of words, whereby each report was converted into a vector of term frequency, for example, Patient1 = (tf_1, tf_2,...,tf_n), where tf_n is the frequency of the nth term in the vocabulary. The processed data were then subjected to two step cluster analysis using the Predictive Analytics Software (PASW) Modeller Program package. The results were then pruned so that the useful ones were considered further. Following initial exploration of clusters, a specific number of clusters was specified in further analysis, based on the non-random variation of as many of the original variables across these clusters as possible, the clinical meaning and heuristic utility of the clusters, and the absence of clusters which could not be interpreted in any way.

In the first analysis, two step cluster analysis was conducted to investigate and explore the distribution characteristics of frequently occurring words in medical reports for patients who were admitted for suicide attempts. Two-step cluster analysis yielded two clusters (Appendix 12A, Figs. 12.1, 12.2, and 12.3). Clusters A and B contained 84.4 % ($n = 353$) and 15.6 % ($n = 65$) of patients, respectively. Cluster A patients were characterized by relatively fewer reports of borderline personality disorder and psychotic symptoms, such as 'hallucinations',

Fig. 12.1 Two-step clustering model summary showing the number of clusters, features used, and the quality of the clustering. Two-step clustering analysis results on the frequently occurring words in medical and psychiatric reports

Model Summary

Algorithm	TwoStep
Input Features	31
Clusters	2

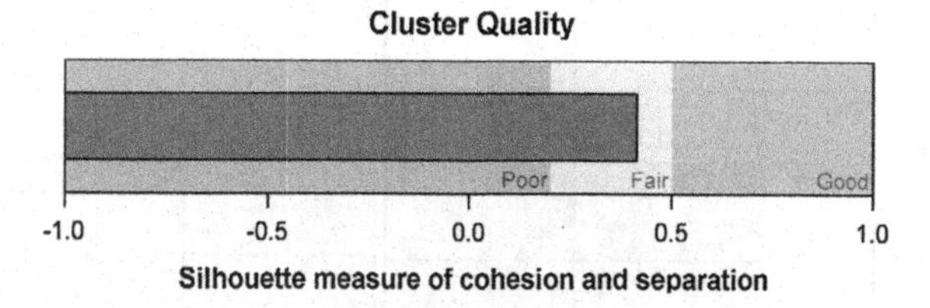

Fig. 12.2 Summary of the two-step clustering

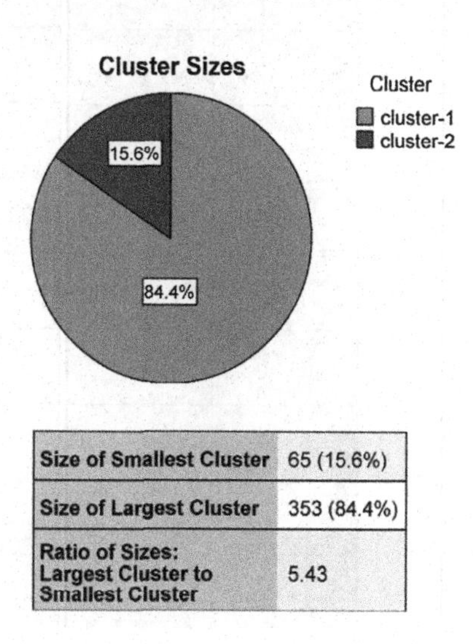

Size of Smallest Cluster	65 (15.6%)
Size of Largest Cluster	353 (84.4%)
Ratio of Sizes: Largest Cluster to Smallest Cluster	5.43

psychosomatic symptoms of 'insomnia', 'headache', less reports of repeated multiple attempts or admissions, less negative feelings, such as 'upset', 'angry', 'frustration', 'depression', 'stress', less cases of unemployment, divorce and quarrel, less reports of 'alcohol' and beer, and less reports of 'overdose' with 'benzodiazepine' and 'paracetamol'. Cluster B patients were characterized by relatively more reports of Borderline Personality Disorder, psychotic symptoms of hallucination, symptoms of 'insomnia', 'headache', more repeated 'multiple' attempts or admissions, more negative feelings including 'upset', 'angry', 'frustration', 'depressed', 'stress', 'pain', more cases of unemployment, divorce and quarrel, and more reports of 'alcohol', 'beer', 'overdose' with 'benzodiazepine' and 'paracetamol'. Within Cluster B, the results of the clustering analysis seemed to be supported by weak but significant ($p < 0.001$) positive correlations between unemployment and lethality ($r = 0.21$), unemployment and living alone ($r = 0.21$), unemployment and alcohol abuse ($r = 0.16$), unemployment and

Clusters

Feature Importance

■1.0 ■0.9 ■0.8 □0.7

Cluster	cluster-1	cluster-2
Label		
Description		
Size	84.4% (353)	15.6% (65)
Features		
chines	0.32	1.40
depress	0.46	3.62
femal	0.36	1.32
hallucin	0.01	0.55
multipl	0.13	1.42
overdos	0.65	2.88
work	0.15	1.32
male	0.18	0.80
upset	0.03	0.31
intent	0.32	0.97
unemploi	0.01	0.32
angri	0.01	0.34
wrist	0.11	0.95
frustrat	0.01	0.23
alcohol	0.31	1.22
borderlin	0.02	0.54
problem	0.23	1.23
drink	0.05	0.55
schizophrenia	0.03	0.54
divorc	0.05	0.29
benzodiazepin	0.10	0.58
beer	0.07	0.32
quarrel	0.13	0.45
indian	0.16	0.55
insomnia	0.08	0.34
argument	0.04	0.14
repeat	0.08	0.23
stress	0.29	0.54
pain	0.68	1.12
headach	0.13	0.23

Fig. 12.3 Importance of features in each cluster. The features characterize the clusters

mental illness ($r = 0.25$), and unemployment and lack of emotional support ($r = -0.20$), as well as weak but significant ($p < 0.001$) positive correlations between mental illness and lack of confidantes ($r = 0.18$), mental illness and alcohol abuse ($r = 0.15$), mental illness and poor coping ($r = 0.27$), and mental illness and lack of emotional support ($r = 0.15$). Cluster B patients seemed to represent a group with poor prognosis and Cluster A patients represented a group with good prognosis.

In the second analysis, cluster analysis was conducted to investigate and explore the distribution characteristics of frequently occurring words recorded as suicide risk factors and precipitants in the psychiatric assessment reports. The raw textual data extracted from the assessment forms were collated for each patient. The data were then converted into a string of words for each patient. These data were then filtered. This process ensured that only the significant and meaningful attributes were retained for cluster analysis. The Word Intersection program was used to filter out "word fillers" such as "and", and rarely occurring words. After the filtering process was completed, the data were subjected to two step cluster analysis using the Predictive Analytics Software (PASW) Modeller Program package.

Two-step cluster analysis yielded two clusters (Appendix 12B, Figs. 12.4, 12.5, and 12.6). Clusters C and D described 53.9 % ($n = 188$) and 46.1 % ($n = 161$) of patients, respectively. Cluster C patients were characterised by the common occurrence of the words 'boyfriend', 'husband', 'feels' and 'quarrel'. Scanning of the textual data indicated that most of the relevant cases reported negative feelings, such as hopelessness, anger, unhappiness, and depression from interpersonal conflicts with their husbands or boyfriends. Cluster D patients were characterized

Model Summary

Algorithm	TwoStep
Input Features	4
Clusters	2

Cluster Quality

Poor Fair Good

-1.0 -0.5 0.0 0.5 1.0

Silhouette measure of cohesion and separation

Fig. 12.4 Two-step clustering model summary showing the number of clusters, features used, and the quality of the clustering

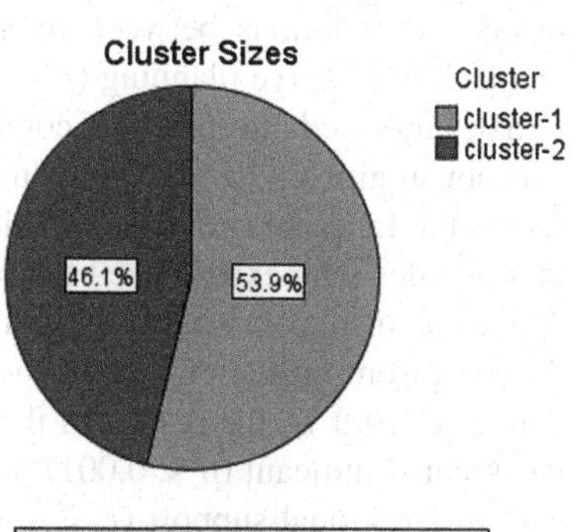

Size of Smallest Cluster	161 (46.1%)
Size of Largest Cluster	188 (53.9%)
Ratio of Sizes: Largest Cluster to Smallest Cluster	1.17

Fig. 12.5 Summary of the two-step clustering

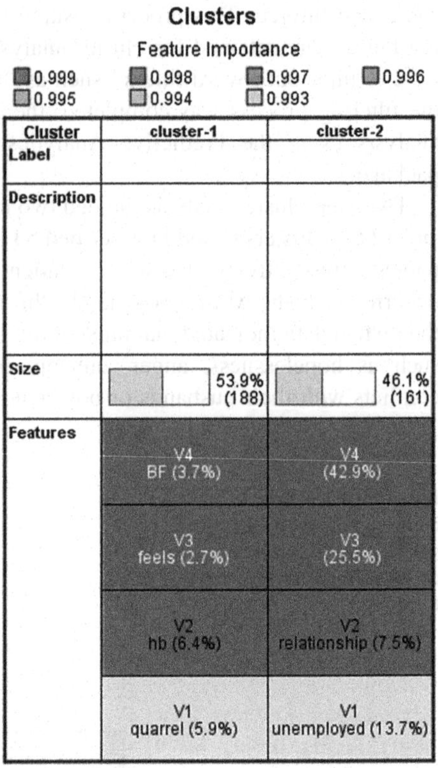

Fig. 12.6 Importance of features in each cluster. The features characterize the clusters

Clusters

Feature Importance

0.999 0.998 0.997 0.996
0.995 0.994 0.993

Cluster Label	cluster-1	cluster-2
Description		
Size	53.9% (188)	46.1% (161)
Features	V4 BF (3.7%)	V4 (42.9%)
	V3 feels (2.7%)	V3 (25.5%)
	V2 hb (6.4%)	V2 relationship (7.5%)
	V1 quarrel (5.9%)	V1 unemployed (13.7%)

by the common occurrence of the words 'unemployment' and 'relationship'. Scanning of the textual data indicated that most of these relevant cases reported unemployment and poor family relationships. Within Cluster C, the results of the clustering analysis seemed to be supported by weak but significant ($p < 0.001$) positive correlations between interpersonal conflict and poor coping ($r = 0.18$) and lack of positive planning ($r = -0.07$). Chi square analysis revealed that more females reported interpersonal conflict, compared to males, although the difference was not significant ($p > 0.05$). Cluster C appeared to contain more female patients due to the frequent occurrence of the words 'boyfriend' and 'husband', suggesting that females who experienced the precipitating risk factor of interpersonal conflict and were also overwhelmed with negative feelings formed a cluster that was different from those in Cluster D, which described patients who were unemployed. Within Cluster D, the results of the clustering analysis seemed to be supported by weak but significant ($p < 0.001$) positive correlations between unemployment and lack of emotional support ($r = -0.20$).

Analysis of the risk factors and precipitants recorded in the psychiatric risk assessment reports showed that for one of the clusters, suicide attempts were precipitated by quarrels with the attempters' boyfriends and husbands which precipitated negative emotions, such as feel 'hopeless', 'unhappy', 'angry' and 'depressed'. For the other cluster, the suicide attempts were precipitated by 'unemployment' accompanied by relationship problems and the feeling that families were not supportive.

12.5 Discussion and Conclusions

Two-step cluster analysis uncovered underlying patterns of risk factors that characterized patients who had multiple suicide attempts and those with single suicide attempts. Two-step cluster analysis also uncovered underlying patterns of risk factors that characterised patients who reported the precipitants of interpersonal conflicts and those who were unemployed.

Textual analysis of medical records revealed that a minority of the cases had a number of recognized risk factors that placed them at higher risk of repeated admissions for multiple suicide attempts. Symptoms of psychotic illness, borderline personality disorder, and affective disorder with psychosomatic complaints of insomnia and headaches, reports of adverse life events, such as unemployment, divorce and quarrels, experience of negative feelings, and usage alcohol, were associated with risk of repeated overdoses with and paracetamol. For the majority of the cases, the incidence of repeated attempts was lower, and they had fewer recognized risk factors, including the demographic, clinical, and psychosocial variables named above. This is consistent with previous studies which reported that multiple attempters had a more severe and complex clinical picture [20].

As this was an exploratory study, more research should be conducted to analyze the differences between the suicide clusters and to make comparisons with matched controls in the normal population. The results could be used to identify the individuals at risk of repeated attempts and to tailor more targeted interventions for these at risk individuals. More analysis should be conducted for suicide risk factors that tend to occur together and more targeted follow up work should be done to reduce the cumulative effects of suicide risk factors.

References

1. Allen, I., Seaman, C.: Data mining for quality. American society for quality control (2006)
2. Arenson, E., Kerkhof, A.: Classification of attempted suicide: A review of empirical studies. Suicide Life Threat. Behav. **26**, 47–67 (1996)
3. Bagley, C., Ramsay, R.: Suicidal Behaviour in Adolescents and Adults. Ashgate, Vermont (1997)
4. Beautrais, A.: Risk factors for serious suicide attempts among young people: A case control study. In: Suicide Prevention: The Global Context. Plenum Press, New York (1998)
5. Brent, D.A., Johnson, B., Bartle, S., Bridge, J., Rather, C., Matta, J., Connolly, J., Constantine, D.: Personality disorder, tendency to impulsive violence, and suicidal behavior in adolescents. J. Am. Acad. Child Adolesc. Psychiatry **32**(1), 69–75 (1993)
6. Busch, K., Fawcet, J., Jacobs, D.: Clinical correlates of inpatient suicide. J. Clin. Psychiatry **64**(1), 14–19 (2003)

7. Chen, E.Y.H., Chan, W.S.C., Chan, S.S.M., Liu, K.Y., Chan, C.L.W., Wong, P.W.C., Law, Y.W., Yip, P.S.F.: A cluster analysis of the circumstances of death in suicides in Hong Kong. Suicide Life-Threat. Behav. **37**(5), 576–584 (2007)
8. Corcoran, P., Kelleher, M.J., Keeley, H.S., Byrne, S., Burke, U., Williamson, E.: A preliminary statistical model for identifying repeaters of parasuicide. Arch. Suicide Res. **3**(1), 65–74 (1997)
9. Diederich, J., Al-Ajmi, A., Yellowlees, P.: Ex-ray: Data mining and mental health. Appl. Soft Comput. J. **7**(3), 923–928 (2007)
10. Eapen, A.G., Ponnambalam, K., Arocha, J.F., Shioda, R., Smith, T.F., Poss, J., Hirdes, J.: Data mining in mental health. Modeling and simulation. In: Proceedings of the 17th IASTED International Conference on Modelling and Simulation, pp. 122–127. Montreal, Canada (2006)
11. Fawcett, J., Scheftner, W.A., Fogg, L., Clark, D.C., et al.: Time-related predictors of suicide in major affective disorder. Am. J. Psychiatry **147**(9), 1189–1194 (1990)
12. Goldney, R., Spence, N.: Is suicide predictable? Aust. N. Z. J. Psychiatry **21**, 3–4 (1987)
13. Goldstein, R.B., Black, D.W., Nasrallah, A., Winokur, G.: The Prediction of Suicide: Sensitivity, Specificity, and Predictive Value of a Multivariate Model Applied to Suicide Among 1906 Patients with Affective Disorders, vol. 48 (1991) First published. doi:10.1001/archpsyc.1991.01810290030004
14. Hadzic, M., Hadzic, F., Dillon, T.: Tree mining in mental health domain. In: Proceedings of the Annual Hawaii International Conference on System Sciences (2008)
15. Hawton, K., Fagg, J.: Repetition of attempted suicide: The performance of the Edinburgh predictive scales in patients in Oxford. Arch. Suicide Res. **1**, 261–272 (1995)
16. Kreitman, N., Foster, J.: Construction and selection of predictive scales, with special reference to parasuicide. Br. J. Psychiatry **159**, 185–192 (1991)
17. Kurz, A., Moller, H., Baindl, G., Burk, F., Tohorst, A., Wachtler, C., Lauter, H.: Classification of parasuicide by cluster analysis: Types of suicidal behaviour, therapeutic and prognostic implications. Br. J. Psychiatry **150**, 520–525 (1987)
18. Laroose, D.: Discovering Knowledge in Data Mining. Wiley, NJ (2005)
19. Maltsberger, J.T., Hendin, H., Haas, A.P., Lipschitz, A.: Determination of precipitant events in the suicide of psychiatric patients. Suicide Life Threat. Behav. **33**(2), 111–121 (2003)
20. Mann, J.J., Water-naux, C., Haas, G., Malone, K.M.: Towards a clinical model of suicidal behaviour in psychiatric patient. Am. J. Psychiatry **156**(2), 181–189 (1999)
21. Nordstrone, P., Asberg, M., Asberg-Wistedt, A., Nordin, C.: Attempted suicide pre-dicts suicide risk in mood disorders. Acta Psychiatr. Scand. **92**, 345–350 (1995)
22. Peake, K., Surko, M., Epstein, I., Medeiros, D.: Data mining concerns in adolescent mental health services: Clinical and program implications. Soc. Work. Mental Health **3**, 287–304 (2005)
23. Pfeffer, C.: The Suicidal Child. Guilford, New York (1986)
24. Pokorny, A.D.: Prediction of Suicide in Psychiatric Patients: Report of a Prospective Study, vol. 40 (1983) First published. doi:10.1001/archpsyc.1983.01790030019002
25. Rudd, M., Berman, A., Joiner, T., Nock, M., Sliverman, M., Mandrusiak, M., Van Orden, K., Witte, T.: Warning signs for suicide: Theory, research, and clinical applications. Suicide Life Threat. Behav. **36**(3), 255–262 (2006)
26. Rudd, M.D., Joiner, T., Rajad, M.H.: Relationships among suicide ideators, attempters, and multiple attempters in a young-adult sample. J. Abnorm. Psychol. **105**(4), 541–550 (1996)
27. Safinovsky, I., Roberts, R., Brown, Y., Cummings, C., James, P.: Problem resolution and repetition of parasuicide. Br. J. Psychiatry **156**, 395–399 (1990)
28. Sederer, L.: Managing Suicidal Inpatients. Treatment of Suicidal People. Taylor and Francis, Washington (1994)
29. Thuraisingham, B.: Data mining: Technologies, Techniques, Tools and Trends. CRC Press, Florida (1999)
30. Yu, L.-C., Wu, C.-H., Jang, F.-L.: Psychiatric document retrieval using a discourse-aware model. Artif. Intell. **173**(7–8), 817–829 (2009)

Chapter 13
Using Diagnostic Information to Develop a Machine Learning Application for the Effective Screening of Autism Spectrum Disorders

Tze Jui Goh, Joachim Diederich, Insu Song and Min Sung

13.1 Introduction

Recent studies have found an increase in the prevalence of Autism Spectrum Disorders [7, 22, 53]. In the United States, the [6] estimated the overall prevalence rate to be 9 per 1,000. In the United Kingdom, a rate of 11.6 per 1,000 was found by, [2], of which childhood autism was estimated to range between 2.48 to 3.89 per 1,000. These figures emphasize the pertinence of ASD, especially when the impairments associated with the disorder are all-encompassing and impact the quality of life of individuals with ASD and their families. The increasing numbers can be attributed to greater awareness of the disorder, thereby resulting in reclassification of previously 'mis-diagnosed' cases and also improved efficiency in identifying individuals with ASD. A broadening definition of ASD, i.e., inclusion of Asperger Disorder and Pervasive Developmental Disorders-Not Otherwise Specified (PDD-NOS), in addition to Autism in the Diagnostic and Statistical Manual (DSM-IV, 1994) and International Statistical Classification of Diseases and Related Health Problems—10th edition (ICD-10) [63] is also a fundamental contributing factor [59].

T. J. Goh (✉) · M. Sung
Institute of Mental Health, Singapore, Singapore
e-mail: Tze_Jui_Goh@imh.com.sg

M. Sung
e-mail: Min_Sung@imh.com.sg

J. Diederich
School of Information Technology and Electrical Engineering,
The University of Queensland, Brisbane Q4072, Australia
e-mail: j.diederich@uq.edu.au

I. Song
School of Business and IT, James Cook University, Singapore Campus,
Singapore 574421, Singapore
e-mail: insu.song@jcu.edu.au

M. Lech et al. (eds.), *Mental Health Informatics*,
Studies in Computational Intelligence 491, DOI: 10.1007/978-3-642-38550-6_13,

Autism is characterized by a triad of impairments [61] in the areas of reciprocal social interaction, communication, and repetitive and stereotyped behaviours. Asperger Disorder is similar to Autism but requires no deviance or delay in language development, according to the DSM-IV-TR (1994). PDD-NOS is diagnosed when there are significant impairments in the areas similar to Autism, but the individuals do not fulfil sufficient criteria for the diagnosis of such.

Although the [18] and [33] guidelines are helpful to clinicians in the diagnostic process, the effectiveness of their utilization depends on the experience of the clinicians [38]. A brief examination of both traditional diagnostic systems reveals that the diagnostic criteria of the disorders are general descriptions of behavioural indicators which are open to the subjective interpretation, clinical observations and accuracy of reporting by informants [43]. The manifestation of symptoms also varies across different individuals and across different chronological and developmental levels [9], all of which form the spectrum nature of ASD. In addition, the definition of ASD is evolving with advances in the knowledge and understanding of its symptomatology. While many models of ASD and possibly the presence of sub-types within the disorder have been postulated, the different methodologies employed and inconsistency in findings [3, 12, 23, 34, 43, 49, 58] result in a lack of consensus on these issues. Although ASD is currently widely accepted as a neuro-developmental disorder with an underlying genetic component, the specific etiology remains elusive. Even in the presence of concrete biological markers, behavioural indicators and phenotypical presentation are still important in order to elucidate the role of environmental factors in the disorder.

A multi-disciplinary approach is recommended for the assessment and diagnosis of ASD [20, 36, 37, 54]. This involves a systematic collection of information regarding the developmental history, behavioural presentation, clinical observations, and an assessment of the cognitive and daily functioning of children by trained professionals. Other assessments, such as medical check-ups or skills assessments (e.g., language, motor, or sensory) may also be conducted to elucidate possible medical conditions (e.g. epilepsy) and to obtain comprehensive profiles for treatment recommendations or education planning. Clinicians are aided by standardized instruments in the assessment process and utilize their clinical judgment to formulate the overall diagnosis. To date, the most comprehensive and reliable standardized instruments used in such an assessment are the Autism Diagnostic Interview - Revised (ADI-R) [52] and the Autism Diagnostic Observation Schedule (ADOS) [15, 31, 44, 47, 54]. The ADI-R is an extended set of standard protocols consisting of 93 items administered in a semi-structure interview with the children's caregivers to obtain detailed information about developmental history and day-to-day behaviours. The three domains of the protocol, namely reciprocal social interactions, language/communication, and restricted, repetitive and stereotyped behaviours correspond with the diagnostic criteria of the DSM-IV [40, 57]. The ADOS is a semi-structured but standardised instrument which consists of four modules. Each module has its own set of protocols, and only one module is selected for administration based on the children's language and developmental level during each assessment. The ADOS allows direct observation in a natural setting and has demonstrated excellent psychometric properties [17, 29, 30, 42].

The timely and accurate diagnosis of the disorder is imperative. It allows access to appropriate treatment, services, and management plans for the individuals and reduces the anguish and stress faced by the families. Studies have also demonstrated that early diagnosis can lead to better prognosis for children with ASD [9, 41]. However, most children get diagnosed only upon entering the school environment when the behavioural difficulties become more prominent. Howlin and Moore [32] reported that most children were diagnosed only when they were 6 years old. Even when parents were concerned about their children's development, they experienced delays in the diagnosis process [27, 64]. Hence, the implementation of early surveillance and screening is crucial to identify children at-risk for ASD at an earlier stage [20, 21, 35].

Fillipek et al. [20, 21] advocated a three-step assessment practice in the diagnosis of children with ASD: identification of children at-risk of developmental disorders by primary care providers, screening for ASD for these at-risk children, and referral for full comprehensive assessment of ASD if the screen is positive. Johnson et al. [35, 36] recommended ASD screening for children during their routine developmental surveillance at the level of primary care providers. While this approach may identify more children at-risk of ASD, its implementation is difficult in the community. Primary care providers may lack experience and expertise in administering the screening tools and may also be reluctant to do so, given practical considerations of time and cost of administering the screening tools.

Early surveillance and screening are often facilitated by chapter and pencil screening instruments, usually rating scales to be completed by caregivers or administered by clinicians. They are easy to administer, take shorter time to complete, and allow a large number of children to be assessed. However, their efficacy also depends on the experience and interpretation of the clinicians. Although several screening instruments have been developed, they vary in their psychometric properties and lack clear evidence of validity [46, 48]. Nonetheless, amongst these screening instruments, there are some that show promise.

The Social Communication Questionnaire (SCQ) [51], previously known as the Autism Screening Questionnaire [4], is the most researched. It has demonstrated good sensitivity (>0.74) and specificity (>0.54) across different studies [1, 4, 8, 10, 14, 19, 62]. Goin-Kochel and Cohen [26] also reported 89 % agreement in classification outcomes between the SCQ and the DSM-IV-TR. The Social Responsiveness Scale (SRS) [11] is a relatively new instrument but has also demonstrated good sensitivity (>0.75) and specificity (>0.67) in the two studies [10, 13] that compared its classification outcomes with diagnosis confirmation based on the ADI-R, ADOS, and clinical consensus. Another pair of instruments, Gilliam Autism Rating Scale (GARS) [24] and the revised Gilliam Autism Rating Scale-Second Edition (GARS-2) [25] have been widely used but lacked empirical evidence of validity. While [19] found good sensitivity (0.83) and specificity (0.68), [39, 45, 56] only established a sensitivity between 0.38 to 0.48 in their studies. This instrument would require further research and validation.

Norris and Lecavalier [46] highlighted the importance of utilizing valid and empirically sound screening tools to identify children at-risk of ASD. They suggested further evaluations of existing instruments by comparing them with control groups and other differential diagnoses. Diagnosis ascertainment is also necessary when comparing classification outcomes between instruments. Other factors, such as raters' interpretation of the items in the screening tools, can also influence classification accuracy. Screening instruments should also be compared within a single sample employing consistent methodology.

The current study takes into consideration the need for an objective screening instrument which has wide applicability and aims to develop a classification model—Support Vector Machine (SVM) application based on machine learning techniques to screen for ASD. Extensive text information gathered from diagnostic assessments is used as reference for the development and training of the model. The classification performance of the resulting 2-Class SVM application is examined.

13.2 Study Design and Method

The study involved three phases. The first phase involved the analysis of text reports generated from comprehensive diagnostic assessments that utilised standardised instruments and clinical evaluations for case formulation, to develop the 2-Class SVM classification model (SVM-2C). The text reports were represented as attribute-value vectors ("bag of words" representation) where each distinct word corresponded to a feature whose value was the frequency of the word in the document. Values were transformed with regard to the length of the sample. In summary, input vectors for machine learning consisted of attributes (the words used in the sample), values (the transformed frequency of the words), and corresponding class labels (autism versus control). The input vectors were then used to generate the SVM-2C. Outputs of the SVM-2C were autism versus control, that is, a binary classification task was learned. The classification performance of the SVM-2C on a recruited sample of participants was then compared to other screening instruments in the second phase. In the third phase, a 1-Class SVM classification model (SVM-1C) was generated using only positive cases (i.e., autism cases). The SVM-2C was then compared to the 1-Class SVM classification models (SVM-1C) to examine the utility of the SVM application with a skewed population, whereby the likelihood of the membership in one category was higher than in the other. The final SVM classification model is also presented.

13.2.1 Phase 1

Phase 1 of the study involved the development of an SVM application by means of machine learning techniques for the classification of ASD (yes or no), so as to facilitate screening procedures for the disorder.

13.2.1.1 Method

Procedure. Two hundred and five diagnostic assessment reports from Autism Clinic @ Child Guidance Clinic, Institute of Mental Health (IMH) in Singapore were subjected to text analysis. All names and identifiers were removed before the reports were included in the study. Children were referred for a comprehensive diagnostic assessment when they were suspected to have an ASD. The assessment comprised administrations of the ADI-R, ADOS, and a cognitive assessment (the type of assessment depended on the chronological and adaptive functioning level of the children) and clinical case formulation, so as to arrive at a diagnostic conclusion. Reports of assessments conducted between the periods of 2006 to 2010 were included. The sample consisted of 188 (91.7 %) positive cases (diagnosis of ASD—Autism, Asperger's Syndrome or PDD-NOS) and 17 (8.3 %) negative cases (not-ASDs), of which 23 were females (11.2 %) and 182 were males (88.8 %). Children were assessed between the ages of 52 (4.3 years) and 229 months (19.0 years). Mean age of the sample was 133.5 months (11.1 years, SD = 36.0). Descriptions of the children's diagnoses and age in months in the text reports are summarised in Table 13.1.

Data Analysis. The text reports were pre-processed to remove formatting and general structural headings. Identifiers (all names) and personal information not relevant to diagnostic decisions were also removed. The text reports were in the ASCII format and frequent words were removed. The text reports were subjected to filtering and clustering techniques, and a 2-Class SVM classification model was generated. For a description of SVM core techniques application in mental health, please refer to [16]. Receiver Operating Curve (ROC), Area Under Curve (AUC) analysis, and other test properties indicative of classification performance were generated.

13.2.1.2 Results

There were no group differences found between the children with different diagnoses. The 2-Class SVM classification model (SVM-2C) was utilized with the 205 text reports, and decision values were generated for each report. A decision value

Table 13.1 Description of children's diagnoses and age in months in text reports at phase 1

Diagnostic category	N	Age in months			
		Mean	SD	Min	Max
Positive: autism spectrum disorders (ASD)	188	133.9	35.9	52	229
Autism	76	135.7	37.6	52	229
Asperger's syndrome	57	132.4	35.6	72	210
Pervasive developmental disorders—not otherwise specified	55	132.8	34.0	77	216
Negative (not ASD)	17	129.5	39.6	81	209
Total	205	133.5	36.1	52	229

Table 13.2 Description of calculation of test properties

Classification results	Actual clinical classification		
	Positive (ASD)	Negative (not ASD)	Total
Positive (ASD)	A	B	A + B
Negative (not ASD)	C	D	C + D
Total	A + C	B + D	N

Sensitivity = A/(A + C), Specificity = D/(B + D), [a] Precision = A/(A + B), Accuracy = (A + D)/N

[a] Also known as positive predictive value

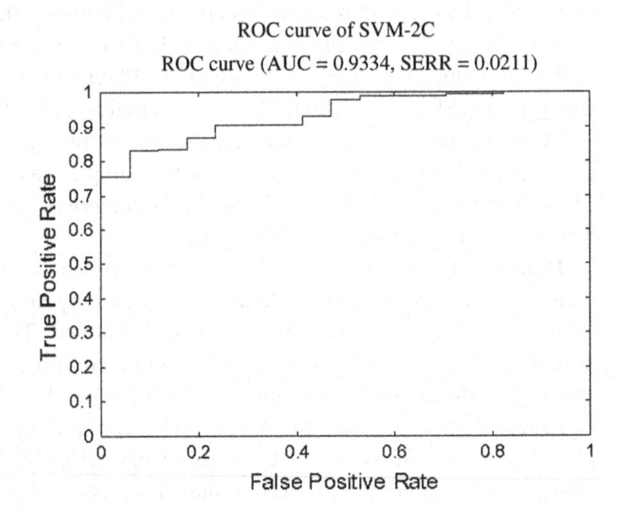

Fig. 13.1 ROC *curve* of the SVM-2C with AUC of 0.9334

of 0.791 was set as the optimal cut-off, i.e., reports with values above 0.791 were classified as positive (ASD), and reports with values of 0.79 and below were classified as negative (not-ASD). One hundred and seventy-two children were classified correctly on the SVM-2C, yielding an accuracy rate of 83.9 %. One hundred and fifty-six children with a positive diagnosis (ASD) and 16 children with a negative diagnosis (not-ASD) were correctly classified. 16.1 % of the children (32 children with an ASD and 1 child without an ASD) were incorrectly classified. Sensitivity was 0.829 and specificity was 0.941. The SVM-2C obtained a precision of 0.993 and AUC of 0.9334. Refer to Table 13.2 for a description of the calculation of test properties. The ROC curve is presented in Fig. 13.1.

13.2.1.3 Discussion

The SVM-2C appears to have good classification psychometric properties and shows promise for use as a screening tool for ASD. It presents as a novel approach to the issue of screening and surveillance of ASD. The classification model is based on directly observed or reported symptoms of children, and its classification parameters are not driven by subjective interpretation of researchers. Furthermore, it is not limited by the current approaches or concepts of ASD, as it allows continuous refinement of its parameters by inputs of accumulated information and knowledge.

However, there are limitations in the current development of the SVM-2C. Although the training dataset is comprised of diagnostic reports with extensive information about the children, the sample is uneven. The ratio of positive to negative cases is large. The sample is also a 'screened' population—referral for the comprehensive assessment was made when the clinical presentation of the children was unclear. Children with clear ASD symptomatology may not have been referred, while neuro-typical children with no issues in their development or behaviours did not attend the clinic. The application of SVM-2C in a skewed population needs to be evaluated. In addition, the reports were written by a select group of clinicians (single site, less than 10 clinicians in total), albeit they were experienced professionals in the field; hence, the reports may reflect bias in interpretation and approach. SVM-2C still requires further validation and research.

13.2.2 Phase 2

The SVM-2C was applied to a separate sample of children and its classification performance was compared with other available screening instruments of ASD. Phase 2 presents a preliminary analysis of the validity of the SVM-2C.

13.2.2.1 Method

Participants Participants were the parents of 16 children (16 males, 0 females) who had presented with socio-emotional or behavioural difficulties and were referred to the Autism Clinic @ Child Guidance Clinic (IMH) for a comprehensive assessment for ASD. The mean age of the parents (3 fathers, 13 mothers) was 41.75 years old (SD = 7.7), with a range of 33 to 63 years. Nine of the 16 parents (56.3 %) had at least pre-university education. The sample consisted of 68.75 % Chinese, 12.5 % of Malays, and 18.75 % Indians. The mean age of the children was 141.6 months (11 years, 9 months, SD = 32.9), with a range of 96 (8 years) to 195 months (16 years,3 months). 93.8 % (15 children) were diagnosed as having an ASD and one was not. Descriptions of the children's diagnosis are summarised in Table 13.3.

Instruments Gillian Autism Rating Scale—Second Edition (GARS-2). The GARS-2 [25] is a 42-item questionnaire that contains three subscales: stereotyped behaviours, communication, and social interaction, as well as a parent interview. Each subscale is comprised o 14 items, and the respondents are asked to rate each item from 0 ('never observed') to 3 ('frequently observed') using a 6 h period as a

Table 13.3 Description of child's diagnosis at phase 2

Diagnostic category	N	Age in months			
		Mean	SD	Min	Max
Positive: autism spectrum disorders (ASD)	188	133.9	35.9	52	229
Autism	76	135.7	37.6	52	229
Asperger's syndrome	57	132.4	35.6	72	210
Pervasive developmental disorders—not otherwise specified	55	132.8	34.0	77	216
Negative (not ASD)	17	129.5	39.6	81	209
Total	205	133.5	36.1	52	229

reference for observations. Raw scores are then computed for each subscale and converted to standard scores. The sum of the standard scores is then tabulated and converted to an Autism Index, which is reported to have a coefficient alpha of 0.94. An Autism Index score above 70 is indicative of 'possibly ASD.'

Social Communication Questionnaire (SCQ)—Lifetime version. The SCQ [4, 51] is a 40-item parent questionnaire that measures symptoms associated with Autism disorders. It was developed based on the ADI-R and is validated for children above 4 years old. The first nineteen items measure current behaviours, and the twentieth item is a qualitative term to indicate the communication level of the child. The other twenty items measure behaviours during the 4-year to 5-year old period. Items describe behaviours and respondents respond 'yes' or 'no' if the descriptions apply to the children. Each item-response is then converted to 0 or 1 and a total score is obtained. The total score has an alpha coefficient of the total score of 0.90. The recommended cut-off score of 15 suggests the possibility of an ASD.

Social Responsiveness Scale (SRS). The SRS [11] is a 65-item questionnaire that assesses children on five subscales: social awareness, social cognition, social communication, social motivation, and autistic mannerisms. Respondents are asked to recall the children's behaviours over the last 6 months and rate each item from 0 ('never true') to 3 ('almost always true'). Raw scores are computed for each subscale and summed to obtain a total raw score. Subscale and total raw scores are converted to a standardised total score. The standardised total score can range from 0 to 195 and has an alpha coefficient of 0.90. A cut-off of 55 and above suggests the possibility of a mild to moderate ASD.

2-Class SVM classification model (SVM-2C). The SVM-2C classification parameters developed in phase 1 was tested and cross-validated on the diagnostic assessment reports of the participants.

Procedure. An invitation letter and study information were sent to parents of children who had undergone the comprehensive diagnostic assessment for ASD at the Child Guidance Clinic/IMH. The assessment includes the ADI-R, ADOS, a cognitive assessment, and clinical evaluation and concludes with a diagnostic formulation. These children were identified via medical records. Parents who were interested in participating in the study contacted the researcher for an appointment at the Child Guidance Clinic. Parents and children gave consent for participating in the study. The instruments were administered via parent-interview in the privacy of the researcher's office. Parent-interview administration was chosen because it allowed the assessor to clarify the interpretation and understanding of the items with the respondents. For all cases, the children stayed in the office with the parents and the researcher during the session. Upon completion of the session, parents were presented with S$50 to compensate them for their time and transport expenses to visit the clinic.

The diagnostic assessment reports on the children who were enrolled in this phase of the study were excluded from the previous phase, i.e., not included in the training dataset of 205 diagnostic assessment reports for generation of the SVM-2C in phase 1.

Data Analysis. The classification performance of each instrument was examined by means of sensitivity, specificity, precision, and accuracy (Table 13.2). The SVM-2C was further cross-validated with the text reports derived from the diagnostic assessment reports of the 16 children. An ROC curve was not generated in view of the small sample size. In addition, logistic regression was conducted to examine the relationship between the cases' classification of each instrument and the actual diagnostic category. Differences between the classification accuracy of the SVM-2C and the SCQ, SRS, and GARS, respectively were assessed by transforming the binomial distributions and applying independent t-tests using manual calculations.

13.2.2.2 Results

Participant (parents and children) characteristics were compared. The mean age (in months) of Chinese children (M = 124.1, SD = 21.9) enrolled was significantly lower, $t\ (11) = -3.77$, $p = 0.003$, than the mean age of Malay children (M = 184.5, SD = 2.12), and also lower than, $t\ (12) = -3.82$, $p = 0.002$, the mean age of Indian children (M = 177.0, SD = 18.0) enrolled in the study. Malay and Indian children did not differ significantly in their mean ages. There were no other significant group differences in the sample.

Classification Performance. Comparing the classification performance of the GARS-2 with the actual diagnoses of the 16 children, GARS-2 correctly classified 12 out of 15 children with an ASD. It misclassified 1 negative case as positive and 3 positive cases as positive? Hence, it obtained a sensitivity of 0.080, specificity of 0.000, and a precision value of 0.923. The accuracy was 0.750. The SCQ and SRS were comparable in their classification performance. Both correctly classified 13 out of 15 children with an ASD correctly but misclassified 2 children with an ASD as negative and 1 negative case as positive. Their sensitivity, specificity, and precision values were 0.866, 0.000, and 0.928, respectively. The accuracy was 0.810.

The SVM-2C was applied to the 16 test data (pre-processed diagnostic reports), and it classified all 15 positive cases correctly. However, it also misclassified the negative case as positive. With SVM Decision values cut-off at 0.791, sensitivity was 0.999, specificity was 0.000 and precision was 0.937. Its accuracy was 0.937.

Table 13.4 Description of calculation of test properties

	Cut-off values	Sensitivity	Specificity	Precision	Accuracy
GARS-2	70	0.800	0.000	0.923	0.750
SCQ	15	0.866	0.000	0.928	0.810
SRS	55	0.866	0.000	0.928	0.810
SVM-2C test performance	0.791	0.999	0.000	0.937	0.937
SVM-2C cross validation	0.919	0.933	1.000	0.999	0.938

Note GARS-2; Gilliams autism rating scale—2nd edition; *SCQ* social communication questionnaire; *SRS* social responsiveness scale; *SVM-2C* 2-class support vector machine application

Table 13.5 Differential predictive ability of the instruments based on logistic regression analysis

	-2 Log likelihood	Cox and snell pseudo *R*-square	Nagelkerke pseudo *R*-square
GARS-2	15.012	0.027	0.043
SCQ	11.780	0.017	0.032
SRS	11.780	0.017	0.032
SVM-2C cross-validated	2.773	0.255	0.683

Note GARS-2; Gilliams autism rating scale—2nd edition; *SCQ* social communication questionnaire; *SRS* social responsiveness scale; *SVM-2C* 2-class support vector machine application

When the SVM-2C was cross-validated with the data from the 16 tests, the cut-off values were adjusted to 0.919, the sensitivity was 0.933, specificity was 1.000, and precision was 0.999, while accuracy was 0.938. AUC was 0.9333. Table 13.4 shows the sensitivity, specificity, precision, and accuracy values for all the instruments.

Logistic Regression. The Cox and Snell Pseudo R-square and the Nagelkerke Pseudo R-square values presented in Table 13.5 highlight the predictive ability of the four instruments in classifying the cases, although none of the four instruments significantly predicted the actual diagnosis of the cases.

The Cox and Snell pseudo R-square was 0.255 for the SVM-2C, which represents a relatively better fit of the model to the data compared to the GARS-2, for which the R-Square was 0.027. SCQ and SRS fared equally poorly with a Cox and Snell pseudo R-square of 0.017. The SVM-2C can predict 68.3 % of the classification outcomes compared to GARS-2 prediction of 4.3 % and SCQ and SRS prediction of 3.2 %.

Test of Differences. Based on the t-tests, there were significant differences between the SVM-2C and the GARS, $t\,(15) = 6.053, p < 0.05$, between the SVM-2C and the SCQ, $t\,(15) = 3.433, p < 0.05$, and between the SVM-2C and the SRS, $t\,(15) = 3.433, p < 0.05$. The SVM-2C application made more accurate classifications than the GARS, SCQ, and SRS.

13.2.2.3 Discussion

Although all four instruments obtained good values for sensitivity, specificity, precision, and accuracy, i.e., they were able to classify the cases reasonably well, in-depth comparison of the instruments was impeded by the small sample size. Nonetheless, the SVM-2C demonstrated its superiority in the classification of ASD children compared to the GARS, SCQ, and SRS; it identified the most number of cases correctly.

Besides the small sample size, the characteristics of the sample were also problematic. The sample was retrospectively recruited and consisted of children and parents as respondents, who presented as a subset population in the clinic. They had undergone the comprehensive assessment previously and may have acquired better skills and knowledge in recognising symptoms of ASD. Furthermore, parents' concerns and observations of their children's behaviours may have altered since the initial assessment. In particular, there was only one negative case within the sample, and its classification singularly impacts the performance of the instruments.

In addition, the administration of the instruments also suggests caution in their comparison. While GARS, SCQ, and SRS were rated on the current responses provided by the parents, the application of the SVM-2C was on the text reports from the initial diagnostic assessment. Significantly more information was provided in the diagnostic assessment that was utilised in the SVM-2C classification. Time factor also needs to be considered. Unfortunately, ratings on the GARS, SRS, and SCQ at the point of initial diagnostic assessment for the sample were not available for comparison.

The results suggest preliminary support for the use of SVM-2C for screening of ASD compared to the traditional paper-and-pencil screening tools. More investigation needs to be done to examine SVM-2C's application in a prospective study and in a bigger non-selected population.

13.2.3 Phase 3

A 1-Class SVM is described to determine the classification performance of the application when only an uneven sample is available to develop the classification model. The SVM-2C is also cross-validated and refined with all information available. A final SVM model is described.

13.2.3.1 Method

Procedure. From the 205 diagnostic assessment reports used in Phase 1, the positive cases were extracted (n = 188) to obtain a 1-Class SVM classification model (SVM-1C). The sample consisted of 19 females (10.1 %) and 169 males

Table 13.6 Description of children's diagnosis and age in months in text reports at phase 3

Diagnostic category	N	Age in months			
		Mean	SD	Min	Max
Positive: autism spectrum disorders (ASD)	203	134.4	35.8	52	229
Autism	82	137.3	37.3	52	229
Asperger's syndrome	62	131.2	35.0	72	210
Pervasive developmental disorders—not otherwise specified	59	133.8	34.2	77	216
Negative (not ASD)	18	129.9	38.4	81	209
Total	221	134.1	35.9	52	229

(88.8 %). Their mean age was 133.8 months (11.1 years, SD = 35.8). There were no group differences found between the children with different ASD diagnoses. The SVM-1C was cross-validated with the 16 text reports obtained in Phase 2 to examine the classification performance of the application in a skewed population.

The 16 text reports were included in a final cross-validation of SVM-2C, and all diagnostic assessments reports (n = 221, 203 positive, 18 negative) were included to refine the classification performance of the SVM application model (SVM). Table 13.6 describes the characteristics of this sample in detail.

13.2.3.2 Results

The SVM-1C cross-validation resulted in an optimal decision value cut-off of 0.012. Fourteen out of 16 children were classified correctly on the SVM-1C, yielding an accuracy of 87.5 %. Two children with a positive diagnosis (ASD) were incorrectly classified as negative. Sensitivity was 0.867, and specificity was 1.00. The SVM-1C obtained a precision of 0.999 and AUC of 0.8667.

The final SVM obtained an accuracy of 83.7 %, with 169 positive cases and 16 negative cases correctly classified. Thirty-four positive cases were misclassified as negative, while 2 negative cases were misclassified as positive. Sensitivity was 0.833, specificity was 0.889, and precision was 0.988, at an optimal decision value cut-off of 0.806. AUC was 0.9100. The ROC curve is presented in Fig. 13.2.

13.2.3.3 Discussion

The SVM-1C demonstrated good classification performance, although it was based on only positive cases. This suggests an applicability of the SVM in a clinical setting, whereby there is a natural selection in the sample, i.e., there is a much higher proportion of children with deviance in behaviours or development than the normal population. It is also useful when a control group for comparison is not available.

The cross-validation of the SVM-2C to obtain the final SVM classification model points to the potential of the application to cope with the continuous

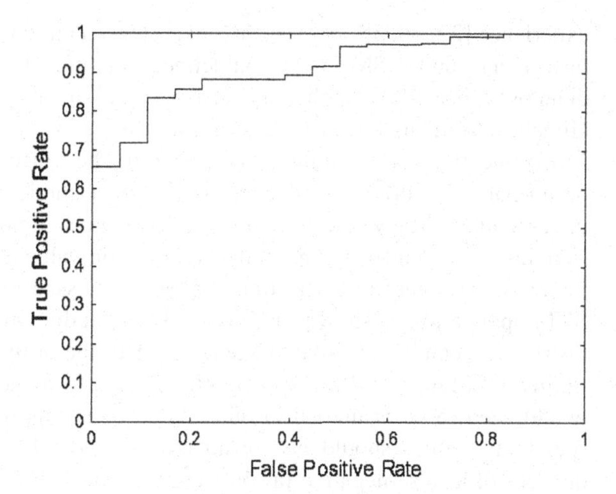

Fig. 13.2 ROC *curve* of the final SVM with AUC of 0.9100

re-definition of the disorder. The final SVM appears to possess excellent classification properties, but it requires more research and validation across different settings and with different populations in a prospective study design.

13.3 Discussion and Conclusions

The objective of the study was to develop and evaluate an objective classification instrument that can improve screening of ASD. A SVM application was developed and compared to other screening instruments currently available. Results showed that performance of the SVM application is encouraging. Although the results of the study are preliminary at most, and the SVM application did not clearly outperform the GARS, SCQ, and SRS in terms of predictive validity for ASD, the SVM application has its advantages even if on par with the other instruments. In medical settings, clinicians take a large amount of notes during consultations and clinical evaluations. Patients also visit medical set-ups,and information on patients accumulates over time. The SVM application is able to process a large quantity of text information and presents an avenue for the use of the information to aid the diagnosis decision-making process. In addition, classification is completed by the application, and the application reduces confounding factors [50], in the screening or diagnosis process. The observations and reporting of presenting behaviours is a necessary process for diagnosis of mental health disorders, especially ASD, but since no rater can be truly objective even with the best of intentions [43], the SVM application provides an 'almost-objective' classification. Although the SVM application is trained on observed behaviours reported by parents or clinicians, new cases are evaluated with reference to presentation of known behaviours and symptoms. The accurate diagnosis of ASD has been shown to rely on clinicians' experience [27, 38, 55, 60]. The less experienced clinicians rely more on screening instruments and DSM-IV-TR guidelines and may be more hesitant to give a diagnosis. The SVM application can be a helpful tool in the absence of expert clinicians to identify children at risk for ASD.

Despite the many limitations present in the current study, it compares the performance of different instruments within a single sample, an area which is under-studied. Many screening instruments were sampled and evaluated on at-risk samples, hence undermining their psychometric value. This may be the reason for lower values found in replicating studies. This issue may be minimised with the SVM application as shown in Phase 3 of the study. On the other hand, screening instruments can be sensitive to age range. The age of the children in the study was limited to a range of 4 to 19 years old. The performance of the SVM application would need to be examined in other age groups. Implications for sensitivity and specificity values should be considered in medical screening, too. The consequences of a false negative far outweigh the cost of a false positive at screening. The SVM application decision values need further research for an optimal cut-off in favour of higher sensitivity rather than higher specificity. In sum, more research is required in the validation of the SVM application, especially in clinical implementation.

The use of machine learning to develop a screening and classification tool, such as the final SVM application described in the present study is a first in the field. The technology can be further developed to be incorporated as a surveillance tool, not only for ASD but also for other psychiatric disorders. The present study also demonstrated the potential use of a novel tool in classification of mental health disorders and concurs with the call for technology to be innovatively applied [5, 28] in medical settings.

References

1. Allen, C.W., Silove, N., William, K., Hutchins, P.: Validity if the social communication questionnaire in assessing risk of autism in preschool children with developmental problems. J. Autism Dev. Disord. **37**, 1272–1278 (2007)
2. Baird, G., Simonoff, E., Pickles, A., Chandler, S., Loucas, T., Meldrum, D.: Prevalence of disorders of the autism spectrum in a population cohort of children in South Thames: The special needs and autism project (SNAP). Lancet **368**, 210–215 (2006)
3. Beglinger, L.J., Smith, T.H.: A review of subtyping in autism and pro-posed dimensional classification model. J. Autism Dev. Disord. **31**(4), 411–422 (2001)
4. Berument, S.K., Rutter, M., Lord, C., Pickles, A., Bailey, A.: Autism screening questionnaire: Diagnostic validity. Br. J. Psychiatry. **175**, 444–451 (1999)
5. Bölte, S., Golan, O., Goodwin, M.S., Zwaigenbaum, L.: Editorial: What can innovative technologies do for autism spectrum disorders? Autism **14**(3), 155–159 (2010)
6. Centre for Disease Control: Prevalence of autism spectrum disorders—autism and developmental disabilities monitoring network. Morb. Mortal. Wkly. Rep. Surveill. Summ. **56**, 1–28 (2007)

7. Chakrabarti, S., Fombonne, E.: Pervasive developmental disorders in preschool children: Confirmation of high prevalence. Am. J. Psychiarty. **162**, 1133–1141 (2005)
8. Chandler, S., Charman, T., Baird, G., Simonoff, E., Loucas, T., Meldrum, D.: Validation of the social communication questionnaire in a population cohort of children with autism spectrum disorder. J. Am. Acad. Child Adolesc. Psychiatry **46**(10), 1324–1332 (2007)
9. Charman, T., Baird, G.: Practitioner review: Diagnosis of autism spectrum disorders in 2- and 3-year-old children. J. Child Psychol. Psychiatry **43**(3), 289–305 (2002)
10. Charman, T., Baird, G., Simonoff, E., Loucas, T., Chandler, S., Meldrum, D.: Efficacy of three screening instruments in the identification of autistic spectrum disorder. Br. J. Psychiatry **191**, 554–559 (2007)
11. Constantino, J.N., Gruber, C.P.: Social Responsiveness Scale (SRS). Western Psychological Services, Los Angeles (2005)
12. Constantino, J.N., Gruber, C.P., Davis, S., Hayes, S., Passanante, N., Przybeck, T.: The factor structure of autistic traits. J. Child Psychol. Psychiatry **45**(4), 719–726 (2004)
13. Constantino, J.N., LaVesser, P.D., Zhang, Y., Abbacchi, A.G.T., Todd, R.D.: Rapid quantitative assessment of autistic social impairment by classroom teachers. J. Am. Acad. Child Adolesc. Psychiatry **46**, 1668–1676 (2007)
14. Corsello, C., Hus, V., Pickles, A., Risi, S., Cook, J.E.H., Leventhal, B.L.: Between a ROC and a hard place: Decision making and making decisions about using the SCQ. J. Child Psychol. Psychiatry. **48**, 932–940 (2007)
15. De bildt, A., Sytema, S., Ketelaars, C., Kraijer, D., Mulder, E., Volkmar, F.: Interrelationship between autism diagnostic observation schedule-generic (ADOS-G), autism diagnostic interview-revised (ADI-R), and the di-agnostic and statistical manual of mental disorders (DSM-IV-TR) classification in children and adolescents with mental retardation. J. Autism Dev. Disord. **34**(2), 129–137 (2004)
16. Diederich, J., Al-Ajmi, A., Yellowlees, P.: Ex-ray: Data mining and mental health. Appl. Soft Comput. **7**(3), 923–928 (2007)
17. DiLavore, P.C., Lord, C., Rutter, M.: The pre-linguistic autism diagnostic observation schedule. J. Autism Dev. Disord. **25**(4), 355–379 (1995)
18. DSM-IV.: Diagnostic and Statistical Manual of Mental Disorders. American Psychiatric Association (1994)
19. Eaves, L.C., Wingert, H., Ho, H.H.: Screening for autism. Autism **10**, 229–242 (2006)
20. Filipek, P.A., Accardo, P.J., Ashwal, S., Baranek, G.T., Cook, E.H., Dawson, G., Gordon, B., Gravel, J.S., Johnson, C.P., Kallen, R.J., Levy, S.E., Minshew, N.J., Ozonoff, S., Prizant, B.M., Rapin, I., Rogers, S.J., Stone, W.L., Teplin, S.W., Tuchman, R.F., Volkmar, F.R.: Practice parameter: Screening and diagnosis of autism. **55**. First published
21. Filipek, P.A., Accardo, P.J., Baranek, G.T., Cook Jr, E.H., Dawson, G., Gordon, B., Gravel, J.S., Johnson, C.P., Kallen, R.J., Levy, S.E., Minshew, N.J., Prizant, B.M., Rapin, I., Rogers, S.J., Stone, W.L., Teplin, S., Tuchman, R.F., Volkmar, F.R.: The screening and diagnosis of autistic spectrum disorders. J. Autism Dev. Disord. **29**(6), 439–484 (1999)
22. Fombonne, E.: Epidemiological surveys of autism and other pervasive developmental disorders: An update. J. Autism Dev. Disord. **33**(4), 365–381 (2003)
23. Georgiades, S., Szatmari, P., Zwaigenbaum, L., Duku, E., Bryson, S., Roberts, W.: Structure of the autism symptom phenotype: A proposed multidimensional model. J. Am. Acad. Child Adolesc. Psychiatry **43**(2), 188–196 (2007)
24. Gilliam, J.E.: Gilliam Autism Rating Scale. PRO-ED, Austin (1995)
25. Gilliam, J.E.: Gilliam Autism Rating Scale–Second Edition. PRO-ED, Austin (2006)
26. Goin-Kochel, R.P., Cohen, R.: Screening cases within a statewide autism registry. Focus Autism Other Dev. Disabil. **23**(3), 148–154 (2008)
27. Goin-Kochel, R.P., Mackintosh, V., Myers, B.J.: How many doctors does it take to make an autism spectrum diagnosis? Autism **10**, 439–451 (2006)
28. Goodwin, M.S.: Enhancing and accelerating the pace of autism research and treatment: The promise of developing innovative technology. Focus Autism Other Dev. Disabil. **23**, 125–128 (2008)

29. Gotham, K., Risi, S., Dawson, G., Tager-Flusberg, H., Joseph, R., Carter, A.: A replication of the autism diagnostic observation schedule (ADOS) revised algorithm. J. Am. Acad. Child Adolesc. Psychiatry **47**(6), 642–651 (2008)
30. Gotham, K., Risi, S., Pickles, A.: The autism diagnostic observation schedule: Revised algorithm for improved diagnostic validity. J. Autism Dev. Disord. **37**, 613–627 (2007)
31. Gray, K.M., Tonge, B.J., Sweeney, D.J.: Using the autism diagnostic interview-revised and the autism diagnostic observation schedule with young children with developmental delay: Evaluating diagnostic validity. J. Autism Dev. Disord. **38**, 657–667 (2008)
32. Howlin, P., Moore, A.: Diagnosis of autism: A survey of over 1200 patients in the UK. Autism **1**, 135–162 (1997)
33. ICD10.: International Statistical Classification of Disease and Related Health. World Health Organization, Geneva (1992)
34. Ingram, D.G., Takahashi, T.N., Miles, J.H.: Defining autism subgroups: A taxometric solution. J. Autism Dev. Disord. **38**, 950–960 (2008)
35. Johnson, C.P., Myers, S.M., Lipkin, P.H., Cartwright, J.D., Desch, L.W., Duby, J.C., Elias, E.R., Levey, E.B., Liptak, G.S., Murphy, N.A., Tilton, A.H., Lollar, D., Macias, M., McPherson, M., Olson, D.G., Strickland, B., Skipper, S.M., Ackermann, J., Del Monte, M., Challman, T.D., Hyman, S.L., Levy, S.E., Spooner, S.A., Yeargin-Allsopp, M.: Identification and evaluation of children with autism spectrum disorders. Pediatrics **120**(5), 1183–1215 (2007)
36. Johnson, C.P., Myers, S.M.: Identification and evaluation of children with autism spectrum disorders. Pediatrics **120**, 1183–1215 (2007)
37. Kabot, S., Masi, W., Segal, M.: Advances in the diagnosis and treatment of autism spectrum disorders. Prof. Psychol. Res. Pract. **34**(1), 26–33 (2003)
38. Klin, A., Lang, J., Cicchetti, D.V., Volkmar, F.R.: Brief report: Interrater reliability of clinical diagnosis and DSM-IV criteria for autistic disorder: Results of the DSM-IV autism field trial. J. Autism Dev. Disord. **30**(2), 163–167 (2000)
39. Lecavalier, L.: An evaluation of the Gilliam autism rating scale. J. Autism Dev. Disord. **35**(6), 795–805 (2005)
40. Lecavalier, L., Aman, M.G., Scahill, L., McDougle, C.J., McCracken, J.T., Vitiello, B.: Validity of the autism diagnostic interview-revised. Am. J. Ment. Retard. **111**(3), 199–215 (2006)
41. Lord, C., Luyster, R.: Early diagnosis of children with autism spectrum disorders. Clin. Neurosci. Res. **6**, 189–194 (2006)
42. Lord, C., Risi, S., Lambrecht, L., Cook, E.H., Leventhal, B.L., DiLavore, P.C.: The autism diagnostic observation schedule-generic: A standard measure of social and communication deficits associated with the spectrum of autism. J. Autism Dev. Disord. **30**(3), 205–223 (2000)
43. Lord, C., Risis, S.: Frameworks and methods in diagnosing autism spectrum disorders. Ment. Retard. Dev. Disabil. Res. Rev. **4**, 90–96 (1998)
44. Lord, C., Rutter, M., DiLavore, P.C., Risi, S.: Autism Diagnostic Observation Schedule. Western Psychological Services, Los Angeles (2002)
45. Mazefsky, C.A., Oswald, D.P.: The discriminative ability and diagnostic utility of the ADOS-G, ADI-R, and GARS for children in a clinical setting. Autism **10**, 533–549 (2006)
46. Norris, M., Lecavalier, L.: Screening accuracy of level 2 autism spectrum disorder rating scales: A review of selected instruments. Autism **14**(4), 263–284 (2010)
47. Noterdame, M., Mildenberger, K., Sitter, S.H.A.: Parent information and direct observation in the diagnosis of pervasive and specific develop-mental disorders. Autism **6**(2), 159–168 (2002)
48. Oosterling, I.J., Swinkels, S.H., Van der Gaag, R.J., Visser, J.C., Dietz, C., Buitelaar, J.K.: Comparative analysis of three screening instruments for autism spectrum disorders in toddlers at high risk. J. Autism Dev. Disord. **39**, 897–909 (2009)

49. Prior, M., Eisenmajer, R., Leekam, S., Wing, L., Gould, J., Ong, B.: Are there subgroups within the autistic spectrum? A cluster analysis of a group of children with autistic spectrum disorders. J. Child Psychol. Psychiatry **39**(6), 893–902 (1998)
50. Rosenberg, R.E., Daniels, A.M., Law, J.K., Law, P.A., Kaufmann, W.E.: Trends in autism spectrum disorder diagnoses: 1994–2007. J. Autism Dev. Disord. **39**, 1099–1111 (2009)
51. Rutter, M., Bailey, A., Lord, C.: Social Communication Questionnaire. Western Psychological Services, Los Angeles (2003)
52. Rutter, M., Le Couteur, A., Lord, C.: Autism Diagnostic Interview-Revised. Western Psychological Services, Los Angeles (2003)
53. Saracino, J., Noseworthy, J., Steiman, M., Reisinger, L., Fombonne, E.: Diagnostic and assessment issues in autism surveillance and prevalence. J. Dev. Phys. Disabil. **22**, 317–330 (2010)
54. Scahill, L.: Diagnosis and evaluation of pervasive developmental disorders. J. Clin. Psychiatry **66**, 19–25 (2005)
55. Skellern, C., Schluter, P., McDowell, M.: From complexity to category: Responding to diagnostic uncertainties of autistic spectrum disorders. J. Paediatr. Child Health **41**, 407–412 (2005)
56. South, M., Williams, B.J., McMahon, W.M., Owley, T., Filipek, P.A., Shernoff, E.: Utility of the Gilliam autism rating scale in research and clinical populations. J. Autism Dev. Disord. **32**, 593–599 (2002)
57. Tadevosyan-Leyer, O., Dowd, M., Mankoski, R., Winklosy, B., Putnam, S., Mcgrath, L.: A principal components analysis of the autism diagnostic interview-revised. J. Am. Acad. Child Adolesc. Psychiatry **42**(7), 864–872 (2003)
58. Volkmar, F.R., State, M., Klin, A.: Autism and autism spectrum disorders: Diagnostic issues for the coming decade. J. Child Psychol. Psychiatry **50**, 108–115 (2009)
59. Wazana, A., Bresnahan, M., Kline, J.: The autism epidemic: Fact or artefact? J. Am. Acad. Child Adolesc. Psychiatry **43**(6), 721–730 (2007)
60. Williams, M.E., Atkins, M.T.S.: Assessment of autism in community settings: Discrepancies in classification. J. Autism Dev. Disord. **39**(4), 660–669 (2008)
61. Wing, L., Gould, J.: Severe impairments of social interaction and associated abnormalities in children: Epidemiology and classification. J. Autism Dev. Disord. **9**(1), 11–29 (1979)
62. Witwer, A.N., Lecavalier, L.: Autism screening tools: An evaluation of the social communication questionnaire and the developmental behaviour checklist-autism screening algorithm. J. Intell. Dev. Disabil. **32**(3), 179–187 (2007)
63. World Health Organisation: The ICD-10 classification of mental and behavioural disorders: Clinical descriptions and diagnostic guidelines. World Health Organization, Geneva (1992)
64. Young, R.L., Brewer, N., Pattison, C.: Parental identification of early behavioural abnormalities in children with autistic disorder. Autism **7**(2), 125–143 (2003)

Conclusion

Insu Song

Every year on the 10th of October, The World Health Organization joins in celebrating the World Mental Health Day. The theme of the day in 2012 was "Depression: A Global Crisis," as depression alone affects more than 350 million people of all ages, in all communities [1]. Mental health has not only become a significant contributor to the global burden of disease, but has also become one of the five most costly medical conditions in developed countries, with costs doubling in the 10 years from 1996 to 2006 [2]. An example of the seriousness of depression can be seen in the fact that, suicide is among the top 20 leading causes of death globally for all ages [3]. Every year, nearly one million people die from suicide and twenty million suicide attempts are made [3]. The condition is worse in developing countries, due to problems accessing treatment, and fewer than 10 % of those who need treatment for depression are able to receive it [1].

Recognizing the urgent need for action in solving the global mental health crisis, WHO launched Mental Health Gap Action Programme (mhGAP) Intervention Guide (mhGAP-IG) for the following priority conditions: depression, psychosis, bipolar disorders, epilepsy, developmental and behavioral disorders in children and adolescents, dementia, alcohol use disorders, drug use disorders, self-harm/suicide, and other significant emotional or medically unexplained complaints [1].

At the same time, we are experiencing this mental health crisis, we are also witnessing a great paradigm shift in technology. The rapid proliferation of cell phones and connectivity now offers an unprecedented opportunity to improve scalability and accessibility of mental health care, particularly for developing countries. Low-cost cell phones now have enough computational power to provide cost effective ways to collect data and provide health care services remotely in the developing world.

In this global context, this book has provided timely information to health-care providers, decision-makers, and Non-Governmental Organizations (NGOs) for scaling up care for people with mental disorders. The chapters of this book have broadly covered modern technologies in use that can scale up care for the priority mental health conditions, including depression (Chaps. 8 and 10), psychosis and

M. Lech et al. (eds.), *Mental Health Informatics*,
Studies in Computational Intelligence 491, DOI: 10.1007/978-3-642-38550-6,

bipolar disorders (Chaps. 5, 8, and 11), and developmental and behavioral disorders in children (Chaps. 6, 7, and 13). Chapters 1, 2, 3, and 4 examined innovative uses of modern technology and contemporary issues in mental health and how technology is changing the way health care services are delivered and how the relationship between patients and health care providers is changing. These studies all strongly indicate the potential power of each of the approaches in solving current mental health care problems: scaling up the care for mental disorders.

The text data mining and analysis tools described in Chaps. 5, 6, 7, 8, 11, and 13 can be used with low-cost 2G cell-phones using Short Messaging Service (SMS). Most developing countries now provide more advanced messaging services, such as Multimedia Messaging Service (MMS) which costs around US$0.01 per message in Bangladesh. Voice analysis technologies, described in Chaps. 9 and 10, can be readily used with MMS or using Automated Voice Response (AVR) systems over Voice Over IP (VoIP) technology to rapidly assess depression and general well-being of mental states. Image analysis and explanation technology explained in Chap. 7 analyzes images and videos collected using MMS to assist health care providers. Cell-phones equipped with more advanced text and image display interfaces can be leveraged to provide Person-Centered Healthcare (Chap. 2), Technology now allows compassionate societies to provide Anytime and Anywhere care (Chap. 3) and to enhance the quality of clinical care (Chap. 4).

The mobile technology ready computerized automated assessment methods detailed in these pages can be integrated into the clinical practices documented in the mhGAP Intervention Guide. As the mhGAP-IG is to be implemented primarily by non-specialists, the integration of the assisted mobile mental health technology will have significant impact in scaling up mental health care for both developing and developed worlds. Within five years, most Africans will have access to cell-phone networks. WHO is about to launch a comprehensive mental health action plan 2013–2020 to address the global mental health crisis and the lack of care, especially in low- and middle-income countries, for people suffering from mental, neurological, and substance use disorders. This action plan presents unique challenges but also great opportunities for IT and health care professionals and activists.

References

1. WHO: WHO mental health gap action programme (mhGAP) intervention guide (2010)
2. Soni, A.: The five most costly conditions, 1996 and 2006: estimates for the U.S. civilian noninstitutionalized population medical expenditure panel survey. Agency for Healthcare Research and Quality (2009)
3. Marcus, M., Yasamy, M.T., Ommeren, M.V., Chisholm, D., Saxena, S.: Depression: a global public health concern (2012)

Index

M. Lech et al. (eds.), *Mental Health Informatics*, Studies in Computational Intelligence 491, DOI: 10.1007/978-3-642-38550-6,

Printed in the United States
By Bookmasters

Printed in the United States
By Bookmasters